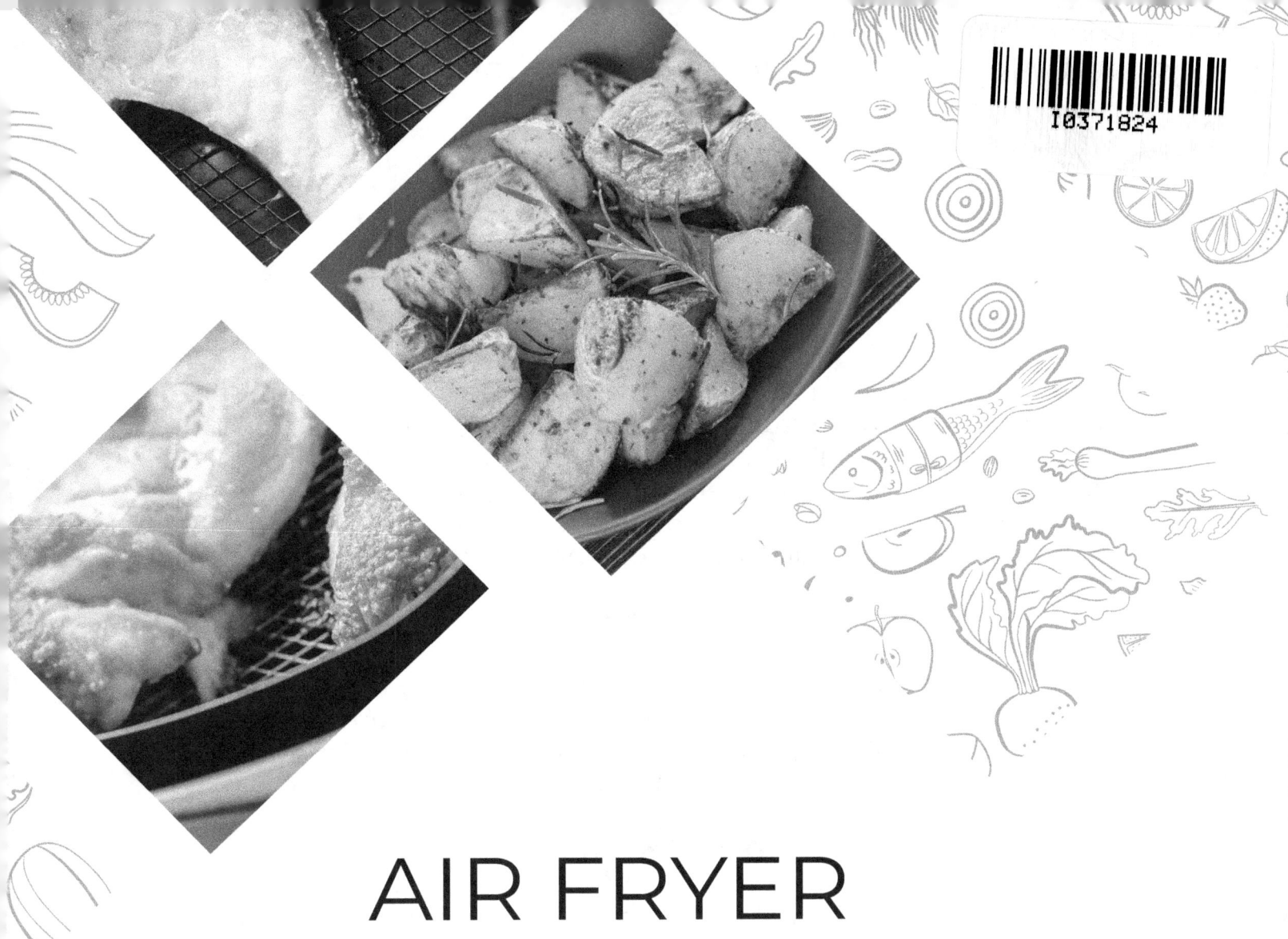

AIR FRYER
Cookbook

600 QUICK AND EASY RECIPES FOR TASTY AND HEALTHIER MEALS. 4-WEEK MEAL PLAN.

Vivian Bayne

Air Fryer Cookbook

Copyright - 2020 - All rights reserved.

The content contained within this book may not be reproduced, duplicated or transmitted without direct written permission from the author or the publisher. Under no circumstances will any blame or legal responsibility be held against the publisher, or author, for any damages, reparation, or monetary loss due to the information contained within this book. Either directly or indirectly.

Legal Notice:

This book is copyright protected. This book is only for personal use. You cannot amend, distribute, sell, use, quote or paraphrase any part, or the content within this book, without the consent of the author or publisher.

Disclaimer Notice:

Please note the information contained within this document is for educational and entertainment purposes only. All effort has been executed to present accurate, up to date, and reliable, complete information. No warranties of any kind are declared or implied. Readers acknowledge that the author is not engaging in the rendering of legal, financial, medical or professional advice. The content within this book has been derived from various sources. Please consult a licensed professional before attempting any techniques outlined in this book.

By reading this document, the reader agrees that under no circumstances is the author responsible for any losses, direct or indirect, which are incurred as a result of the use of information contained within this document, including, but not limited to, - errors, omissions, or inaccuracies.

TABLE OF CONTENTS

INTRODUCTION	5
HOW TO USE AN AIR FRYER	8
BENEFITS OF AIR FRYING	11
BASIC CARE AND CLEANING	13
HOW TO PREPARE YOUR KITCHEN TO AIR FRY	15
USEFUL TIPS ON HOW TO BEST COOK WITH AN AIR FRYER	17
WHAT ARE THE BEST AND WORST FOOD TO AIR FRY	19
AIR FRYING COOKING CHARTS	21
4-WEEK MEAL PLAN	24
BREAKFAST	27
SNACKS	62
SIDE DISHES	94
POULTRY	117
MEAT	144
BONUS KETO AIR FRYER RECIPES	202
VEGETABLES AND VEGETARIAN	222
SWEETS AND DESSERTS	250
CONCLUSION	274
INDEX OF RECIPES	275

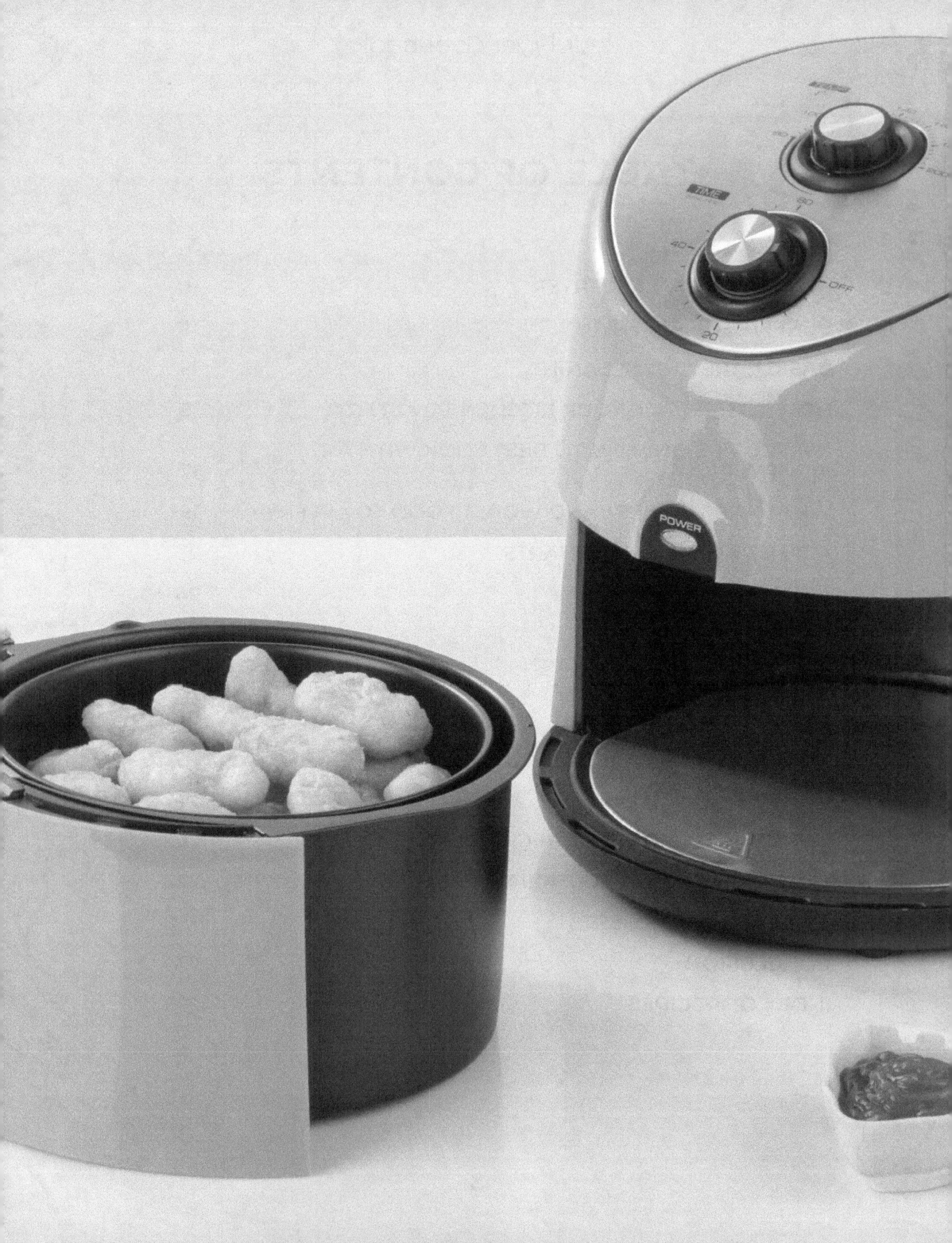

INTRODUCTION

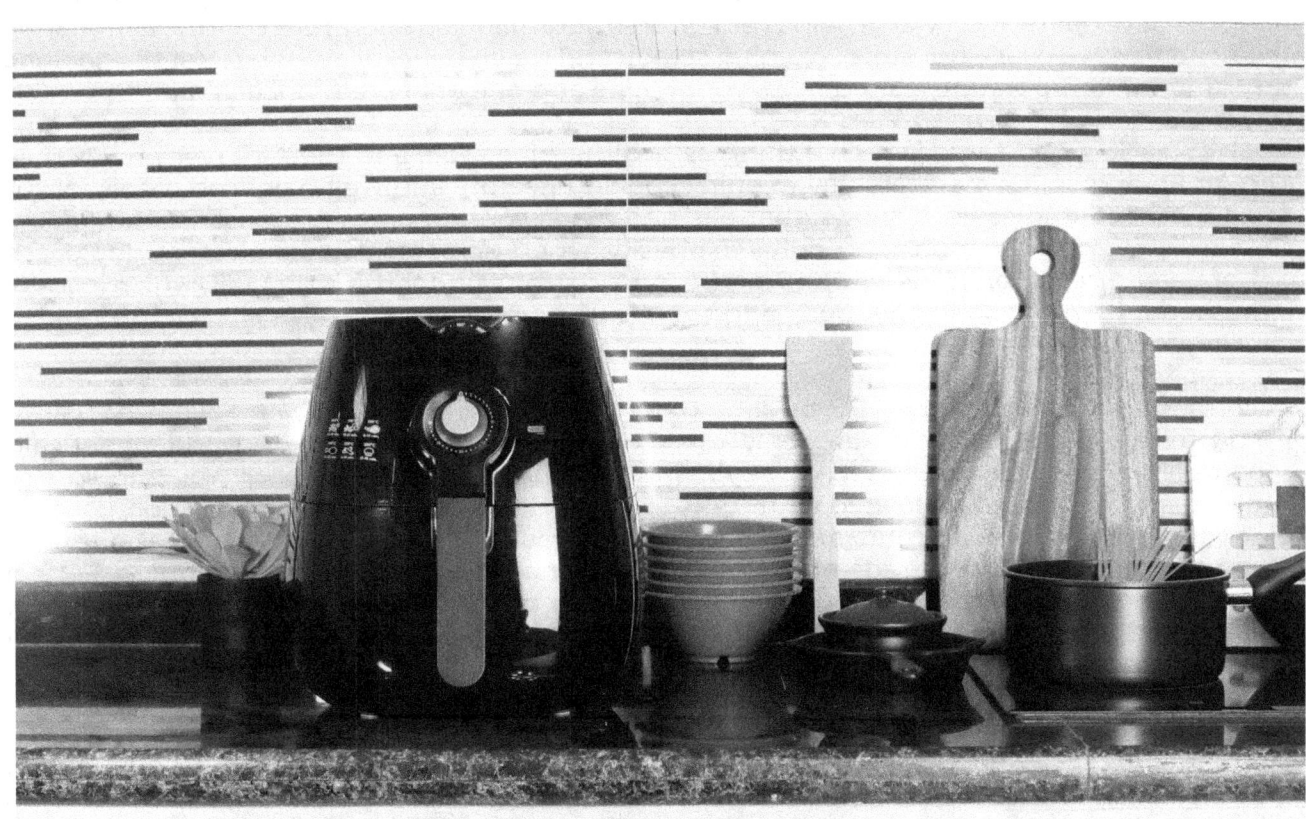

If you're reading this cookbook, you probably already know what an Air Fryer is, but in case you don't, let me introduce you to the wonders of my favorite kitchen gadget. The Air Fryer is an "all-in-one" kitchen appliance that promises to replace a deep fryer, convection oven, and microwave; it also lets you sauté your foods. The Air Fryer is a unique kitchen gadget designed to fry food in a special chamber using super-heated air. In fact, the hot air circulates inside the cooking chamber using the convection mechanism, cooking your food evenly from all sides. It uses the so-called Maillard effect, a chemical reaction that gives fried food that distinctive flavor. Simply put, thanks to the hot air, your foods get that crispy exterior and a moist interior and does not taste like the fat.

Why use an Air Fryer? I'm asked this question time and time again, so my answer is always the same: it all boils down to versatility, health, and speed. It means that I can "set it and forget it" until it is done. Unlike most cooking methods, there's no need to keep an eye on it. I can pick the ingredients, turn the machine on and walk away – no worries about overcooked or burned food. Another great benefit of using an Air Fryer is that unlike the heat in your oven or on a stovetop, the cooking chamber's heat is constant and allows your food to cook evenly. Plus, it is energy-efficient and a space-saving solution.

Is an Air Fryer worth buying? It is a personal matter. You should keep in mind personal factors such as your kitchen equipment, counter space, budget, cooking preferences, and your family's size. However, there are numerous benefits you'll get from using an Air Fryer.

Air Fryer Cookbook

Here are the top three benefits of using an Air Fryer.

Fast cooking and convenience. The Air Fryer is an electric device, so you just need to press the right buttons and go about your business. It heats up in a few minutes so it can cut down cooking time; further, hot air circulates around your food, cooking it quickly and evenly. Roast chicken is perfectly cooked in 30 minutes, baby back ribs in less than 25 minutes, and beef chuck or steak in about 15 minutes. You can use dividers and cook different foods at the same time. The Air Fryer is a real game-changer, it is a cost-saving solution in many ways. I also use my Air Fryer to keep my food warm. Air Fryer features automatic temperature control, eliminating the need to slave over a hot stove. A digital screen and touch panel allow you to set the cooking time and the temperature according to your recipe and personal preferences.

Healthy eating. Yes, there is such a thing as healthy fried food, and the Air Fryer proves that! The Air Fryer inspires me every day to enjoy cooking healthy and well-balanced meals for my family. Recent studies have shown that air-fried foods contain up to 80% less fat than deep-fried foods. Deep-fried food contributes to obesity, type 2 diabetes, high cholesterol, increased risk of heart disease, etc. Plus, fats and oils become harmful under the high heat, which leads to increased inflammation in your body and speeds up aging. Further, these oils release cancer-causing toxic chemicals.

According to the leading experts, you should not be afraid of healthy fats and oils, especially if you follow a diet like the ketogenic diet. Avoid partially hydrogenated and genetically modified oils such as cottonseed oil, soybean oil, corn oil, and rice bran oil. You should also avoid margarine since it is loaded with trans-fats. Good fats and oils include olive oil, coconut oil, avocado oil, sesame oil, nuts and seeds. Air-fried foods are delicious and have the texture of regular fried food, but they do not taste like fat. French fries are only the beginning. Perfect ribs, hearty casseroles, fast snacks, and delectable desserts turn out great in this revolutionary kitchen gadget. When it comes to healthy dieting that does not compromise flavor, the Air Fryer is a real winner.

The ultimate solution for losing pounds and maintaining a healthy weight.
One of the greatest benefits of owning an Air Fryer is the possibility to maintain an ideal weight in a comfortable and healthy way. The best part is that you do not have to give up fried fish fillets, saucy steaks, and scrumptious desserts. Choosing a healthy-cooking technique is the key to success. Air frying requires less fat compared to many other cooking methods, making your weight loss diet more achievable.

To compare: Hot oil conducts heat very well and cooks food quickly. When you put food into a deep-fat fryer, the water on the food's surface instantly evaporates. Water from inside the food is released, which rapidly moves the oil around, causing the oil's bubbling action. The food's interior is cooked as the heat moves through the food. The crust starts to brown due to a chemical reaction called the Maillard reaction, in which sugars and proteins on the crust break down and recombine to form compounds that look brown and taste great.

Hot air cooks food more slowly because it does not conduct heat as well as oil or water. To understand the difference, think of how you can put your hand into a 350°F oven for a few seconds, but you cannot put it into boiling water (212°F). To mimic deep-frying, but without all the unhealthy oil, an Air Fryer uses a fan to push the air around the food to dramatically speed the cooking process. So, just as in a deep-fat fryer, in an Air Fryer, the surface of the food dehydrates, water is released, and the interior cooks in a few minutes. Foods cooked in an Air Fryer cook 25 percent faster than foods cooked in a conventional oven.

And because little or no oil is used, cooking with an Air Fryer is a much more versatile way to cook food than cooking with a deep fryer. You can bake, roast, grill, stir-fry, and even steam foods in an Air Fryer. So instead of just cooking alternatives to fried foods, use this appliance to make foods without those hundreds of added fat calories; it actually will help improve your health and well-being.

Although Air Fryer cooking seems new, professional chefs have been using it for decades in

Air Fryer Cookbook

commercial kitchens for its speed and cooking and browning features. Today these ovens are widely available to home cooks at affordable prices.

There are millions of Air Fryers in private homes today, but people have had to figure out on their own how to adapt their favorite recipes, with various degrees of success. This book is here to help!

While other Air Fryer cookbooks offer recipes that are certainly healthier than their deep-fried counterparts, this book is one of the few that offers truly healthy recipes. I developed the recipes in this book to be as low in fat, sodium, and sugars as possible, and high in vitamins and fiber.

Air Fryer Step-by-Step:
You can think of an Air Fryer as a miniature convection oven. Inside the Air Fryer, a heater underneath the food heats the air. A slotted pan over the heater lets the superheated air move quickly around the food. A fan keeps the air circulating, and a vent pulls moisture and cooler air out of the appliance, so the temperature inside stays high and constant.

Just as in deep-frying, a crust immediately forms on the food in the Air Fryer. This helps seal in moisture so the interior of the food can cook. The starches inside the food gelatinize, the proteins denature, and the fiber softens as the outside browns—all fancy terms meaning the food cooks as it heats.

Most recipes for Air Fryers are very similar to recipes cooked in ovens or deep-fried in oil. But there are some essential differences.

Batter: Hot oil instantly solidifies a batter. But in an Air Fryer, the liquid runs off in the few seconds intakes for the air to heat it. Wet foods will not work in an Air Fryer.

Shape: Cut foods into similarly sized pieces, so everything cooks evenly in your Air Fryer.

Coatings: Foods coated with bread crumbs, ground nuts, or grated cheeses should be moist enough to ensure those small particles stay on the food and do not drop off into the Air Fryer and burn.

Once the food is prepared according to the recipe, the Air Fryer is usually preheated, following the directions that came with your appliance. The food is placed in a basket and inserted into the Air Fryer before you start timing. In just a few minutes, the outcome is a perfectly cooked, hot, crisp food that is ready to eat.

HOW TO USE AN AIR FRYER

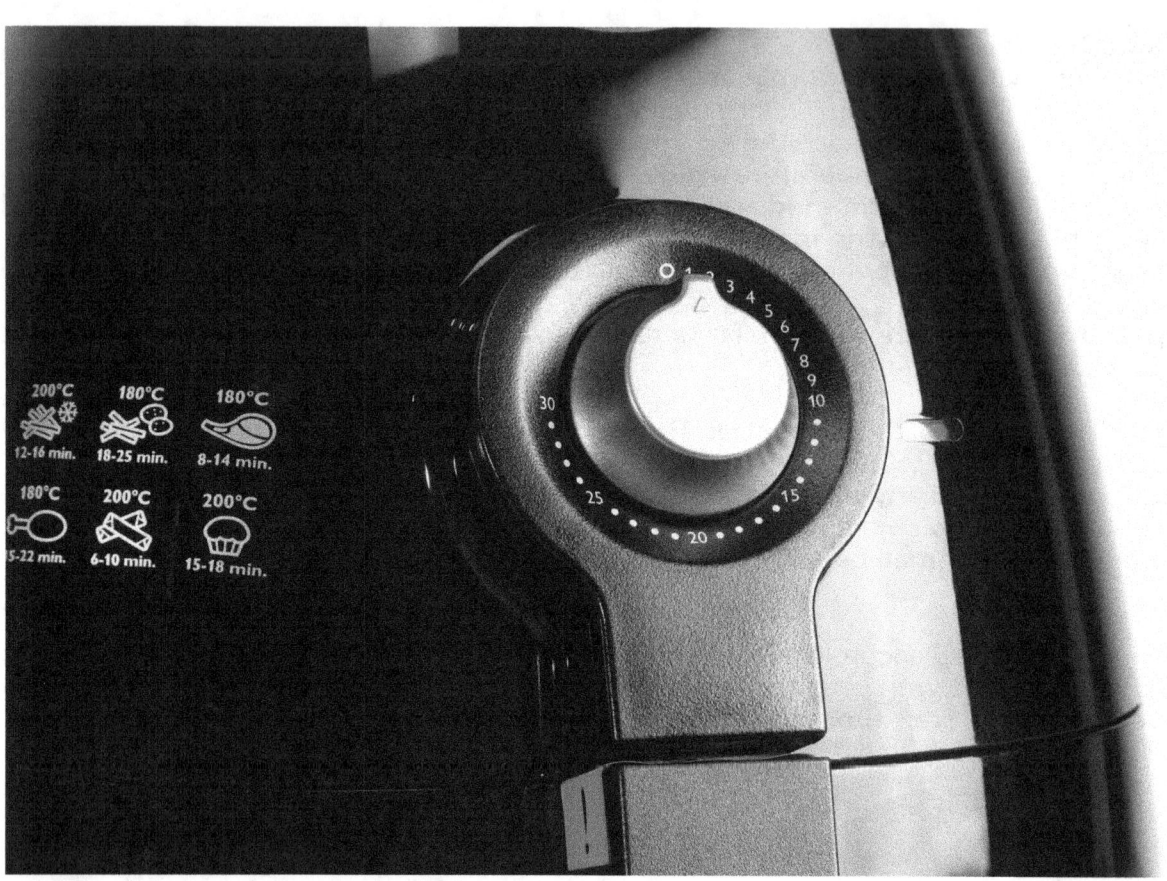

A n Air Fryer uses superheated air in the same way a convection oven works. While conventional ovens simply heat the air, convection ovens blow the air around with a fan.

These days, most new full-size and built-in Air Fryer toaster ovens come with an Air Fryer function, but here's a sad truth: most people don't use the Air Fryer function on their ovens. Why? Because they don't know how to.
Air circulation doesn't just heat the food faster; it also accelerates all the chemical reactions that occur in cooking. The bits of butter in a pastry crust, for example, melt faster, which means they release steam more quickly, which leads to more air between layers - in other words, a flakier crust. When roasting meats, the fat is rendered and the skin is browned more quickly, sealing in juices. The meat, because it cooks faster, stays moist, retaining its juicy flavor. The same is true of vegetables: the dry environment created by the fan's air circulation means the sugars caramelize more quickly, locking in moisture and providing deep, round flavor.

HOW TO PERFECTLY USE AN AIR FRYER ROASTER OVEN
Before you use any function to prepare your food, note that you shouldn't use kitchen foil to cover any of the Air Fryer toast oven accessories as it could stop fat dripping to the pullout tray, and an accumulation of fat on the kitchen foil could start a fire.

Air Fryer Cookbook

Air Fry Function
When you think air fry, think of crunchier, healthier and tastier deep frying. When using the Air Fryer, place the basket in the baking pan and place these in the lower rack position. Select Air Fry on the function dial and set the temperature according to your recipe. Turn on the ON/Oven Timer and set to the cooking time that your recipe specifies. The power light will come on and once you're cooking time elapses the ringer will go off once and the oven will automatically shut itself.

Bake Function
For foods that require gentle baking, such as cakes, muffins, and other pastries, use the bake function. However, if you are looking for extra browning or extra crunch, use convection bake which is ideal for bread, scones, pizza, veggies and roasts.
You can make pizza on the baking pan, or you can alternatively buy a pizza stone instead.
Fit your rack and baking pan into your recipe's recommended position and select bake or convection bake. Set the ON/Oven Timer dial to your recipe's time. When baking pastries, it is recommendable to preheat your oven for 5 minutes before the actual cook time.
The power light will come on to signify the beginning of cooking. The timer will go off once the cooking time is over, and the oven will automatically turn itself off.

Toast Function
Select the toast function and place your food item at the center for even cooking.
Place your rack in the lower position and center the food items. Select toast on your function dial and select Toast/Broil to set your temperature. Turn the ON/Toast Timer to your level of desired brownness to start toasting.
The power light will come on and once the cycle is over, the ringer will go off once before the oven automatically goes off.

Broil Function
The broil function is perfect for top browning of casseroles, gratins, pies, meats and veggies. You can use the convection broil for meats and fish as it gives a deeper browning.
Gently place the Air Fryer toast oven basket in the baking pan and either select Broil or Convection Broil. For the temperature, either set it to Broil/Toast. Next, turn on the ON/Oven Timer dial to your recipe's specification, then start broiling. The power light will come on. Once the cooking is done, the timer will go off once and the oven will automatically turn off.
Note: Do not use glass dishes to broil.

Warm Function
Position the baking pan or oven rack on the lower rack position, set your temperature to warm and choose warm on your function dial. Next, set your ON/Oven Timer to the desired time. The power light will come on and the ringer will go off once the time you set elapses. The oven will automatically shut itself.

AIR FRYER PARTS AND BUTTONS
Note: there are many types and brands of Air Fryers in the market. Below I'm listing the parts and buttons that you would usually find in the most common Air Fryers. For specific instructions, you should read your appliance's manual.

ON/Toast Timer Dial
This allows you to select how light or dark you want your toast to be. By turning this button on, you start the toasting process for one cycle, after which it will power itself off.

ON/Oven Timer Dial
This dial sets the entire unit on apart from the toast. By turning this button on, you start the cooking cycle, which automatically turns itself off once done.

Function Dial
This is where you select your cooking method. It could either be bake, toast, broil, convection bake, convection broil or warm.

Air Fryer Cookbook

Power Light
This light comes on when the unit is in use.

Oven Temperature Dial
You'll use this to set the temperature you need.

Air Fryer Toast Oven Basket
Always use the oven basket when using the air fry function for optimal results.

Pullout Tray
This is used to catch the drippings from the food you are cooking. It's removable for easier cleaning.

Cord Storage
This is located at the back of the oven and it's used for neatly tucking away the cord when the unit is off.

Oven Rack
This gives you the perfect room for baking.
Auto-shut feature the Air Fryer toast oven automatically turns itself off when a cooking or toasting cycle is complete.

TIPS AND TRICKS

Lightly Splash Food with Oil
You will require your cooking splash when using your Air Fryer as it helps keep food from adhering to the bin. Shower the food gently, or you could simply include a smidgen of oil.

Dry Your Food
Pat dry the food before cooking, especially marinated meals. Doing this will prevent an excess of smoke and splattering. Foods that contain high-fat substances, for example, chicken bosom and wings, for the most part store fat when cooking. Therefore, ensure you clean the fat from the base of the Air Fryer on occasion.

Batch Cook
The Air Fryer has a cooking limit. If you're cooking for many people, you should cook in batches.

Shake Your Container While Cooking
Open the Air Fryer at regular intervals and shake around the food in the bin. Chips, French fries, and other small food items can pack; shaking around prevents that. Shake the food on the bin every 5 to 10 minutes to allow it to cook and shape well.

Distribute Evenly
Overcrowding is a no-no with the Air Fryer. If you need your food to cook well, give it a lot of room so that air can flow well. You need to appreciate the firmness of your dinners, isn't that so? Congestion keeps air from distributing over the food. So, make sure to space it out.

Set Fryer to Preheat Before Cooking
Preheat the Air Fryer when it has not been used for some time. Preheat for 3-5 minutes to allow it to heat up appropriately.

BENEFITS OF AIR FRYING

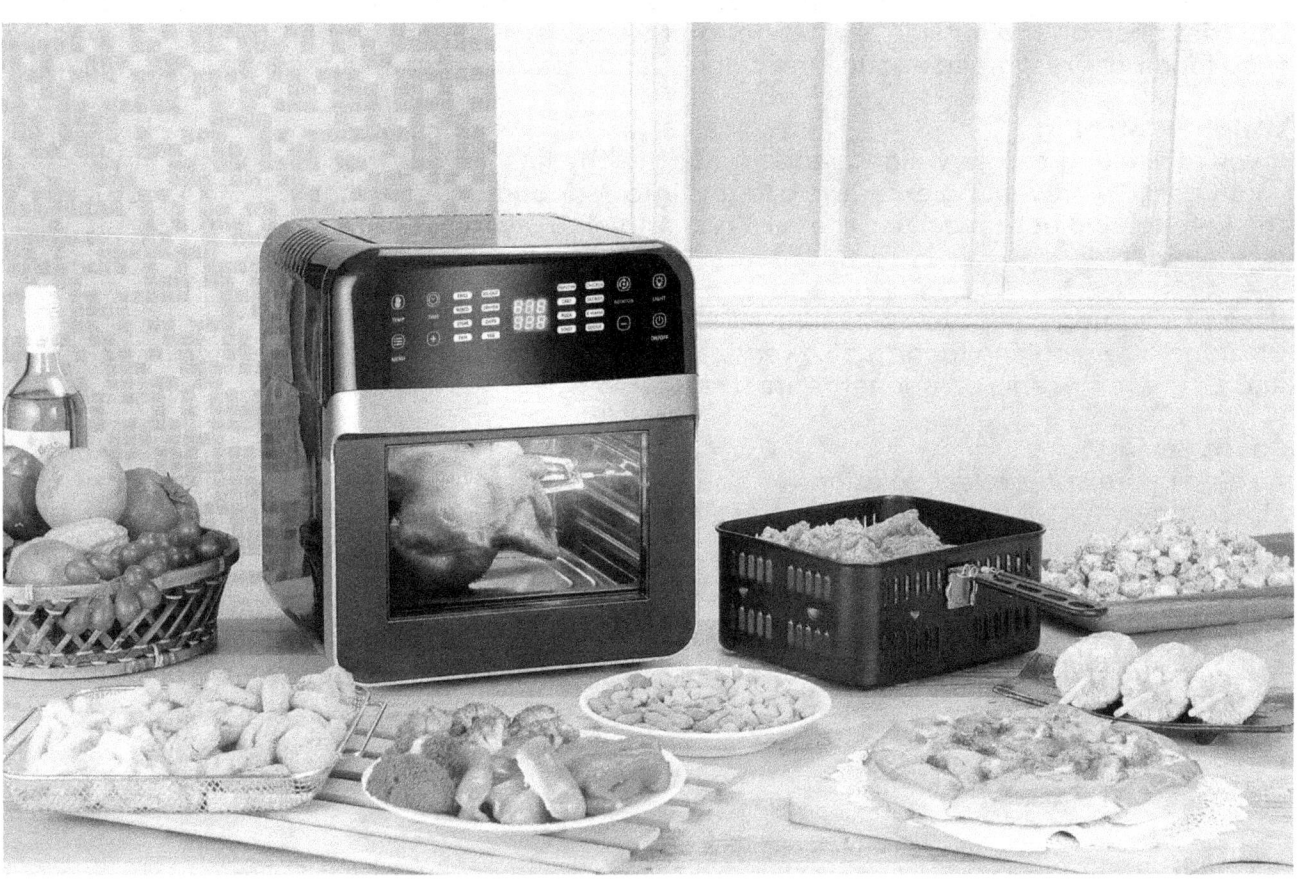

A ir Fryers have many benefits to offer when it comes to improving quality of life. It helps in maintaining your wellness and fitness.

Time-saving
Free time has become a luxury in our fast-paced lifestyles. Air Fryers are designed to save you time by serving you crunchy snacks and fried cuisines in a matter of minutes. If you are always on a tight schedule, an Air Fryer is no less than a time saver.

Superfast heating
Unlike traditional frying and baking methods, Air Fryers take only a few minutes to heat and prepare foods. They are always ready to make meals whenever you crave fried foods. Most Air Fryer models get ready in only 3 minutes to heat up properly.

Versatile options
Air Fryers allow you to cook a diverse range of foods, be it chicken tenders, mushrooms, crispy fries, fried shrimp, mozzarella sticks, or grilled vegetables. You want to grill, fry, roast, or bake your foods? Air Fryers are there to prepare them in no time. Specific ultra-modern range of Air Fryers also allow you to make many recipes in a single cooking session.

Air Fryer Cookbook

Natural food taste
It's quite common for anyone to worry about their food's ability to delight them with their mouthwatering flavors. When it comes to Air Fryers, things are no different. Air Fryers prepare meals without compromising on their taste profile. As far as the taste is concerned, they can easily be compared with deep-fried foods.

Healthy and Fatty Foods
Air Fryers work with transfer technology. They blow hot air into the cooking pan to cook food quickly and evenly on all sides. When frying your food in an Air Fryer, you need a tablespoon or less than a tablespoon of oil. One bowl of fries requires only one tablespoon of oil and makes the fries crisp on the outside and tender on the inside. If you are among the people who like fried food but are worried about extra calories and fats, this kitchen appliance is for you.

Weight Watching
If you're seeking to lose weight, reducing unhealthy fats in your food is a quick way to reach your goals. By preventing excessive bad fats into your body, weight loss is more effective. Even the ketogenic diet appreciates the Air Fryer and allows you to eat healthy fatty foods cooked by the Air Fryer.

Ease of cleaning
Cleaning after cooking foods is also very easy as Air Fryers are designed for effortless cleaning and all the removable components are dishwasher safe.

Space Saving
Air Fryers are the perfect solution for households with small counter space. They can fit in almost any area: tabletop, fridge top and even on the dinner table if you are the kind who likes to cook and eat simultaneously.

Energy Saving
I saved the best for the last. With the entire world going crazy about saving energy, the Air Fryer is one to count down those numbers. They use lesser electric power than regular electric ovens and do not heat up spaces.

Air Fryer Cookbook

BASIC CARE AND CLEANING

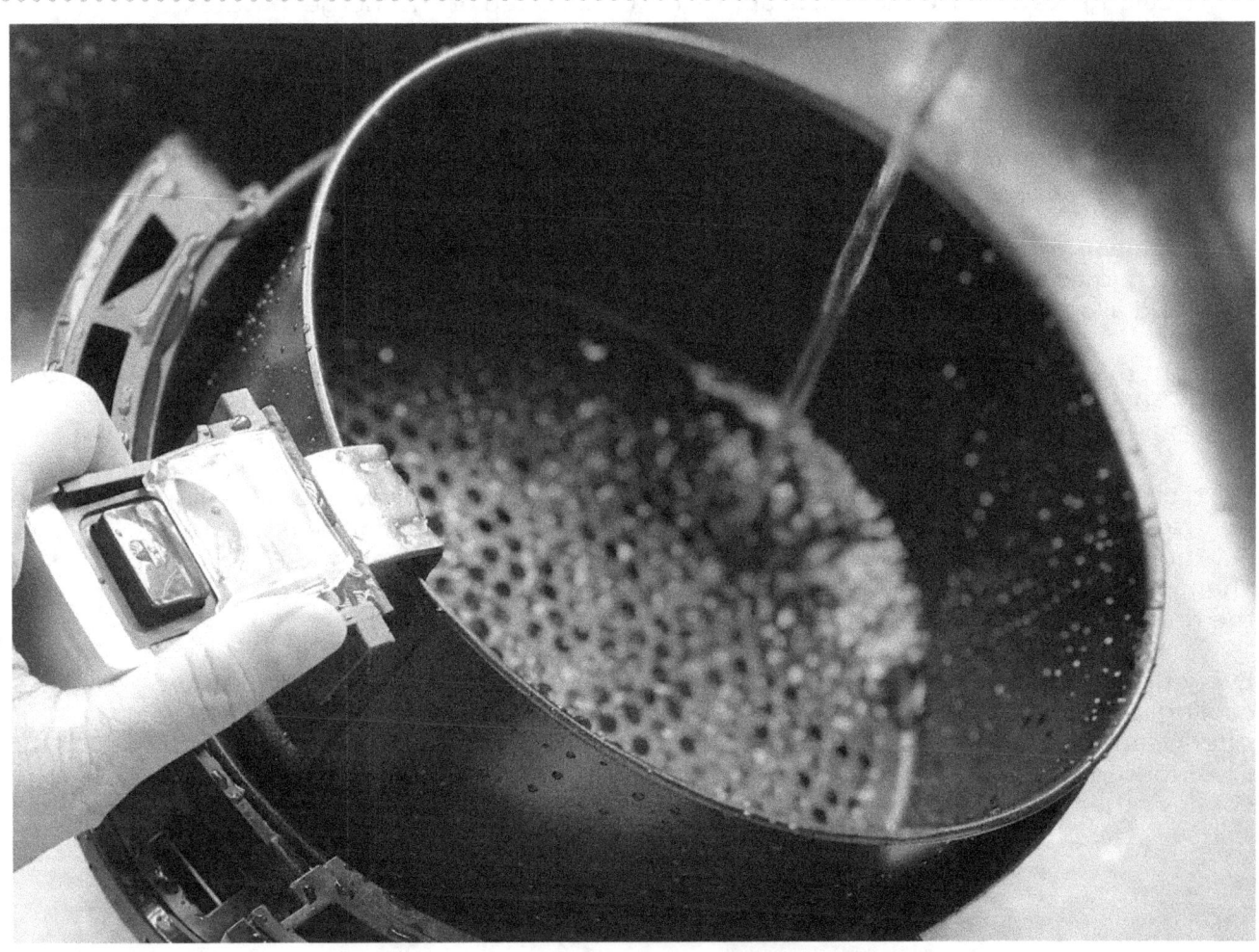

One of the other aspects I love of Air Fryer cooking is that it is "no mess, no fuss." Is there anything as off-putting as having to clean a mountain of greasy and sticky dishes after you're done preparing a delicious meal?

When using an Air Fryer, you'll most of the time only need a saucepan, mixing bowl, and a spoon in addition to your Air Fryer. What's more, the air fry basket and cooking tray are made of nonstick material, which makes cleaning a breeze. All you need is some warm soapy water and a dishcloth. Also, if food particles are stuck to the cooking tray or basket, you can just soak it for a while.

Don't forget that you also won't have to wipe down any areas around the Air Fryer - there won't be oil splatter everywhere as with normal deep frying. Everything happens in a closed container.

Overall, cleaning your Air Fryer is straightforward, but here is my cleaning routine for

Air Fryer Cookbook

reference.
1. Always make sure your Air Fryer is completely cooled down before attempting to clean it.
2. Never use any scouring pads, harsh chemicals, or powders on the in or outside of your Air Fryer.
3. Remove the cooking tray and air fry basket. You can soak the tray in warm water if it is too dirty just to wipe down. Alternatively, place the cooking tray in the dishwasher for a quick clean. You can spray the tray, basket, and cooking chamber with a mixture of baking soda and vinegar to remove stubborn food particles.
4. Clean the air fry basket and the outside of the Air Fryer with a soft wet cloth and dry to avoid streaking. Never rinse the whole appliance under a tap or submerge in water.
5. Unplug the appliance and make sure there isn't any grease or food debris inside. Use a soft cloth to clean the inside. In hard-to-reach areas, I always use a cleaning brush to remove debris.
6. Let all the parts dry entirely and then reassemble. You can cover your Air Fryer with a cover to avoid any dust from settling on it - but I know you'll be using it too often for that to happen!

How to clean the machine
When it comes to cleaning the Air Fryer Toast Oven, the general rule of thumb is to un-plug the fryer and allow it to cool completely.

Take out the baking pan, Air Fryer toast oven basket, oven rack and tray and hand wash these in warm-hot water with liquid soap. You can either use a nylon brush to clean them or a scouring pad. Do not put them in your dish washer at all.

Next, clean the interior walls using a clean damp cloth or sponge with a bit of liquid soap. Do not use any abrasive materials or corrosive products as these will damage the walls.
For the exterior part, use a clean damp cloth with a bit of liquid soap and it will clean up easily. Then just use a soft dry cloth to dry it completely. Avoid abrasive materials to avoid damaging the finish of the Air Fryer toast oven.

Every time you cook a greasy meal, clean the top interior part of the oven immediately after cooling. Doing this on a regular basis will ensure your Air Fryer performs very efficiently.
After cleaning, use the storage cleats, located at the back of the oven to store the cord of the Air Fryer toast oven. Do not wrap the cord around its body as this can damage it.
For any other kind of maintenance or servicing, take your unit to authorized service personnel.

Air Fryer Cookbook

HOW TO PREPARE YOUR KITCHEN TO AIR FRY

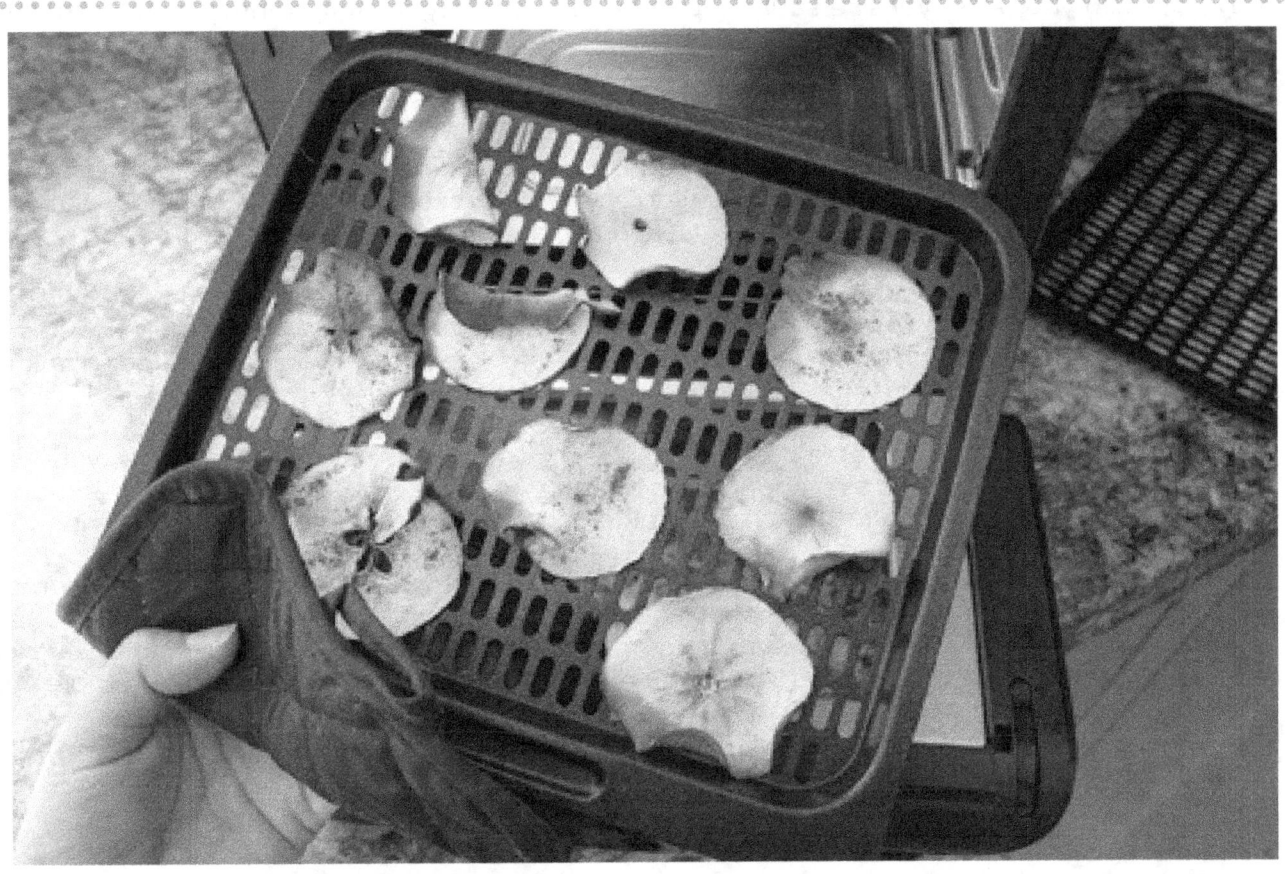

There are some tools I suggest you add to your kitchen arsenal so that you'll be able to cook anything your heart desires in your Air Fryer.

But before you go out looking for accessories, there are a few things you have to keep in mind.

Keep the size of the Air Fryer in mind. If you own a 4-1 Instant Vortex Air Fryer for example, I recommend not purchasing any pans or items larger than 8 ½ inches deep by 9 ½ inches wide. A square 8x8 pan will fit perfectly! If you own an Instant Pot, most of the items that are suitable for that appliance will work in the Vortex Air Fryer and other Air Fryers.

Don't forget the air space. Before buying deep items, keep in mind that there should be space at the top and bottom of the item for air to circulate.

Pay attention to the materials. A lot of items claim to be oven-safe, but that is not always the case. The quick heating of the air and the speedy circulation may cause glass dishes to crack or break. Where possible, don't use glass as all but choose stainless steel, aluminum, or ceramic items. If you have to use glass, make sure it's from a reputable brand known for its oven safety.

Okay, let's look at the top six Air Fryer accessories I recommend.

1. **Parchment Liners**

Air Fryer Cookbook

Who has time to clean food stuck to the fry basket? Air Fryer liners will cut your clean-up process in half. Don't use just any liners. Look for ones with holes in to help air circulate, and even then, you have to make sure the parchment paper is weighed down with something heavy, or the air will pick it up and whirl it around.

2.   Baking Pan

You can bake sweet and savory dishes in a baking pan; cake, monkey bread, macaroni, and cheese, etc. The fact that you can cook so many dishes in a baking pan makes it one of those must-have accessories.

3.   Grill Pan

Why not push your Air Fryer's versatility up a notch further by turning it into a grill? With this basic item, you'll be able to make burgers, grill steak, chicken, seafood, and anything else you can toss onto a grill.

4.   Cooking Rack with Skewers

A raised cooking rack is essential if you plan on using your Air Fryer for cooking larger foods. Air Fryers work by circulating heat around the food. If you place something down on the surface, the air won't be able to move around it, leaving you with uneven crispness. By using a cooking rack, the food is elevated, and air can circulate freely; the result is an even, crisp coating.

5.   Silicone Oven Mitts

I suppose you can use traditional oven mitts, but I'd highly recommend getting the silicone kind. They're not bulky, do a better job of protecting you from heat, but most importantly, they have a better grip than fabric mitts. You don't want a basket with hot food slipping and falling on you, your child, or pet. Personally, I see these as essential.

6.   Waffle Molds

Do your kids love waffles for breakfast each Saturday morning? The good news is, you can make them in the Air Fryer in a fraction of the time it would take you making it the traditional way. All you need are some Air Fryer waffle molds, and you're well on your way to winning the parent of the year award.

For those of you who use your Air Fryer the most out of all your other appliances, you may consider buying a full Air Fryer accessories pack. They include almost everything you need to ensure your Air Fryer success. You can also compare different versions to make sure you get one that contains items you think you'll use the most. With your kitchen all kitted out, there will be nothing you can't give a crispy coating.

Air Fryer Cookbook

USEFUL TIPS ON HOW TO BEST COOK WITH AN AIR FRYER

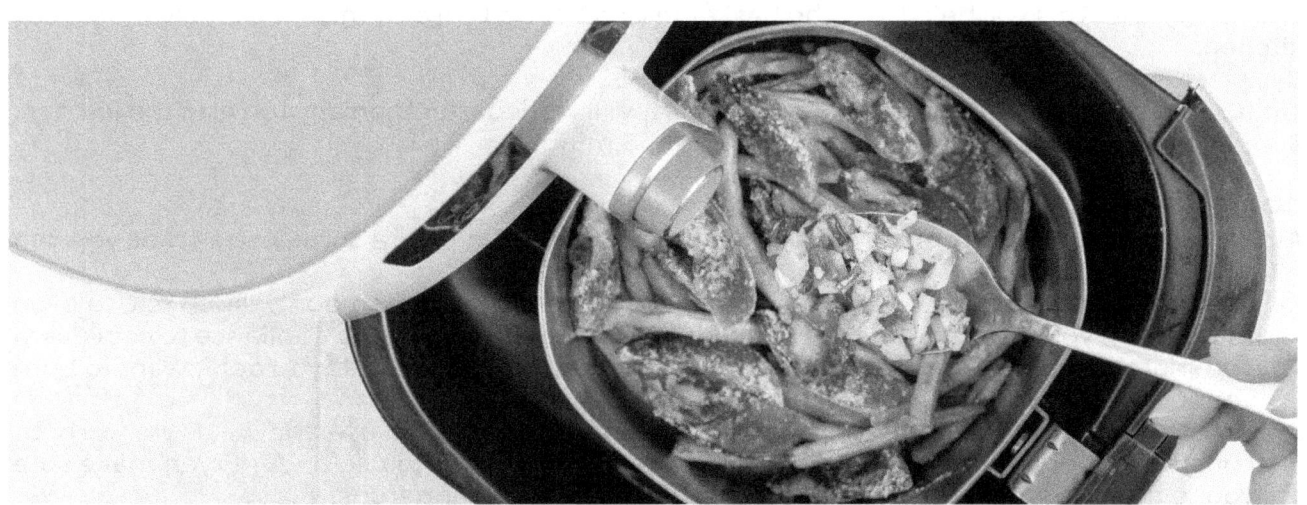

The following tips are ways to get the most from your Air Fryer and help you incorporate it into an everyday use appliance.

Tip 1: Placement of your Air Fryer is important; be sure it is placed on a heat-resistant countertop allowing five inches of space on all sides of the Air Fryer. This is to allow for proper venting of your Air Fryer during cooking.

Tip 2: Pre-Heat! Always before frying, bring your basket and inside of the Air Fryer up to temp. This is simple to do: just set your Air Fryer to the desired temperature and then turn it on for 3 minutes. When the timer sounds, the fryer is heated and you are ready to cook.

Tip 3: Invest in a hand pump kitchen spray bottle. This is a must-have when air frying. While you can brush or drizzle oil onto your food, a spray bottle gives more even coverage. Why not just use spray cans? The spray cans contain different aerosol agents that could break down the non-stick surface of your Air Fryer. With the hand-pump bottle, you can feel comfortable to spray right inside your basket and give your food the perfect coating.

Tip 4: What's fried food without breading? While you don't have to add breading to some items like chicken wings, there are many that like to. The key to breading in your Air Fryer is being diligent and not skipping steps. Always coat food with flour first, then egg, then breadcrumbs. Payi close attention to ensure that the breadcrumbs are pressed into the food. The Air Fryer is a convection oven so it has a really powerful fan and if the bread crumbs haven't adhered well, they will come off.

Tip 5: Overcrowding is not good. It is tempting to toss a few extra pieces in, but doing this makes it so that the air cannot fully circulate around what you are cooking. Overcrowding will also make the process take more time.

Air Fryer Cookbook

Tip 6: Use a little water in the bottom under the basket when cooking bacon or other fatty foods. This helps prevent the grease from getting too hot and smoking. Just enough water to slightly cover the bottom but not so much that it's coming up into the basket.

Tip 7: Use toothpicks to hold food in place. Light foods sometimes can fly around inside the Air Fryer. Using a toothpick to hold the bread on top of your grilled cheese sandwich, so it stays in place.

Tip 8: Always remove the basket from the drawer. If you pull the drawer and basket from the Air Fryer the grease and drippings are still at the bottom of the drawer. Removing the basket allows you to not include any unwanted grease on the plate before serving.

Tip 9: Clean up. Just like any other kitchen appliance, it is important to clean up the basket after every use. This will help keep the basket in good condition and the fried smell out of your kitchen.

Tip 10: Self-drying. Use the Air Fryer to dry itself; it will work better than any towel in the kitchen. Simply just set the fryer to 300 and turn it on for 3 minutes.

DOs and DON'Ts
Although your Air Fryer comes with built-in safety features, here are some extra steps you can follow to ensure safe use.
1. The Air Fryer gets really hot while working its air frying magic, so don't touch it. Use oven mitts when you slide out the air fry basket or, better yet, wait for the appliance to cool down completely. Also, keep an eye out for steam escaping from the vents; you don't want to burn your hands or face.
2. You shouldn't let anyone with physical or mental disabilities use the Air Fryer without constant supervision. The same goes if a person has no idea to use an Air Fryer; make sure you're there that they're not doing something wrong or dangerous.
3. Always place your Air Fryer out of reach of children. Make sure not to let the cord dangle from the countertop where a toddler can grab it and pull the warm appliance on to themselves.
4. Do not use your Air Fryer if you notice that its power cord is damaged.
5. Air Fryers are indoor appliances, so don't use it outside.
6. Never place your Air Fryer near a hot gas or an electric burner. It should be stable and secure on a dry, flat surface.
7. Make sure the air fry basket is locked in place before you use your fryer.
8. Don't tip the air fry basket to remove the food. The liquid inside may splash on you and cause burns.

WHAT ARE THE BEST AND WORST FOOD TO AIR FRY

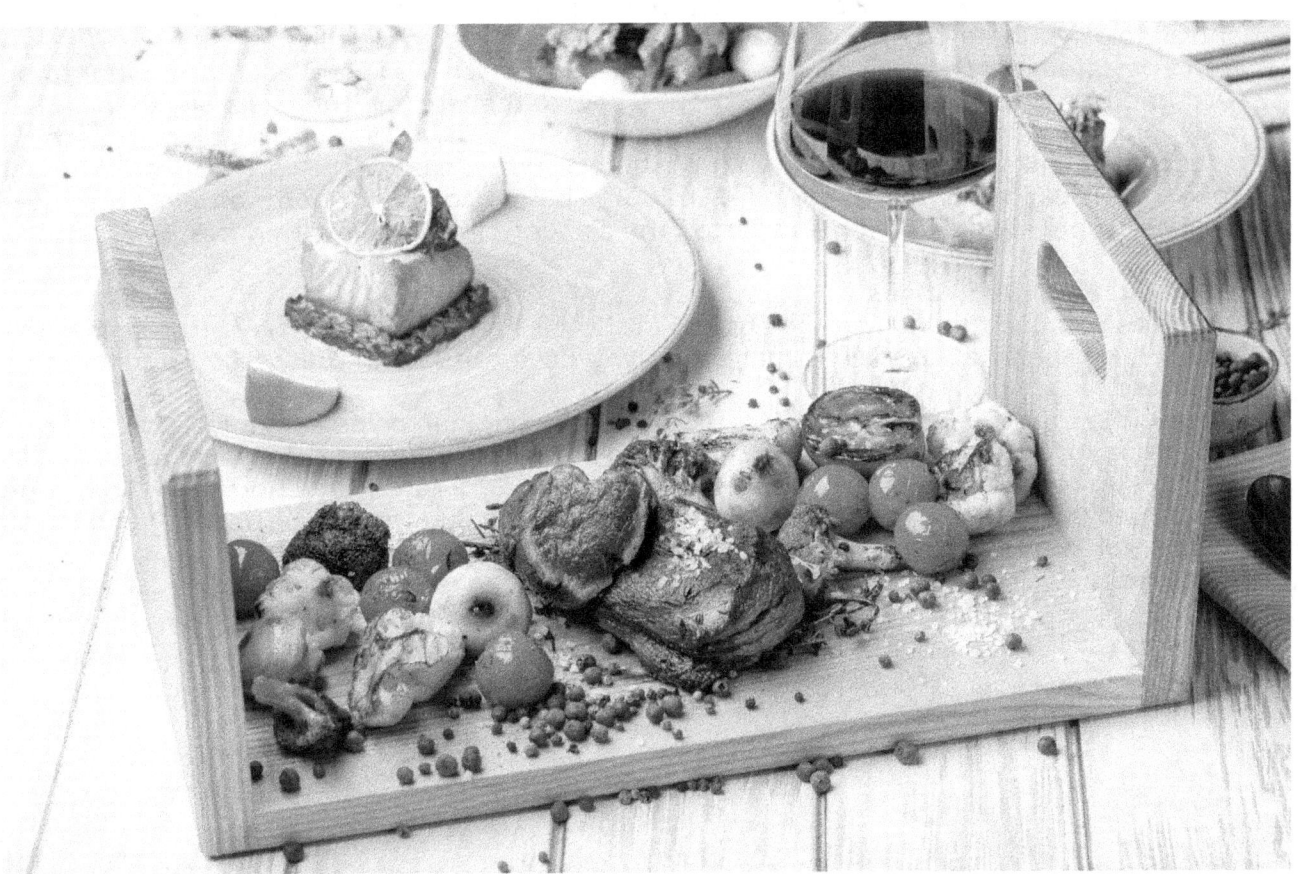

It goes without saying that with an Air Fryer, you can fry the foods that you always enjoyed deep-fried. They may even end up tasting better! Here are some things you need to keep in mind when it comes to ingredients.

The Best
- You can cook all vegetables in your Air Fryer. Cover it generously in batter and pop it in the Air Fryer. Crumbed beans with a tomato salsa are one of my favorite appetizers to serve to guests.
- You can cook meat, fish, and poultry in your Air Fryer any way you like: grill, roast, or fry. What are you in the mood for?
- Baking frozen foods in your Air Fryer will give it extra crunch than a standard convection oven would.
- If you fancy yourself a baker, you'd be happy to know that there won't be any temperature fluctuations in the Air Fryer. So, no more flopped souffle, cakes, or muffins.

Air Fryer Cookbook

The Worst

The Air Fryer is not meant for wet ingredients. The fan is mighty, and soups and sauces will just end up splattered all over. The same goes for food covered in wet batter. You'll end up with a ruined recipe and a big mess to clean.

Also, consider if the food you plan on making requires a lot of stirring. Pasta, for instance, will not cook well in an Air Fryer since it requires not only a lot of liquid to cook but also regular stirring.

How to Save Time Cooking

The Air Fryer will already cut your cooking time in half, but there are ways that you can get out of the kitchen even quicker. I enjoy cooking mouth-watering meals, but some days I want to get in and out as quickly as possible to spend time with my friends and family.

Here are some things I do to save time in the kitchen.
- Prepare ingredients. This is also known as mise en place. It is where you dice, cut, marinate, and prep all your ingredients before you start cooking.
- Don't deviate from the recipe. I know there are times when you feel you know what to do next and forget to check the recipe. If you're new to the kitchen, there is a big chance that you'll end up using too much or little of something, and you'll end up doing something wrong. It will take extra time to fix your mistake or, worst-case scenario, start from scratch.
- Take your meat out of the fridge a few minutes before cooking. Room temperature meat will cook more evenly, and it may shorten the cooking time by a few minutes.

Convert Your Favorite Recipes

Most recipes you can think of can be cooked in the Air Fryer. You'll only have to consider the size of the air fry basket, as well as make sure you have the required accessories for baking, sautéing, etc.

You'll also have to air fry food for 20% less time than the original recipe calls for, as the Air Fryer gets significantly hotter than the traditional convection oven. This means you'll also have to adjust the suggested temperature. I always set it to 25-50°F less than suggested. The same applies to packaged foods. For example, if the instructions on a packet of frozen French fries say to cook for 18 minutes at 450°F, then you'll air fry it for 15 minutes at 400°F.

It's as easy as that! Now it is up to you to find new and exciting recipes to try in your Air Fryer. You can start by browsing the collection of recipes in this cookbook. I am sure you'll see something that gets you salivating!

AIR FRYING COOKING CHARTS

The following charts provide a guide for cooking times and temperatures for your Air Fryer. These times assume that the basket is shaken to redistribute or items are flipped halfway through the cooking time.

BEEF	Portions	Time (mins)	Temp (F)
Hamburger	5 oz.	14	370°F
Stake, Filet Mignon	6 oz.	14	400°F
Steak, Flank	1 ½ lbs.	12	400°F
Meatball	1-inch rounds	7	370°F
Meatballs	3-inch rounds	10	380°F
Ribeye – with bone	1-inch thick, 8 oz.	10 to 14	400°F
Steak, Sirloin	1-inch thick, 12 oz.	9 to 14	400°F

CHICKEN	Portions	Time (mins)	Temp (F)
Breasts –with bone	1 ¼ lbs.	25	370°F
Breasts, w/o bone	4 oz.	12	380°F
Drumstick	2 lbs.	18	375°F
Thighs – with bone	2 lbs.	22	380°F
Thighs, boneless	1 lbs.	18	380°F
Legs – with bone	1 ¾ lbs.	30	380°F
Wings, drumette	2 lbs.	14	400°F
Game Hen	2 lbs. - halved	20	390°F
Whole Chicken	Whole	75	360°F
Tenders	Tenders	8 to 10	360°F

FISH AND SEAFOOD	Portions	Time (mins)	Temp (F)
Fish Fillet	8 oz. – 1 inch.	10	400°F
Salmon, fillet	8 oz.	13	375°F
Swordfish steak	8 oz.	10	400°F
Calamari	8 oz.	4	400°F
Tuna, Steak	8 oz.	7 to 10	400°F
Scallops	8 oz.	5 to 7	400°F
Shrimp	8 oz.	5	400°F

FROZEN FOODS	Portions	Time (mins)	Temp (F)
Thin Fries	20 oz.	14	400°F
Thick Fries	17 oz.	18	400°F
Mozzarella - Sticks	11 oz.	8	400°F
Fish Sticks	10 oz.	10	400°F
Fish Fillets	½-inch, 10 oz.	14	400°F
Onion Rings	12 oz.	8	400°F
Chicken Nuggets	12 oz.	10	400°F
Breaded Shrimp	Breaded Shrimp	9	400°F

PORK AND LAMB	Portions	Time (mins)	Temp (F)
Loin	2 lbs.	55	360°F
Pork Chops, bone in	1-inch, 6 ½ oz.	12	400°F
Tenderloin	1 ½ – 2 lbs.	15	370°F
Bacon	regular	5 to 7	400°F
Bacon	thick-cut	6 to 10	400°F
Sausages	regular	15	380°F
Lamb Chop	1-inch thick	8 to 12	400°F
Lamb - Rack	1 ½ – 2 lbs.	22	380°F

Air Fryer Cookbook

VEGETABLES	Portions	Time (mins)	Temp (F)
Asparagus	1-inch sliced	5	400°F
Beets	whole	40	400°F
Broccoli	florets	6	400°F
Brussel Sprouts	halved	15	380°F
Carrots	1-inch sliced	15	380°F
Cauliflower	florets	12	400°F
Corn on the cob	cob	6	390°F
Eggplant	1 ½ -inch cubed	15	400°F
Fennel	quartered	15	370°F
Mushrooms	1/4-inch sliced	5	400°F
Onions	pearl	10	400°F
Peppers	1-inch chunks	15	400°F
Potatoes	1 ½ lb. small baby	15	400°F
Potatoes	1-inch chunks	12	400°F
Potatoes	Whole - baked	40	400°F
Squash	1/2-inch chunks	12	400°F
Sweet Potato	baked	30 to 35	380°F
Tomatoes	cherry	4	400°F
Tomatoes	halves	10	350°F
Zucchini	1/2-inch sticks	12	400°F

4-WEEK MEAL PLAN

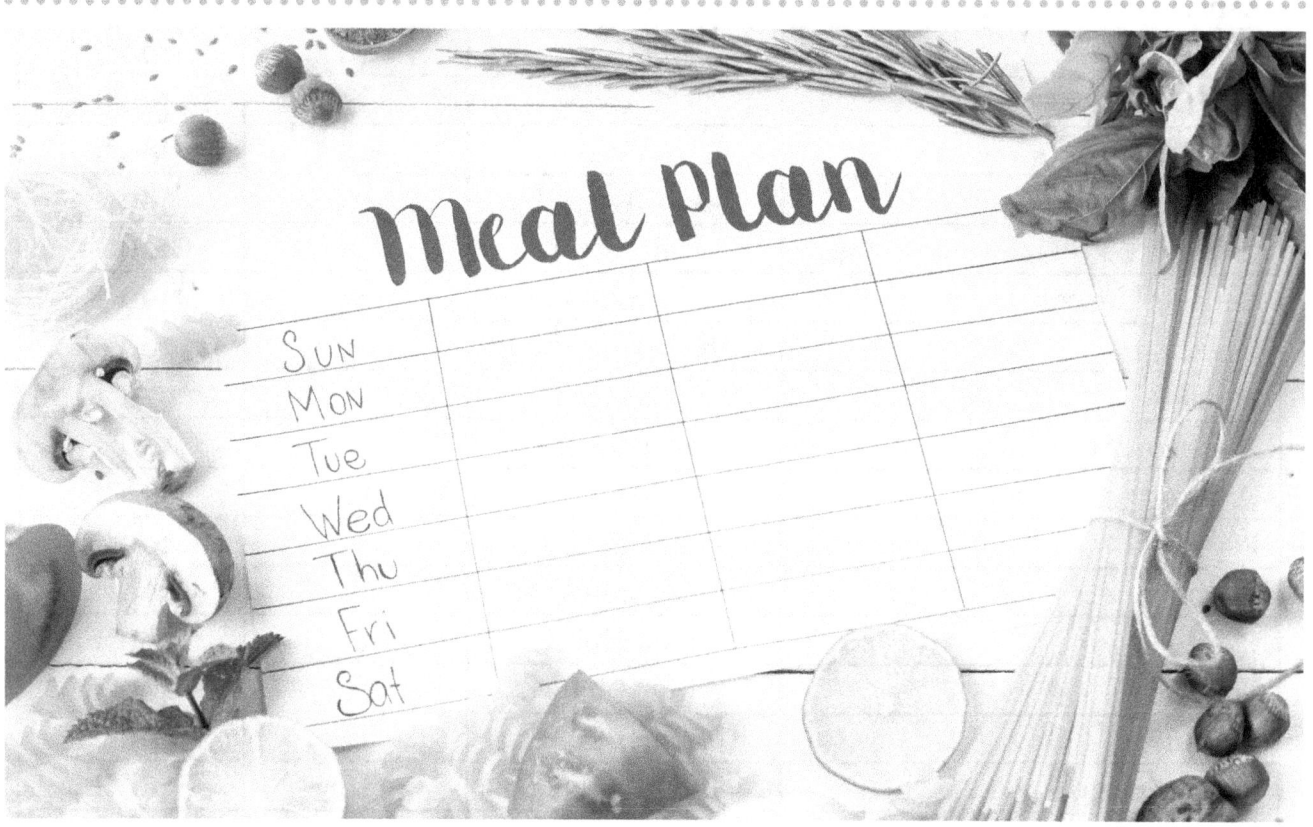

A month comprises weeks, so starting off with planning your meals for a week can serve as a guideline for you. Here are some tips on how to go about it.

Set aside time before the week starts to plan your meals
This saves you a lot of compromises. Setting time aside makes you plan with your diet regime in mind, the time you have to cook, the available groceries at home, what you wish to buy and can afford all at the same time. Fridays and Saturdays are good days for this.

Check your Calendar for the week
Events can actually interfere with your planning, so use your calendar to determine what time you will or will not be cooking, and how much food you need or shopping you will have to do.
Consider the people you will be feeding
Children, aged persons, and young adults need to be considered when planning meals in terms of calories needed, food items to deal with, and exactly what they like and do not like.

Add leftovers to your plan
If you are cooking for a large family, kids or guests, chances are there will be leftovers. What happens to them? Well, they save you from cooking a new meal every time you know how to treat them right. So yes, include them.

Cultivate Good Food Storage Habits
Learn to store food properly. That way, some meals can end up becoming cornerstone ingredients for another superb meal.
Take your favorite traditional method recipes and convert them over to amazing air frying creations. Virtually anything you have a recipe to cook in the oven, you can convert to cook

Air Fryer Cookbook

in the Air Fryer. Remember: the Air Fryer heat is significantly more intense than a standard oven, so start by reducing the suggested temperature by 25°F to 50°F and reduce the time by approximately 20%.

If the recipe calls for something to be baked at 425°F for 60 minutes you would air fry it at 400°F for 48 minutes, timing may vary. Always feel free to open the Air Fryer and check for doneness. Cooking packaged foods can also apply to the same rules as above. For example, if you are cooking frozen fries, the bag suggests 450°F for 18 minutes then cook the fries at 400°F for 15 minutes. Remember to shake the basket with items like French fries to help with the cooking process and evenly browning.

The Air Fryer is not a complicated appliance, but there are some tips I picked up that I want to share with you. But, before I do, let's look at things to keep in mind to ensure your safety.

Choosing the Right Cooking Mode

All cooking programs are essentially the same. The only difference is the temperature the mode heats to, as well as the cooking time. In the beginning, I didn't know this, and, unfortunately, the manual doesn't tell you. The different programs are only there for your convenience—you don't have to manually set the time and temperature; you just press one button.

Once you have the food you want to eat, the next step is to make sure that you are cooking it the way you want. There are some different methods that you should use. The first is that you want to make sure that you are going one of three ways. The best methods are using an Air Fryer, the stovetop, or firing up the grill.

There are lots of interesting ideas as well. When you reflect on where you were and how far you have come, you will notice that you were eating a bunch of starches, including pasta, rice, mac and cheese, baked potatoes, etc. The Air Fryer is one of the best ways to prepare food in a healthy way, making life so much easier.

Here is a 4-week meal plan example to help you plan your meals throughout the month. The number between brackets indicates the recipe's number, so that you can easily locate it in the book.

Days	Breakfast	Lunch	Dinner	Dessert
1	Zucchini Muffins (1)	Turkey Breasts (201)	Rolled Salmon Sandwich (75)	Cocoa Pudding (558)
2	Jalapeno Breakfast Muffins (2)	Salmon Patties (388)	Vegetable Egg Rolls (190)	Blueberry Coconut Crackers (559)
3	Simple Egg Soufflé (3)	Ketogenic Mach and Cheese (460)	Tomato & Feta Shrimp (441)	Cauliflower Pudding (560)
4	Vegetable Egg Soufflé (4)	Pork Joint (312)	Chicken Fillets, Brie & Ham (218)	Sweet Vanilla Rhubarb (561)
5	Asparagus Frittata (5)	Zucchini Curry (490)	Roast Beef (284)	Shortbread fingers (562)
6	Breakfast Scramble Casserole (21)	Pesto Gnocchi (196)	Rotisserie Chicken (203)	Fruit Crumble Pie (563)
7	Breakfast Grilled Ham and Cheese (22)	Honey Duck Breasts (208)	Crispy Keto Pork Bites (423)	Chocolate Mug Cake (564)
8	Zucchini Noodles (8)	Lamb Burgers (296)	Duck Thighs from the Air Fryer (488)	Fried Peaches (565)
9	Mushroom Frittata (9)	Roasted Chicken (442)	Fish Nuggets (407)	Coconut Donuts (543)
10	Blueberry Breakfast Cobbler (10)	Sauteed Trout with Almonds (371)	Potato Gratin (478)	Apple Pie (567)
11	Yummy Breakfast Italian Frittata (11)	Chicken Meatballs (228)	Wild Caught Salmon (422)	Cinnamon Rolls (568)
12	Savory Cheese and Bacon Muffins (12)	Beef Rolls (281)	Rice Flour Coated Shrimp (400)	Cherries and Rhubarb Bowls (569)
13	Best Air-Fried English Breakfast (13)	Chicken Casserole (467)	Chinese Style Cod (343)	Pumpkin Bowls (570)
14	Sausage and Egg Breakfast Burrito (14)	Air Fryer Baby Back Ribs (309)	Codfish Nuggets (357)	Apple Jam (571)

Days	Breakfast	Lunch	Dinner	Dessert
15	French Toast Sticks (15)	Honey Glazed Salmon (373)	Beef and Broccoli (325)	Yogurt and Pumpkin Cream (570)
16	Home-Fried Potatoes (16)	Beef Balls with Mixed Herbs (132)	Salt and Pepper Wings (266)	Raisins Rice Mix (571)
17	Homemade Cherry Breakfast Tarts (17)	Chopped Bondiola (489)	Spicy Mackerel (341)	Orange Bowls (572)
18	Sausage and Cream Cheese Biscuits (18)	Flying Fish (417)	Buffalo Chicken Tenders (210)	Strawberry Jam (573)
19	Classic Hash Brown (23)	Hot Chicken Wingettes (96)	Light Herbed Meatballs (323)	Caramel Cream (574)
20	Cheesy Tater Tot Breakfast Bake (20)	Buttery Cod (389)	Tilapia and Chives Sauce (346)	Wrapped Pears (575)
21	Radish Hash Brown (25)	Easy Lemon Chicken Thighs (214)	Perfect Chicken Thighs Dinner (269)	Perfect Cinnamon Toast (576)
22	Vegetable Egg Cups (26)	Simple Beef Patties (278)	Teriyaki Wings (211)	Angel Food Cake (579)
23	Spinach Frittata (27)	Lemon Butter Scallops (339)	Air Fryer Fish Tacos (418)	Apple Dumplings (580)
24	Omelette Frittata (28)	Cajun Pork Steaks (328)	Adobo Chicken (440)	Chocolate Donuts (581)
25	Coconut Porridge with Flax Seed (31)	Garlic Lemon Shrimp (404)	Fish with Chips (382)	Apple Hand Pies (582)
26	Baked Berry Oatmeal (36)	Greek Vegetable Skillet (322)	Italian Shredded Chicken (444)	Sweet Cream Cheese Wontons (583)
27	Pancakes (41)	Chicken Parmesan Wings (205)	Egg Roll Pizza Sticks (480)	French Toast Bites (584)
28	Eggs on the Go (45)	Beef Tenderloin (292)	Spicy Zucchini (471)	Cinnamon Sugar Roasted Chickpeas (585)

BREAKFAST

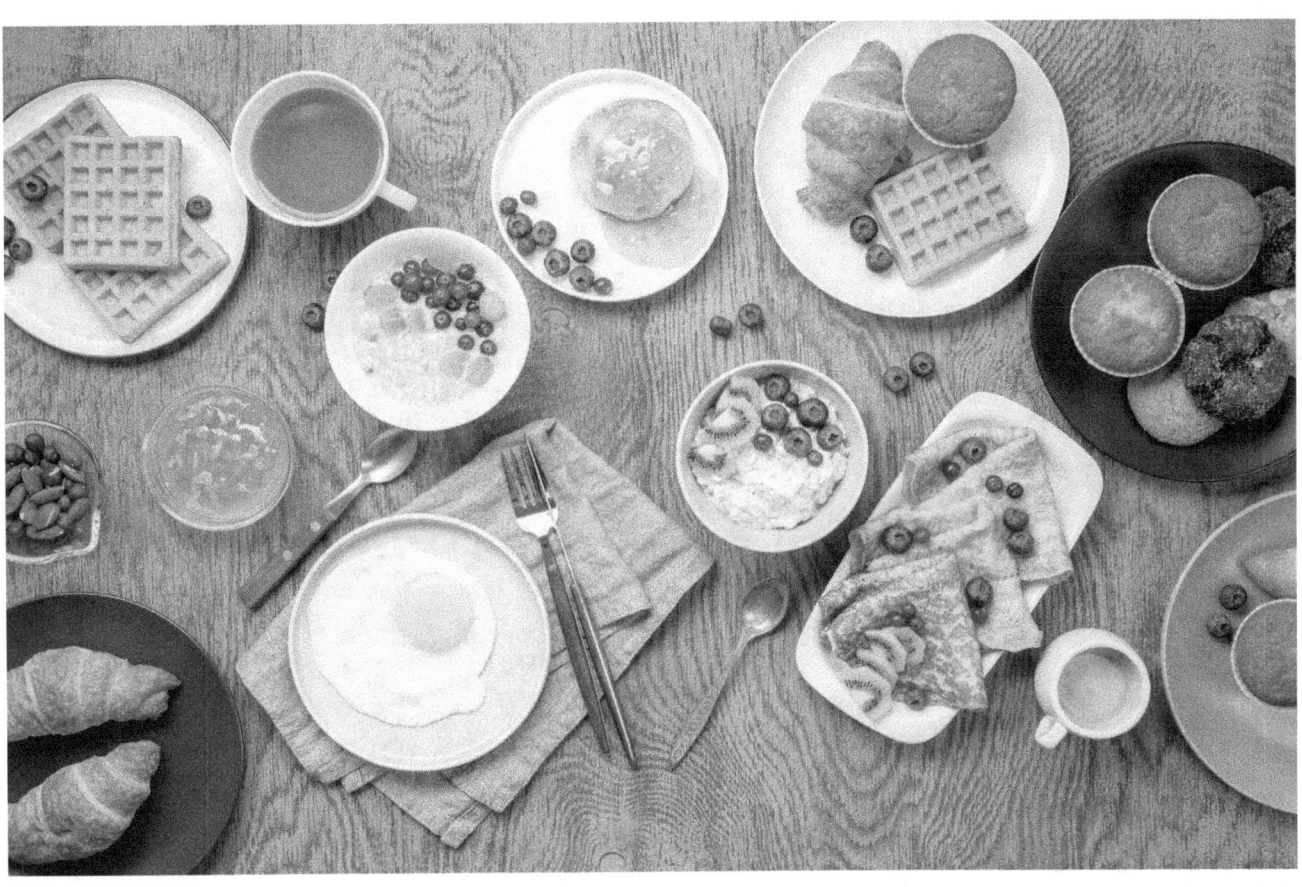

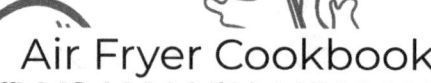

Air Fryer Cookbook

1. ZUCCHINI MUFFINS

PREPARATION: 10 MIN   **COOKING:** 20 MIN   **SERVINGS:** 8

INGREDIENTS

- 6 eggs
- 4 drops stevia
- 1/4 cup swerve
- 1/3 cup coconut oil, melted
- 1 cup zucchini, grated
- 3/4 cup coconut flour
- 1/4 tsp. ground nutmeg
- 1 tsp. ground cinnamon
- 1/2 tsp. baking soda

Nutrition: *Calories 136, Fat 12g, Carbs 1g, Protein 4g*

DIRECTIONS

1. Preheat the Air Fryer to 325°F.
2. Add all ingredients except zucchini in a bowl and mix well.
3. Add zucchini and stir well.
4. Pour batter into the silicone muffin molds and place into the Air Fryer basket.
5. Cook muffins for 20 minutes
6. Serve and enjoy.

2. JALAPENO BREAKFAST MUFFINS

PREPARATION: 10 MIN   **COOKING:** 15 MIN   **SERVINGS:** 8

INGREDIENTS

- 5 eggs
- 1/3 cup coconut oil, melted
- 2 tsp. baking powder
- 3 tbsp. erythritol
- 3 tbsp. jalapenos, sliced
- 1/4 cup unsweetened coconut milk
- 2/3 cup coconut flour
- 3/4 tsp. sea salt

Nutrition: *Calories 125, Fat 12g, Carbs 7g, Protein 3g*

DIRECTIONS

1. Preheat the Air Fryer to 325°F.
2. In a large bowl, mix together coconut flour, baking powder, erythritol, and sea salt.
3. Stir in eggs, jalapenos, coconut milk, and coconut oil until well combined.
4. Pour batter into the silicone muffin molds and place into the Air Fryer basket.
5. Cook muffins for 15 minutes
6. Serve and enjoy.

3. SIMPLE EGG SOUFFLÉ

PREPARATION: 5 MIN   **COOKING:** 8 MIN   **SERVINGS:** 2

INGREDIENTS

- 2 eggs
- 1/4 tsp. chili pepper
- 2 tbsp. heavy cream
- 1/4 tsp. pepper
- 1 tbsp. parsley, chopped
- Salt

Nutrition: *Calories 116, Fat 10g, Carbs 1.1g, Protein 6g*

DIRECTIONS

1. In a bowl, whisk eggs with remaining gradients.
2. Spray two ramekins with cooking spray.
3. Pour egg mixture into the prepared ramekins and place into the Air Fryer basket.
4. Cook soufflé at 390°F for 8 minutes
5. Serve and enjoy.

4. VEGETABLE EGG SOUFFLÉ

PREPARATION: 10 MIN **COOKING:** 20 MIN **SERVINGS:** 4

INGREDIENTS

- 4 large eggs
- 1 tsp. onion powder
- 1 tsp. garlic powder
- 1 tsp. red pepper, crushed
- 1/2 cup broccoli florets, chopped
- 1/2 cup mushrooms, chopped

DIRECTIONS

1. Sprinkle four ramekins with cooking spray and set aside.
2. In a bowl, whisk eggs with onion powder, garlic powder, and red pepper.
3. Add mushrooms and broccoli and stir well.
4. Pour egg mixture into the prepared ramekins and place ramekins into the Air Fryer basket.
5. Cook at 350°F for 15 minutes. Make sure soufflé is cooked. If soufflé is not cooked, then cook for 5 minutes more.
6. Serve and enjoy.

Nutrition: *Calories 91 Fat 5.1g Carbs 4.7g Protein 7.4g*

5. ASPARAGUS FRITTATA

PREPARATION: 10 MIN **COOKING:** 10 MIN **SERVINGS:** 4

INGREDIENTS

- 6 eggs
- 3 mushrooms, sliced
- 10 asparagus, chopped
- 1/4 cup half and half
- 2 tsp. butter, melted
- 1 cup mozzarella cheese, shredded
- 1 tsp. pepper
- 1 tsp. salt

DIRECTIONS

1. Toss mushrooms and asparagus with melted butter and add into the Air Fryer basket. Cook mushrooms and asparagus at 350°F for 5 minutes. Shake basket twice.
2. Meanwhile, in a bowl, whisk together eggs, half and half, pepper, and salt. Transfer cook mushrooms and asparagus into the Air Fryer baking dish. Pour egg mixture over mushrooms and asparagus.
3. Place dish in the Air Fryer and cook at 350°F for 5 minutes or until eggs are set. Slice and serve.

Nutrition: *Calories 211 Fat 13g Carbs 4g Protein 16g*

7. BROCCOLI STUFFED PEPPERS

PREPARATION: 10 MIN **COOKING:** 40 MIN **SERVINGS:** 2

INGREDIENTS

- 4 eggs
- 1/2 cup cheddar cheese, grated
- 2 bell peppers cut in half and remove seeds
- 1/2 tsp. garlic powder
- 1 tsp. dried thyme
- 1/4 cup feta cheese, crumbled
- 1/2 cup broccoli, cooked
- 1/4 tsp. pepper
- 1/2 tsp. salt

DIRECTIONS

1. Preheat the Air Fryer to 325°F.
2. Stuff feta and broccoli into the bell peppers halved.
3. Beat egg in a bowl with seasoning and pour egg mixture into the pepper halved over feta and broccoli.
4. Place bell pepper halved into the Air Fryer basket and cook for 35-40 minutes
5. Top with grated cheddar cheese and cook until cheese melted.
6. Serve and enjoy.

Nutrition: Calories 340 Fat 22g Carbs 12g Protein 22g

8. ZUCCHINI NOODLES

PREPARATION: 10 MIN **COOKING:** 44 MIN **SERVINGS:** 3

INGREDIENTS

- 1 egg
- 1/2 cup parmesan cheese, grated
- 1/2 cup feta cheese, crumbled
- 1 tbsp. thyme
- 1 garlic clove, chopped
- 1 onion, chopped
- 2 medium zucchinis, trimmed and spiralized
- 2 tbsp. olive oil
- 1 cup mozzarella cheese, grated
- 1/2 tsp. pepper
- 1/2 tsp. salt

DIRECTIONS

1. Preheat the Air Fryer to 350°F.
2. Add spiralized zucchini and salt in a colander and set aside for 10 minutes. Wash zucchini noodles and pat dry with a paper towel.
3. Heat the oil in a pan over medium heat. Add garlic and onion and sauté for 3-4 minutes
4. Add zucchini noodles and cook for 4-5 minutes or until softened.
5. Add zucchini mixture into the Air Fryer baking pan. Add egg, thyme, cheeses. Mix well and season.
6. Place pan in the Air Fryer and cook for 30-35 minutes
7. Serve and enjoy.

Nutrition: Calories 435 Fat 29g Carbs 10.4g Protein 25g

9. MUSHROOM FRITTATA

PREPARATION: 10 MIN   **COOKING:** 13 MIN   **SERVINGS:** 1

INGREDIENTS

- 1 cup egg whites
- 1 cup spinach, chopped
- 2 mushrooms, sliced
- 2 tbsp. parmesan cheese, grated
- Salt

DIRECTIONS

1. Sprinkle pan with cooking spray and heat over medium heat. Add mushrooms and sauté for 2-3 minutes Add spinach and cook for 1-2 minutes or until wilted.
2. Transfer mushroom spinach mixture into the Air Fryer pan. Beat egg whites in a mixing bowl until frothy. Season it with a pinch of salt.
3. Pour egg white mixture into the spinach and mushroom mixture and sprinkle with parmesan cheese. Place pan in Air Fryer basket and cook frittata at 350°F for 8 minutes
4. Slice and serve.

Nutrition: *Calories 176 Fat 3g Carbs 4g Protein 31g*

10. BLUEBERRY BREAKFAST COBBLER

PREPARATION: 10 MIN   **COOKING:** 15 MIN   **SERVINGS:** 4

INGREDIENTS

- ⅓ cup whole-wheat pastry flour
- ¾ tsp. baking powder
- Dash sea salt
- ½ cup 2% milk
- 2 tbsp. pure maple syrup
- ½ tsp. vanilla extract
- Cooking oil spray
- ½ cup fresh blueberries
- ¼ cup Granola, or plain store-bought granola

DIRECTIONS

1. In a medium bowl, whisk the flour, baking powder, and salt. Add the milk, maple syrup, and vanilla and gently whisk, just until thoroughly combined.
2. Preheat the unit in bake mode, setting the temperature to 350°F, and setting the time to 3 minutes.
3. Spray a 6-by-2-inch round baking pan with cooking oil and pour the batter into the pan. Top evenly with the blueberries and granola.
4. Once the unit is preheated, place the pan into the basket and cook for 15 minutes.
5. When the cooking is complete, the cobbler should be nicely browned and a knife inserted into the middle should come out clean. Enjoy plain or topped with a little vanilla yogurt.

Nutrition: *Calories 112 Fat 1g Carbs 23g Protein 3g*

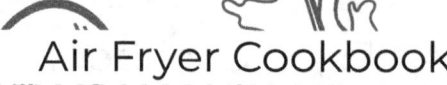
Air Fryer Cookbook

11. YUMMY BREAKFAST ITALIAN FRITTATA

PREPARATION: 5 MIN   **COOKING:** 10 MIN   **SERVINGS:** 6

INGREDIENTS

- 6 eggs
- 1/3 cup of milk
- 4 oz. of chopped Italian sausage
- 3 cups of stemmed and roughly chopped kale
- 1 red deseeded and chopped bell pepper
- ½ cup of a grated feta cheese
- 1 chopped zucchini
- 1 tbsp. of freshly chopped basil
- 1 tsp. of garlic powder
- 1 tsp. of onion powder
- 1 tsp. of salt
- 1 tsp. of black pepper

DIRECTIONS

1. Turn on your Air Fryer to 360°F.
2. Grease the Air Fryer pan with a nonstick cooking spray.
3. Add the Italian sausage to the pan and cook it inside your Air Fryer for 5 minutes
4. While doing that, add and stir in the remaining ingredients until it mixes properly.
5. Add the egg mixture to the pan and allow it to cook inside your Air Fryer for 5 minutes
6. Thereafter carefully remove the pan and allow it to cool off until it gets chill enough to serve.
7. Serve and enjoy!

Nutrition: *Calories 225 Fat 14g Carbs 4.5g Protein 20g*

12. SAVORY CHEESE AND BACON MUFFINS

PREPARATION: 5 MIN   **COOKING:** 17 MIN   **SERVINGS:** 4

INGREDIENTS

- 1 ½ cup of all-purpose flour
- 2 tsp.s of baking powder
- ½ cup of milk
- 2 eggs
- 1 tbsp. of freshly chopped parsley
- 4 cooked and chopped bacon slices
- 1 thinly chopped onion
- ½ cup of shredded cheddar cheese
- ½ tsp. of onion powder
- 1 tsp. of salt
- 1 tsp. of black pepper

DIRECTIONS

1. Turn on your Air Fryer to 360°F.
2. Using a large bowl, add and stir all the ingredients until it mixes properly.
3. Then grease the muffin cups with a nonstick cooking spray or line it with a parchment paper. Pour the batter proportionally into each muffin cup.
4. Place it inside your Air Fryer and bake it for 15 minutes
5. Thereafter, carefully remove it from your Air Fryer and allow it to chill.
6. Serve and enjoy!

Nutrition: *Calories 180 Fat 18g Carbs 16g Protein 15g*

Air Fryer Cookbook

13. BEST AIR-FRIED ENGLISH BREAKFAST

PREPARATION: 5 MIN **COOKING:** 20 MIN **SERVINGS:** 4

INGREDIENTS

- 8 sausages
- 8 bacon slices
- 4 eggs
- 1 (16-oz.) can of baked beans
- 8 slices of toast

Nutrition: *Calories 850 Fat 40gCarbs 20g Protein 48g*

DIRECTIONS

1. Add the sausages and bacon slices to your Air Fryer and cook them for 10 minutes at a 320°F.
2. Using a ramekin or heat-safe bowl, add the baked beans, then place another ramekin and add the eggs and whisk.
3. Place it inside your Air Fryer and cook it for an additional 10 minutes or until everything is done.
4. Serve and enjoy!

14 SAUSAGE AND EGG BREAKFAST BURRITO

PREPARATION: 5 MIN **COOKING:** 30 MIN **SERVINGS:** 6

INGREDIENTS

- 6 eggs
- Salt
- Pepper
- Cooking oil
- ½ cup chopped red bell pepper
- ½ cup chopped green bell pepper
- 8 oz. ground chicken sausage
- ½ cup salsa
- 6 medium (8-inch) flour tortillas
- ½ cup shredded Cheddar cheese

Nutrition: *Calories 236 Fat 13gCarbs 16g Protein 15g*

DIRECTIONS

1. In a medium bowl, whisk the eggs. Add salt and pepper to taste.
2. Place a skillet on medium-high heat. Spray with cooking oil. Add the eggs. Scramble for 2 to 3 minutes, until the eggs are fluffy. Remove the eggs from the skillet and set aside.
3. If needed, spray the skillet with more oil. Add the chopped red and green bell peppers. Cook for 2 to 3 minutes, once the peppers are soft.
4. Add the ground sausage to the skillet. Break the sausage into smaller pieces using a spatula or spoon. Cook for 3 to 4 minutes, until the sausage is brown.
5. Add the salsa and scrambled eggs. Stir to combine. Remove the skillet from heat.
6. Spoon the mixture evenly onto the tortillas.
7. To form the burritos, fold the sides of each tortilla in toward the middle and then roll up from the bottom. You can secure each burrito with a toothpick. Or you can moisten the outside edge of the tortilla with a small amount of water. I prefer to use a cooking brush, but you can also dab with your fingers.
8. Spray the burritos with cooking oil and place them in the Air Fryer. Do not stack. Cook the burritos in batches if they do not all fit in the basket. Cook for 8 minutes at 345°F
9. Open the Air Fryer and flip the burritos. Heat it for an additional 2 minutes or until crisp.
10. If necessary, repeat steps 8 and 9 for the remaining burritos.
11. Sprinkle the Cheddar cheese over the burritos. Cool before serving.

Air Fryer Cookbook

15. FRENCH TOAST STICKS

PREPARATION: 5 MIN **COOKING:** 15 MIN **SERVINGS:** 12

INGREDIENTS

- 4 slices Texas toast (or any thick bread, such as challah)
- 1 tbsp. butter
- 1 egg
- 1 tsp. stevia
- 1 tsp. ground cinnamon
- ¼ cup milk
- 1 tsp. vanilla extract
- Cooking oil

DIRECTIONS

1. Cut each slice of bread into 3 pieces (for 12 sticks total).
2. Place the butter in a small, microwave-safe bowl. Heat for 15 seconds, or until the butter has melted.
3. Remove the bowl from the microwave. Add the egg, stevia, cinnamon, milk, and vanilla extract. Whisk until fully combined.
4. Sprinkle the Air Fryer basket with cooking oil.
5. Dredge each of the bread sticks in the egg mixture.
6. Place the French toast sticks in the Air Fryer. It is okay to stack them. Spray the French toast sticks with cooking oil. Cook for 8 minutes at 330°F.
7. Open the Air Fryer and flip each of the French toast sticks. Cook for an additional 4 minutes, or until the French toast sticks are crisp.
8. Cool before serving.

Nutrition: Calories 52 Fat 2g Carbs 7g Protein 2g

16. HOME-FRIED POTATOES

PREPARATION: 5 MIN **COOKING:** 25 MIN **SERVINGS:** 4

INGREDIENTS

- 3 large russet potatoes
- 1 tbsp. canola oil
- 1 tbsp. extra-virgin olive oil
- 1 tsp. paprika
- Salt
- Pepper
- 1 cup chopped onion
- 1 cup chopped red bell pepper
- 1 cup chopped green bell pepper

DIRECTIONS

1. Cut the potatoes into ½-inch cubes. Place the potatoes in a large bowl of cold water and allow them to soak for at least 30 minutes, preferably an hour.
2. Dry out the potatoes and wipe thoroughly with paper towels. Return them to the empty bowl.
3. Add the canola and olive oils, paprika, and salt and pepper to flavor. Toss to fully coat the potatoes.
4. Transfer the potatoes to the Air Fryer. Cook for 20 minutes at 350°F, shaking the Air Fryer basket every 5 minutes (a total of 4 times).
5. Put the onion and red and green bell peppers to the Air Fryer basket. Fry for an additional 3 to 4 minutes, or until the potatoes are cooked through and the peppers are soft.
6. Cool before serving.

Nutrition: Calories 279 Fat 8g Carbs 50g Protein 6g

17. HOMEMADE CHERRY BREAKFAST TARTS

PREPARATION: 15 MIN   **COOKING:** 20 MIN   **SERVINGS:** 6

INGREDIENTS

For the tarts:
- 2 refrigerated piecrusts
- ⅓ Cup cherry preserves
- 1 tsp. cornstarch
- Cooking oil

For the frosting:
- ½ cup vanilla yogurt
- 1 oz. cream cheese
- 1 tsp. stevia
- Rainbow sprinkles

Nutrition: *Calories 119 Fat 4g Carbs 19g Protein 2g*

DIRECTIONS

1. To make the tarts:
2. Place the piecrusts on a flat surface. Make use of a knife or pizza cutter, cut each piecrust into 3 rectangles, for 6 in total. (I discard the unused dough left from slicing the edges.)
3. In a small bowl, combine the preserves and cornstarch. Mix well.
4. Scoop 1 tbsp. of the preserve mixture onto the top half of each piece of piecrust.
5. Fold the bottom of each piece up to close the tart. Press along the edges of each tart to seal using the back of a fork.
6. Sprinkle the breakfast tarts with cooking oil and place them in the Air Fryer. I do not recommend piling the breakfast tarts. They will stick together if piled. You may need to prepare them in two batches. Cook for 10 minutes at 350°F
7. Allow the breakfast tarts to cool fully before removing from the Air Fryer.
8. If needed, repeat steps 5 and 6 for the remaining breakfast tarts.
9. To make the frosting:
10. In a small bowl, mix the yogurt, cream cheese, and stevia. Mix well.
11. Spread the breakfast tarts with frosting and top with sprinkles, and serve.

18. SAUSAGE AND CREAM CHEESE BISCUITS

PREPARATION: 5 MIN   **COOKING:** 15 MIN   **SERVINGS:** 5

INGREDIENTS

- 12 oz. chicken breakfast sausage
- 1 (6 oz.) can biscuits
- ⅛ cup cream cheese

Nutrition: *Calories 240 Fat 13g Carbs 20g Protein 9g*

DIRECTIONS

1. Form the sausage into 5 small patties.
2. Place the sausage patties in the Air Fryer. Cook for 5 minutes a at 360°F
3. Open the Air Fryer. Flip the patties. Cook for an additional 5 minutes
4. Remove the cooked sausages from the Air Fryer.
5. Separate the biscuit dough into 5 biscuits.
6. Place the biscuits in the Air Fryer. Cook for 3 minutes
7. Open the Air Fryer. Flip the biscuits. Cook for an additional 2 minutes
8. Remove the cooked biscuits from the Air Fryer.
9. Split each biscuit in half. Spread 1 tsp. of cream cheese onto the bottom of each biscuit. Top with a sausage patty and the other half of the biscuit, and serve.

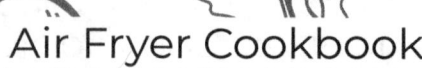

19. FRIED CHICKEN AND WAFFLES

PREPARATION: 10 MIN **COOKING:** 30 MIN **SERVINGS:** 4

INGREDIENTS

- 8 whole chicken wings
- 1 tsp. garlic powder
- Chicken seasoning or rub
- Pepper
- ½ cup all-purpose flour
- Cooking oil
- 8 frozen waffles
- Maple syrup (optional)

Nutrition: *Calories: 51 Fat: 1.1g Carbs: 9g Protein: 2.2g*

DIRECTIONS

1. In a medium bowl, spice the chicken with the garlic powder and chicken seasoning and pepper to flavor.
2. Put the chicken to a sealable plastic bag and add the flour. Shake to thoroughly coat the chicken.
3. Sprinkle the Air Fryer basket with cooking oil.
4. With the use of tongs, put the chicken from the bag to the Air Fryer. It is okay to pile the chicken wings on top of each other. Sprinkle them with cooking oil. Heat for five minutes at 380°F
5. Unlock the Air Fryer and shake the basket. Presume to cook the chicken. Keep shaking every 5 minutes until 20 minutes has passed and the chicken is completely cooked.
6. Take out the cooked chicken from the Air Fryer and set aside.
7. Wash the basket and base out with warm water. Put them back to the Air Fryer.
8. Ease the temperature of the Air Fryer to 370°F.
9. Put the frozen waffles in the Air Fryer. Do not pile. Depends on how big your Air Fryer is, you may need to cook the waffles in batches. Sprinkle the waffles with cooking oil. Cook for 6 minutes
10. If necessary, take out the cooked waffles from the Air Fryer, then repeat step 9 for the leftover waffles.
11. Serve the waffles with the chicken and a bit of maple syrup if desired.

20. CHEESY TATER TOT BREAKFAST BAKE

PREPARATION: 5 MIN **COOKING:** 20 MIN **SERVINGS:** 4

INGREDIENTS

- 4 eggs
- 1 cup milk
- 1 tsp. onion powder
- Salt
- Pepper
- Cooking oil
- 12 oz. ground chicken sausage
- 1-lb. frozen tater tots
- ¾ cup shredded Cheddar cheese

Nutrition: *Calories 518 Fat 30g Carbs 31g Protein 30g*

DIRECTIONS

1. In a medium bowl, whisk the eggs. Add the milk, onion powder, and salt and pepper to taste. Stir to combine.
2. Spray a skillet with cooking oil and set over medium-high heat. Add the ground sausage. Using a spatula or spoon, break the sausage into smaller pieces. Cook for 3 to 4 minutes at 360°F, until the sausage is brown. Remove from heat and set aside.
3. Spray a barrel pan with cooking oil. Make sure to cover the bottom and sides of the pan. Place the tater tots in the barrel pan. Cook for 6 minutes
4. Open the Air Fryer and shake the pan, then add the egg mixture and cooked sausage. Cook for an additional 6 minutes. Open the Air Fryer and sprinkle the cheese over the tater tot bake. Cook for an additional 2 to 3 minutes. Cool before serving.

21. BREAKFAST SCRAMBLE CASSEROLE

PREPARATION: 20 MIN **COOKING:** 10 MIN **SERVINGS:** 4

INGREDIENTS

- 6 slices bacon
- 6 eggs
- Salt
- Pepper
- Cooking oil
- ½ cup chopped red bell pepper
- ½ cup chopped green bell pepper
- ½ cup chopped onion
- ¾ cup shredded Cheddar cheese

DIRECTIONS

1. In a pan, over medium-high heat, cook the bacon, 5 to 7 minutes, flipping to evenly crisp. Dry out on paper towels, crumble, and set aside. In a medium bowl, whisk the eggs. Add salt and pepper to taste.
2. Spray a barrel pan with cooking oil. Make sure to cover the bottom and sides of the pan. Add the beaten eggs, crumbled bacon, red bell pepper, green bell pepper, and onion to the pan. Place the pan in the Air Fryer and cook for 6 minutes at 380°F. Open the Air Fryer and sprinkle the cheese over the casserole. Cook for an additional 2 minutes. Cool before serving.

Nutrition: *Calories 348 Fat 26g Carbs 4g Protein 25g*

22. Breakfast Grilled Ham and Cheese

PREPARATION: 5 MIN **COOKING:** 10 MIN **SERVINGS:** 2

INGREDIENTS

- 1 tsp. butter
- 4 slices bread
- 4 slices smoked country ham
- 4 slices Cheddar cheese
- 4 thick slices tomato

DIRECTIONS

1. Spread ½ tsp. of butter onto one side of 2 slices of bread. Each sandwich will have 1 slice of bread with butter and 1 slice without.
2. Assemble each sandwich by layering 2 slices of ham, 2 slices of cheese, and 2 slices of tomato on the unbuttered pieces of bread. Top with the other bread slices, buttered side up.
3. Place the sandwiches in the Air Fryer buttered-side down. Cook for 4 minutes at 330°F
4. Open the Air Fryer. Flip the grilled cheese sandwiches. Cook for an additional 4 minutes
5. Cool before serving. Cut each sandwich in half and enjoy.

Nutrition: *Calories 525 Fat 25g Carbs 34g Protein 41g*

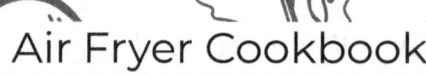
Air Fryer Cookbook

23. CLASSIC HASH BROWNS

PREPARATION: 15 MIN   **COOKING:** 20 MIN   **SERVINGS:** 4

INGREDIENTS

- 4 russet potatoes
- 1 tsp. paprika
- Salt
- Pepper
- Cooking oil

DIRECTIONS

1. Peel the potatoes using a vegetable peeler. Using a cheese grater shred the potatoes. If your grater has different-size holes, use the area of the tool with the largest holes.
2. Put the shredded potatoes in a large bowl of cold water. Let sit for 5 minutes Cold water helps remove excess starch from the potatoes. Stir to help dissolve the starch.
3. Dry out the potatoes and dry with paper towels or napkins. Make sure the potatoes are completely dry.
4. Season the potatoes with the paprika and salt and pepper to taste.
5. Spray the potatoes with cooking oil and transfer them to the Air Fryer. Cook for 20 minutes at 360°F and shake the basket every 5 minutes (a total of 4 times).
6. Cool before serving.

Nutrition: *Calories 150 Fat 9g Carbs 34g Protein 4g*

24. CANADIAN BACON AND CHEESE ENGLISH MUFFINS

PREPARATION: 5 MIN   **COOKING:** 10 MIN   **SERVINGS:** 4

INGREDIENTS

- 4 English muffins
- 8 slices Canadian bacon
- 4 slices cheese
- Cooking oil

DIRECTIONS

1. Split each English muffin. Assemble the breakfast sandwiches by layering 2 slices of Canadian bacon and 1 slice of cheese onto each English muffin bottom. Put the other half on top of the English muffin. Place the sandwiches in the Air Fryer. Spray the top of each with cooking oil. Cook for 4 minutes at 380°F
2. Open the Air Fryer and flip the sandwiches. Cook for an additional 4 minutes
3. Cool before serving.

Nutrition: *Calories 333 Fat 14g Carbs 27g Protein 24g*

25. RADISH HASH BROWNS

PREPARATION: 10 MIN **COOKING:** 13 MIN **SERVINGS:** 4

INGREDIENTS

- 1 lb. radishes, washed and cut off roots
- 1 tbsp. olive oil
- 1/2 tsp. paprika
- 1/2 tsp. onion powder
- 1/2 tsp. garlic powder
- 1 medium onion
- 1/4 tsp. pepper
- 3/4 tsp. sea salt

DIRECTIONS

1. Slice onion and radishes using a mandolin slicer.
2. Add sliced onion and radishes in a large mixing bowl and toss with olive oil.
3. Transfer onion and radish slices in Air Fryer basket and cook at 360°F for 8 minutes Shake basket twice.
4. Return onion and radish slices in a mixing bowl and toss with seasonings.
5. Again, cook onion and radish slices in Air Fryer basket for 5 minutes at 400°F. Shake the basket halfway through.
6. Serve and enjoy.

Nutrition: *Calories 62 Fat 3.7g Carbs 7.1g Protein 1.2g*

26. VEGETABLE EGG CUPS

PREPARATION: 10 MIN **COOKING:** 20 MIN **SERVINGS:** 4

INGREDIENTS

- 4 eggs
- 1 tbsp. cilantro, chopped
- 4 tbsp. half and half
- 1 cup cheddar cheese, shredded
- 1 cup vegetables, diced
- Pepper
- Salt

DIRECTIONS

1. Sprinkle four ramekins with cooking spray and set aside.
2. In a mixing bowl, whisk eggs with cilantro, half and half, vegetables, 1/2 cup cheese, pepper, and salt.
3. Pour egg mixture into the four ramekins.
4. Place ramekins in Air Fryer basket and cook at 300°F for 12 minutes
5. Top with remaining 1/2 cup cheese and cook for 2 minutes more at 400°F.
6. Serve and enjoy.

Nutrition: *Calories 194 Fat 11.5g Carbs 6g Protein 13g*

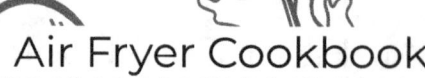
Air Fryer Cookbook

27. SPINACH FRITTATA

PREPARATION: 5 MIN   **COOKING:** 8 MIN   **SERVINGS:** 1

INGREDIENTS

- 3 eggs
- 1 cup spinach, chopped
- 1 small onion, minced
- 2 tbsp. mozzarella cheese, grated
- Pepper
- Salt

DIRECTIONS

1. Preheat the Air Fryer to 350°F. Spray Air Fryer pan with cooking spray.
2. In a bowl, whisk eggs with remaining ingredients until well combined.
3. Pour egg mixture into the prepared pan and place pan in the Air Fryer basket.
4. Cook frittata for 8 minutes or until set. Serve and enjoy.

Nutrition: *Calories 384 Fat 23.3g Carbs 10.7g Protein 34.3g*

28. OMELET FRITTATA

PREPARATION: 10 MIN   **COOKING:** 6 MIN   **SERVINGS:** 2

INGREDIENTS

- 3 eggs, lightly beaten
- 2 tbsp. cheddar cheese, shredded
- 2 tbsp. heavy cream
- 2 mushrooms, sliced
- 1/4 small onion, chopped
- 1/4 bell pepper, diced
- Pepper
- Salt

DIRECTIONS

1. In a bowl, whisk eggs with cream, vegetables, pepper, and salt.
2. Preheat the Air Fryer to 400°F.
3. Pour egg mixture into the Air Fryer pan. Place pan in Air Fryer basket and cook for 5 minutes
4. Add shredded cheese on top of the frittata and cook for 1 minute more.
5. Serve and enjoy.

Nutrition: *Calories 160 Fat 10 Carbs 4g Protein 12g*

29. CHEESE SOUFFLÉS

PREPARATION: 10 MIN **COOKING:** 6 MIN **SERVINGS:** 8

INGREDIENTS

- 6 large eggs, separated
- 3/4 cup heavy cream
- 1/4 tsp. cayenne pepper
- 1/2 tsp. xanthan gum
- 1/2 tsp. pepper
- 1/4 tsp. cream of tartar
- 2 tbsp. chives, chopped
- 2 cups cheddar cheese, shredded
- 1 tsp. salt

DIRECTIONS

1. Preheat the Air Fryer to 325°F.
2. Spray eight ramekins with cooking spray. Set aside.
3. In a bowl, whisk together almond flour, cayenne pepper, pepper, salt, and xanthan gum.
4. Slowly add heavy cream and mix to combine.
5. Whisk in egg yolks, chives, and cheese until well combined.
6. In a large bowl, add egg whites and cream of tartar and beat until stiff peaks form.
7. Fold egg white mixture into the almond flour mixture until combined.
8. Pour mixture into the prepared ramekins. Divide ramekins in batches.
9. Place the first batch of ramekins into the Air Fryer basket.
10. Cook soufflé for 20 minutes
11. Serve and enjoy.

Nutrition: *Calories 210 Fat 16g Carbs 1g Protein 12g*

30. CHEESE AND RED PEPPER EGG CUPS

PREPARATION: 10 MIN **COOKING:** 15 MIN **SERVINGS:** 4

INGREDIENTS

- 4 Large free-range eggs
- 1 cup Shredded cheese
- 1 cup Diced red pepper
- 4 tbsps half and half
- Salt and Pepper.

DIRECTIONS

1. Preheat your Air Fryer to 300°F and grease four ramekins.
2. Grab a medium bowl and add the eggs. Whisk well.
3. Add the red pepper, half the cheese, half and half, salt and pepper. Stir well to combine.
4. Pour the mixture between the ramekins and pop into the Air Fryer.
5. Cook for 15 minutes then serve and enjoy.

Nutrition: *Calories 195 Fat 12g Carbs 7g Protein 13g*

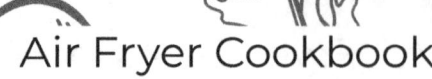

31. COCONUT PORRIDGE WITH FLAX SEED

PREPARATION: 5 MIN **COOKING:** 30 MIN **SERVINGS:** 3

INGREDIENTS

- 1 ½ cup Unsweetened almond milk
- 2 tbsp. Coconut flour
- 2 tbsp. Vegan vanilla protein powder
- ¼ tsp. Powdered erythritol
- 3 tbsp. Golden flaxseed meal

Nutrition: Calories 249 Fats 13.7g Carbs 6g Protein 17g

DIRECTIONS

1. Preheat your Air Fryer at a temperature of about 375°F
2. Combine coconut flour with the golden flaxseed meal and the protein powder in a bowl
3. Spray your Air Fryer with cooking spray, then pour the mixture in the Air Fryer pan
4. Pour the milk and top with chopped blueberries and chopped raspberries
5. Move the pan in the Air Fryer and close
6. Set the temperature at about 375°F and the timer to about 30 minutes
7. When the timer beeps, turn off your Air Fryer and remove the baking pan
8. Serve and enjoy your delicious porridge!

32. EASY CHOCOLATE DOUGHNUT

PREPARATION: 10 MIN **COOKING:** 12 MIN **SERVINGS:** 6

INGREDIENTS

- 3 tbsps Melted unsalted butter
- ¼ cup Powdered sugar
- 8 Refrigerated biscuits
- 48 Semisweet chocolate chips

Nutrition: Calories 393 Fat 17g Carbs 55g Protein 5g

DIRECTIONS

1. Cut the biscuits into thirds then flatten them and place 2 chocolate chips at the center.
2. Wrap the chocolate with dough to seal the edges.
3. Rub each dough hole with some butter.
4. Set the dough into the Air Fryer to cook for 12 minutes at 340°F.
5. Set aside to add powdered sugar.
6. Serve and enjoy.

33. CHEESY SPINACH OMELET

PREPARATION: 5 MIN **COOKING:** 10 MIN **SERVINGS:** 2

INGREDIENTS

- 3 Eggs
- 2 tbsps Chopped fresh spinach
- ½ cup Shredded cheese
- Pepper
- Salt

Nutrition: Calories 209 Fat 15.9g Carbs 1g Protein 15.4g

DIRECTIONS

1. Mix the eggs with pepper and salt then whisk and put in an oven-safe tray.
2. Add spinach and cheese but do not stir.
3. Allow to cook in the Air Fryer for 8 minutes at 390°F.
4. Cook for 2 more minutes to brown the omelet.
5. Serve on plates to enjoy.

34. ROASTED GARLIC AND THYME DIPPING SAUCE

PREPARATION: 5 MIN **COOKING:** 30 MIN **SERVINGS:** 1

INGREDIENTS

- ½ tsp. Minced fresh thyme leaves
- 1/8 tsp. Salt
- ½ cup Light mayonnaise
- 2 tbsps Crushed roasted garlic
- 1/8 tsp. Pepper

DIRECTIONS

1. Wrap garlic in foil. Put it in the cooking basket of the Air Fryer and roast for 30 minutes at 390°F.
2. Combine all the ingredients to serve.

Nutrition: Calories 485 Fat 39.4g Carbs 34.1g Protein 2.2g

35. CHEESY SAUSAGE AND EGG ROLLS

PREPARATION: 15 MIN **COOKING:** 15 MIN **SERVINGS:** 8

INGREDIENTS

- 8 pieces Cooked breakfast sausage links
- 3 Eggs
- Salt and Pepper
- 4 Cheddar cheese slices
- 8 oz. Refrigerated crescent rolls

DIRECTIONS

1. Set the Air Fryer at 325°F to preheat.
2. Beat the eggs; reserve one tbsp. as egg wash and scramble the rest.
3. Halve the cheese slices. Separate the dough into 8 triangles.
4. Fill each triangle with a half-slice of cheese, a tbsp. of scrambled eggs, and a sausage link.
5. Loosely roll up all filled triangles before placing in the Air Fryer basket. Brush with the egg wash that was set aside and sprinkle all over with pepper and salt.
6. Cook for 15 minutes. Serve right away.

Nutrition: Calories 270 Fat 20.0g Protein 10.0g Carbs 13.0g

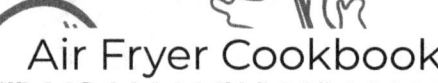
Air Fryer Cookbook

36. BAKED BERRY OATMEAL

PREPARATION: 5 MIN   **COOKING:** 25 MIN   **SERVINGS:** 2-4

INGREDIENTS

- 1 medium-size egg
- 1 cup of whole milk
- 1 cup of rolled oats
- 2½ tbsp. of brown sugar
- ½ tsp. of baking powder
- ½ tsp. of ground cinnamon
- Oil
- 2 cups of divided, mixed berries
- 2 tbsp. of slivered almonds
- Sprinkling of nutmeg

DIRECTIONS

1. In a bowl, combine the egg with the milk, mixing well to combine.
2. In a second bowl, combine the oats with the brown sugar, baking powder, and cinnamon. Mix thoroughly.
3. Spritz your Air Fryer safe pan with oil spray.
4. Add ¼ cup of the mixed berries to the Air Fryer.
5. Pour the oatmeal mixture over the fruit, followed by the egg and milk mixture.
6. Allow to rest for approximately 10 minutes before adding the remaining fruit on top.
7. Scatter the slivered almonds over the berries and season with a sprinkling of nutmeg.
8. Place the pan in your Air Fryer and bake at 320°F, for 10 minutes. Check the progress and either continue to bake or remove from the appliance.
9. Set aside to rest for 4-5 minutes and serve.

Nutrition: *Calories 151 Fat 7.1g Carbs 17.9g Protein 3.6g*

37. BROCCOLI AND CHEDDAR CHEESE QUICHE

PREPARATION: 5 MIN   **COOKING:** 10 MIN   **SERVINGS:** 1

INGREDIENTS

- 1 medium-size egg
- 3-4 tbsp. of heavy cream
- 4-5 very small-size broccoli florets
- 1 tbsp. of finely grated Cheddar cheese

DIRECTIONS

1. In a bowl, whisk the egg along with the heavy cream.
2. Lightly grease a 5" circular, ceramic quiche-style dish.
3. Arrange the broccoli florets evenly on the bottom of the dish.
4. Pour in the egg-cream mixture.
5. Scatter the grated Cheddar cheese over the top and air fry at 325°F for 10 minutes.
6. Serve and enjoy.

Nutrition: *Calories 162 Fat 5.23g Carbs 14.3g Protein 9.4g*

Air Fryer Cookbook

38. EGG AND CHEESE PUFF PASTRY TARTS

PREPARATION: 10 MIN **COOKING:** 20 MIN **SERVINGS:** 4

INGREDIENTS

- All-purpose flour
- 1 (9") square sheet of frozen, thawed puff pastry
- ¾ cup of shredded Cheddar cheese
- 4 large-size eggs
- 1 tbsp. of minced fresh chives

DIRECTIONS

1. Preheat the Air Fryer to 390°F.
2. On a lightly floured clean work surface, unfold the sheet of pastry and cut it into 4 even squares.
3. Put 2 of the pastry squares in the Air Fryer basket, spacing them apart from one another.
4. Air fry until the pastry is a light golden brown, for approximately 10 minutes.
5. Open the basket, and with a metal spoon, press down the middles of each pastry square to create an indentation. Scatter 3 tbsp. of shredded cheese into each indent. Crack an egg carefully into the middle of each pastry.
6. Air fry for 8-10 minutes, until the eggs are cooked to your preferred level of doneness.
7. Transfer the tarts to a wire baking rack set over wax paper and allow it to cool for 4-5 minutes.
8. Repeat Steps 2-4 with the remaining ingredients.
9. Garnish with half of the chives and serve warm.

Nutrition: *Calories 231 Fat 6.5g Carbs 10.3g Protein 6.4g*

39. FRENCH TOAST

PREPARATION: 5 MIN **COOKING:** 3 MIN **SERVINGS:** 4

INGREDIENTS

- 2 medium-size eggs
- ⅔ cup of whole milk
- 1 tbsp. of cinnamon
- 1 tsp. of vanilla extract
- 4 slices of whole wheat bread

DIRECTIONS

1. In a small-size bowl, combine the eggs with the milk, cinnamon, and vanilla extract. Beat to break up the eggs and incorporate them.
2. Dip each side of bread in the egg mixture, shaking off any excess.
3. Add the dipped bread slices into the pan and Air Fryer for a few minutes at 320°F. Flip the bread over and air fry for an additional 3 minutes.
4. Serve.

Nutrition: *Calories 231 Fat 6.3g Carbs 13.6g Protein 4.6g*

40. GRILLED GRUYERE CHEESE SANDWICH

PREPARATION: 5 MIN   **COOKING:** 10 MIN   **SERVINGS:** 1

INGREDIENTS

- 2 oz. of thinly sliced Gruyere cheese
- 2 slices of whole-grain bread
- 1 tbsp. of butter

Nutrition: Calories 151 Fat 7.1g Carbs 17.9g Protein 3.6g

DIRECTIONS

1. Lay the Gruyere cheese between the 2 slices of bread.
2. Butter up the outside of the bread slices.
3. Place the cheese sandwich in the Air Fryer basket. You may need to use toothpicks to secure.
4. Air fry the sandwich for approximately 3-5 minutes at 360°F until the cheese melts.
5. Flip the sandwich over and turn the heat up to 380°F until crisp.
6. Continue to Air Fryer for approximately 5 minutes, until the sandwich is to your desired texture. You will need to check continually that the sandwich doesn't burn.
7. Set to one side to cool slightly before enjoying.

41. PANCAKES

PREPARATION: 5 MIN   **COOKING:** 10 MIN   **SERVINGS:** 2

INGREDIENTS

- 2 tbsps. coconut oil
- 1 tsp. maple extract
- 2 tbsps. cashew milk
- 2 eggs
- 2/3 oz. /20g pork rinds

Nutrition: Calories 280 Carbs 31g Fat 2g Protein 5g

DIRECTIONS

1. Grind up the pork rinds until fine and mix with the rest of the ingredients, except the oil.
2. Add the oil to a skillet. Add a quarter-cup of the batter and fry until golden on each side. Continue adding the remaining batter.

42. BREAKFAST SANDWICH

PREPARATION: 5 MIN   **COOKING:** 5 MIN   **SERVINGS:** 2

INGREDIENTS

- 2 oz. /60g cheddar cheese
- 1/6 oz. /30g smoked ham
- 2 tbsps. butter
- 4 eggs

Nutrition: Calories 180 Carbs 19g Fat 7g Protein 10g

DIRECTIONS

1. Spray your Air Fryer pan with olive oil. Crack the eggs into the pan
2. Air fry for 3 minutes at 370°F, sprinkle pepper and salt on them.
3. Place an egg down as the sandwich base. Top with the ham and cheese and a drop or two of Tabasco.
4. Place the other egg on top and enjoy.

43. EGG MUFFINS

PREPARATION: 10 MIN   **COOKING:** 15-20 MIN   **SERVINGS:** 3

INGREDIENTS

- 1 tbsp. green pesto
- 1/3 cup of shredded cheese
- 1/3 cup of cooked bacon
- 1 scallion, chopped
- 6 Eggs

Nutrition: *Calories 160 Carbs 11g Fat 6g Protein 8g*

DIRECTIONS

1. You should set your fryer to 350°F.
2. Place liners in a regular cupcake tin. This will help with easy removal and storage.
3. Beat the eggs with pepper, salt, and the pesto. Mix in the cheese.
4. Pour the eggs into the cupcake tin and top with the bacon and scallion.
5. Cook for 15-20 minutes, or until the egg is set.

44. BACON & EGGS

PREPARATION: 5 MIN   **COOKING:** 5 MIN   **SERVINGS:** 4

INGREDIENTS

- Parsley
- Cherry tomatoes
- 1/3 oz. /150g bacon
- 6 Eggs

Nutrition: *Calories 150 Carbs 10g Fat 6g Protein 7g*

DIRECTIONS

1. Set your air Fryer at 370°F. Fry up the bacon for 5 minutes and put it to the side with the grease.
2. Spray your Air Fryer pan with olive oil. Crack the eggs into the pan
3. Air fry for 3 minutes at 370°F, sprinkle pepper and salt on them
4. Scramble the eggs in the bacon grease, with some pepper and salt. If you want, scramble in some cherry tomatoes. Sprinkle with some parsley and enjoy.

45. EGGS ON THE GO

PREPARATION: 5 MIN   **COOKING:** 15 MIN   **SERVINGS:** 1

INGREDIENTS

- 110g bacon, cooked
- Pepper
- Salt
- 6 Eggs

Nutrition: *Calories 140 Carbs 10g Fat 5g Protein 7g*

DIRECTIONS

1. You should set your fryer to 370°F.
2. Place liners in a regular cupcake tin. This will help with easy removal and storage.
3. Crack an egg into each of the cups and sprinkle some bacon onto each of them. Season with some pepper and salt.
4. Bake for 15 minutes, or once the eggs are set.

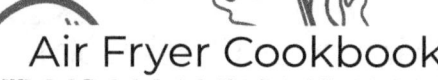

46. PROTEIN BANANA BREAD

PREPARATION: 10 MIN   **COOKING:** 1 H 10 MIN   **SERVINGS:** 6

INGREDIENTS

- 3 eggs
- 1/3 cup coconut flour
- 1/2 cup swerve
- 2 cups almond flour
- 1/2 cup ground chia seed
- 1/2 tsp. vanilla extract
- 4 tbsp. butter, melted
- 3/4 cup almond milk
- 1 tbsp. baking powder
- 1/3 cup protein powder
- 1/2 cup water
- 1/2 tsp. salt

DIRECTIONS

1. Grease loaf pan with butter and set aside.
2. Set temperature 325°F, timer for 1 hour 10 minutes. Press start to preheat the Air Fryer.
3. In a small bowl, whisk together chia seed and 1/2 cup water. Set aside.
4. In a large bowl, mix together almond flour, baking powder, protein powder, coconut flour, sweetener, and salt.
5. Stir in eggs, milk, chia seed mixture, vanilla extract, and butter until well combined.
6. Pour batter into the prepared loaf pan and bake for 1 hour 10 minutes.
7. Sliced and serve.

Nutrition: *Calories 162 Carbs 13.4g Fat 11.2g Protein 5.2g*

47. EASY KALE MUFFINS

PREPARATION: 10 MIN   **COOKING:** 30 MIN   **SERVINGS:** 8

INGREDIENTS

- 6 eggs
- 1/2 cup milk
- 1/4 cup chives, chopped
- 1 cup kale, chopped
- Salt and Pepper

DIRECTIONS

1. Spray 8 cups muffin pan with cooking spray and set aside.
2. Set temperature 350°F, timer for 30 minutes. Press start to preheat the Air Fryer.
3. Add all ingredients into the mixing bowl and whisk well.
4. Pour mixture into the prepared muffin pan and bake for 30 minutes.
5. Serve and enjoy.

Nutrition: *Calories 89 Carbs 2g Fat 3.6g Protein 5g*

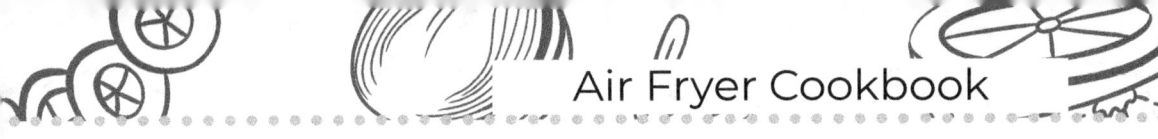

48. MOZZARELLA SPINACH QUICHE

PREPARATION: 10 MIN **COOKING:** 45 MIN **SERVINGS:** 6

INGREDIENTS

- 4 eggs
- 10 oz frozen spinach, thawed
- 1/2 cup mozzarella cheese, shredded
- 1/4 cup parmesan cheese, grated
- 8 oz mushrooms, sliced
- 2 oz feta cheese, crumbled
- 1 cup almond milk
- 1 garlic clove, minced
- Salt and Pepper

DIRECTIONS

1. Spray a pie dish with cooking spray and set aside.
2. Set temperature 350°F, timer for 45 minutes. Press start to preheat the Air Fryer.
3. Spray medium pan with cooking spray and heat over medium heat.
4. Add garlic, mushrooms, pepper, and salt in a pan and sauté for 5 minutes.
5. Add spinach in pie dish then add sautéed mushroom on top of spinach.
6. Sprinkle feta cheese over spinach and mushroom.
7. In a bowl, whisk eggs, parmesan cheese, and almond milk.
8. Pour egg mixture over spinach and mushroom then sprinkle shredded mozzarella cheese and bake for 45 minutes.
9. Sliced and serve.

Nutrition: *Calories 197 Carbs 6.2g Fat 16g Protein 10.4g*

49. FANCY BREAKFAST QUINOA

PREPARATION: 10 MIN **COOKING:** 3 MIN **SERVINGS:** 5

INGREDIENTS

- 1/2 cup walnuts, soaked and chopped
- 4 oz. sesame seeds, soaked
- 2 oz. hemp seeds, soaked overnight
- 1 tsp. date sugar
- 1/2 tsp. ground cinnamon
- 5 oz. quinoa puff
- 1 tsp. hemp seed oil
- 1 cup of coconut milk

DIRECTIONS

1. Take a bowl and mix in all the seeds and spices. Add hemp seed oil
2. Stir well until the mixture is thick. Flatten mixture on your cooking basket
3. Preheat your Air Fryer to 330°F
4. Transfer to your Air Fryer and cook for 2-3 minutes until light brown
5. Transfer mix to a serving bowl. Add quinoa puff, stir well and add coconut milk stir again
6. Serve and enjoy

Nutrition: *Calories 510 Carbs 50 g Fat 8g Protein 21g*

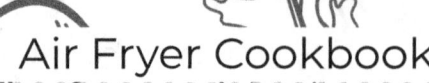

50. FRESH SAUTÉED APPLE

PREPARATION: 10 MIN **COOKING:** 10 MIN **SERVINGS:** 4

INGREDIENTS

- 2 tbsp. olive oil
- 3 apples, peeled, cored and sliced
- 1 tbsp. garlic clove, grated
- 1 tbsp. date sugar
- Pinch of salt

DIRECTIONS

1. Preheat your Air Fryer 300°F. Add coconut oil to the cooking basket, add remaining ingredients and stir well.
2. Transfer to Air Fryer, cook for 5-10 minutes, making sure to shake the basket occasionally until golden. Serve and enjoy!

Nutrition: Calories 32 Carbs 32g Fat 9g Protein 3g

51. PERFECT VEGETABLE ROAST

PREPARATION: 10 MIN **COOKING:** 10 MIN **SERVINGS:** 4

INGREDIENTS

- 2 cups Roma tomatoes
- 1/2 cup mushrooms halved
- 1 red bell pepper, seeded and cut into bite-sized portions
- 1 tbsp. coconut oil
- 1 tbsp. garlic powder
- 1 tsp. salt

DIRECTIONS

1. Preheat your Air Fryer 400°F
2. Take a bowl and add mushrooms, Roma tomatoes, bell pepper, oil, salt, garlic powder and mix well
3. Transfer to Air Fryer cooking basket
4. Cook for 12-15 minutes, making sure to shake occasionally
5. Serve and enjoy once crispy!

Nutrition: Calories 19 Carbs 19g Fat 16g Protein 7g

52. HERB FRITTATA

PREPARATION: 10 MIN **COOKING:** 25 MIN **SERVINGS:** 4

INGREDIENTS

- 2 tbsp. chopped green scallions
- 1/2 tsp. ground black pepper
- 2 tbsp. chopped cilantro
- 1/2 tsp. salt
- 2 tbsp. chopped parsley
- 1/2 cup half and half, reduced-fat
- 4 eggs, pastured
- 1/3 cup shredded cheddar cheese, reduced-fat

DIRECTIONS

1. Switch on the Air Fryer, insert fryer basket, grease it with olive oil, then shut with its lid, set the fryer at 330°F and preheat for 10 minutes.
2. Meanwhile, take a round heatproof pan that fits into the fryer basket, grease it well with oil and set aside until required.
3. Crack the eggs in a bowl, beat in half-and-half, then add remaining ingredients, beat until well mixed and pour the mixture into prepared pan.
4. Open the fryer, place the pan in it, close with its lid and cook for 15 minutes at the 330°F until its top is nicely golden, frittata has set and inserted toothpick into the frittata slides out clean.
5. When Air Fryer beeps, open its lid, take out the pan, then transfer frittata onto a serving plate, cut it into pieces and serve.

Nutrition: *Calories 141 Fat 10g Carbs 2g Protein 8g*

53. ZUCCHINI BREAD

PREPARATION: 25 MIN **COOKING** 40 MIN **SERVINGS:** 8

INGREDIENTS

- ¾ cup shredded zucchini
- 1/2 cup almond flour
- 1/4 tsp. salt
- 1/4 cup cocoa powder, unsweetened
- 1/2 cup chocolate chips, unsweetened, divided
- 6 tbsp. erythritol sweetener
- 1/2 tsp. baking soda
- 2 tbsp. olive oil
- 1/2 tsp. vanilla extract, unsweetened
- 2 tbsp. butter, unsalted, melted
- 1 egg, pastured

DIRECTIONS

1. Switch on the Air Fryer, insert fryer basket, grease it with olive oil, then shut with its lid, set the fryer at 310°F and preheat for 10 minutes.
2. Meanwhile, place flour in a bowl, add salt, cocoa powder, and baking soda and stir until mixed.
3. Crack the eggs in another bowl, whisk in sweetener, egg, oil, butter, and vanilla until smooth and then slowly whisk in flour mixture until incorporated.
4. Add zucchini along with 1/3 cup chocolate chips and then fold until just mixed.
5. Take a mini loaf pan that fits into the Air Fryer, grease it with olive oil, then pour in the prepared batter and sprinkle remaining chocolate chips on top.
6. Open the fryer, place the loaf pan in it, close with its lid and cook for 30 minutes at the 310°F until inserted toothpick into the bread slides out clean.
7. When Air Fryer beeps, open its lid, remove the loaf pan, then place it on a wire rack and let the bread cool in it for 20 minutes.
8. Take out the bread, let it cool completely, then cut it into slices and serve.

Nutrition: *Calories 356 Fat 17g Carbs 49g Protein 5.1g*

54 BLUEBERRY MUFFINS

PREPARATION: 10 MIN   **COOKING:** 30 MIN   **SERVINGS:** 14

INGREDIENTS

- 1 cup almond flour
- 1 cup frozen blueberries
- 2 tsp.s baking powder
- 1/3 cup erythritol sweetener
- 1 tsp. vanilla extract, unsweetened
- ½ tsp. salt
- ¼ cups melted coconut oil
- 1 egg, pastured
- ¼ cup applesauce, unsweetened
- ¼ cup almond milk, unsweetened

DIRECTIONS

1. Switch on the Air Fryer, insert fryer basket, grease it with olive oil, then shut with its lid, set the fryer at 360°F and preheat for 10 minutes.
2. Meanwhile, place flour in a large bowl, add berries, salt, sweetener, and baking powder and stir until well combined.
3. Crack the eggs in another bowl, whisk in vanilla, milk, and applesauce until combined and then slowly whisk in flour mixture until incorporated.
4. Take fourteen silicone muffin cups, grease them with oil, and then evenly fill them with the prepared batter.
5. Open the fryer; stack muffin cups in it, close with its lid and cook for 10 minutes until muffins are nicely golden brown and set.
6. When Air Fryer beeps, open its lid, transfer muffins onto a serving plate and then remaining muffins in the same manner.
7. Serve straight away.

Nutrition: Calories 201 Fat 8.8g Carbs 27.3g Protein 3g

55. BAKED EGGS

PREPARATION: 5 MIN   **COOKING:** 17 MIN   **SERVINGS:** 2

INGREDIENTS

- 2 tbsp. frozen spinach, thawed
- ½ tsp. salt
- ¼ tsp. ground black pepper
- 2 eggs, pastured
- 3 tsp.s grated parmesan cheese, reduced-fat
- 2 tbsp. milk, unsweetened, reduced-fat

DIRECTIONS

1. Switch on the Air Fryer, insert fryer basket, grease it with olive oil, then shut with its lid, set the fryer at 330°F and preheat for 5 minutes.
2. Meanwhile, take two silicon muffin cups, grease them with oil, then crack an egg into each cup and evenly add cheese, spinach, and milk.
3. Season the egg with salt and black pepper and gently stir the ingredients, without breaking the egg yolk.
4. Open the fryer, add muffin cups in it, close with its lid and cook for 8 to 12 minutes until eggs have cooked to desired doneness.
5. When Air Fryer beeps, take out the muffin cups and serve.

Nutrition: Calories 161 Fat 11.4g Carbs 3g Protein 12.1g

56. BAGELS

PREPARATION: 10 MIN **COOKING:** 20 MIN **SERVINGS:** 6

INGREDIENTS

- 2 cups almond flour
- 2 cups shredded mozzarella cheese, low-fat
- 2 tbsp. butter, unsalted
- 1 1/2 tsp. baking powder
- 1 tsp. apple cider vinegar
- 1 egg, pastured
- For Egg Wash:
- 1 egg, pastured
- 1 tsp. butter, unsalted, melted

DIRECTIONS

1. Place flour in a heatproof bowl, add cheese and butter, then stir well and microwave for 90 seconds until butter and cheese has melted.
2. Then stir the mixture until well combined, let it cool for 5 minutes and whisk in the egg, baking powder, and vinegar until incorporated and dough comes together.
3. Let the dough cool for 10 minutes, then divide the dough into six pieces, shape each piece into a bagel and let the bagels rest for 5 minutes.
4. Prepare the egg wash and for this, place the melted butter in a bowl, whisk in the egg until blended and then brush the mixture generously on top of each bagel.
5. Take a fryer basket, line it with parchment paper and then place prepared bagels in it in a single layer.
6. Switch on the Air Fryer, insert fryer, then shut with its lid, set the fryer at 350°F and cook for 10 minutes at the 350°F until bagels are nicely golden and thoroughly cooked, turning the bagels halfway through the frying.
7. When Air Fryer beeps, open its lid, transfer bagels to a serving plate and cook the remaining bagels in the same manner.
8. Serve straight away.

Nutrition: Calories 408 Fat 33.5g Protein 20.3g Carbs 8.3g

57. CAULIFLOWER HASH BROWNS

PREPARATION: 10 MIN **COOKING:** 25 MIN **SERVINGS:** 6

INGREDIENTS

- 1/4 cup chickpea flour
- 4 cups cauliflower rice
- 1/2 medium white onion, peeled and chopped
- 1/2 tsp. garlic powder
- 1 tbsp. xanthan gum
- 1/2 tsp. salt
- 1 tbsp. nutritional yeast flakes
- 1 tsp. ground paprika

DIRECTIONS

1. Switch on the Air Fryer, insert fryer basket, grease it with olive oil, then shut with its lid, set the fryer at 375°F and preheat for 10 minutes.
2. Meanwhile, place all the ingredients in a bowl, stir until well mixed and then shape the mixture into six rectangular disks, each about ½-inch thick.
3. Open the fryer, add hash browns in it in a single layer, close with its lid and cook for 25 minutes at 375°F until nicely golden and crispy, turning halfway through the frying.
4. When Air Fryer beeps, open its lid, transfer hash browns to a serving plate and serve.

Nutrition: Calories 115 Carbs 6.2g Fat 7.3g Protein 7.4g

Air Fryer Cookbook

58. POTATOES WITH BACON

PREPARATION: 10 MIN   **COOKING:** 20 MIN   **SERVINGS:** 2

INGREDIENTS

- potatoes, peeled and cut into medium cubes
- garlic cloves, minced
- bacon slices, chopped
- 2 rosemary springs, chopped
- 1 tbsp. olive oil
- Salt and black pepper to the taste
- 2 eggs, whisked

DIRECTIONS

1. In your Air Fryer's pan, mix oil with potatoes, garlic, bacon, rosemary, salt, pepper and eggs and whisk.
2. Cook potatoes at 400°F for 20 minutes,
3. Divide everything on plates and serve for breakfast. Enjoy!

Nutrition: Calories 211 Fat 6g Carbs 8g Protein 5g

59. ZUCCHINI SQUASH MIX

PREPARATION: 10 MIN   **COOKING:** 44 MIN   **SERVINGS:** 3

INGREDIENTS

- 1 lb. zucchini, sliced
- 1 tbsp. parsley, chopped
- 1 yellow squash, halved, deseeded, and chopped
- 1 tbsp. olive oil
- Pepper
- Salt

DIRECTIONS

1. Place all ingredients into the large bowl and mix well.
2. Transfer bowl mixture into the Air Fryer basket and cook at 400°F for 35 minutes.
3. Serve and enjoy.

Nutrition: Calories 49 Fat 3g Carbs: 4g Protein 1.5g

60. SPECIAL CORN FLAKES CASSEROLE

PREPARATION: 10 MIN **COOKING:** 18 MIN **SERVINGS:** 5

INGREDIENTS

- In a bowl, mix eggs with sugar, nutmeg and milk and whisk well.
- In another bowl, mix cream cheese with blueberries and whisk well.
- Put corn flakes in a third bowl.
- Spread blueberry mix on each bread slice; then dip in eggs mix and dredge in corn flakes at the end.
- Place bread in your Air Fryer's basket; heat up at 400°F and bake for 8 minutes.
- Divide among plates and serve for breakfast.

DIRECTIONS

1. Sprinkle pan with cooking spray and heat over medium heat. Add mushrooms and sauté for 2-3 minutes Add spinach and cook for 1-2 minutes or until wilted.
2. Transfer mushroom spinach mixture into the Air Fryer pan. Beat egg whites in a mixing bowl until frothy. Season it with a pinch of salt.
3. Pour egg white mixture into the spinach and mushroom mixture and sprinkle with parmesan cheese. Place pan in Air Fryer basket and cook frittata at 350°F for 8 minutes
4. Slice and serve.

Nutrition: *Calories 300 Fat 5g Carbs 16g Protein 4g*

61. PROTEIN RICH EGG WHITE OMELET

PREPARATION: 10 MIN **COOKING:** 25 MIN **SERVINGS:** 4

INGREDIENTS

- 1 cup egg whites
- 1/4 cup mushrooms; chopped
- 2 tbsp. chives; chopped
- 1/4 cup tomato; chopped
- 2 tbsp. skim milk
- Salt and black pepper to the taste

DIRECTIONS

1. In a bowl, mix egg whites with tomato, milk, mushrooms, chives, salt and pepper;
2. Whisk well and pour into your Air Fryer's pan. Cook at 320°F, for 15 minutes;
3. Cool omelet down, slice, divide among plates and serve.

Nutrition: *Calories 100 Fat 3g Carbs 7g Carbs 4g*

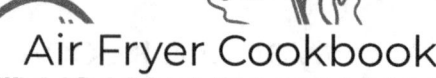

62. SHRIMP SANDWICHES

PREPARATION: 10 MIN **COOKING:** 15 MIN **SERVINGS:** 4

INGREDIENTS

- 1 ¼ cups cheddar; shredded
- 2 tbsp. green onions; chopped.
- whole wheat bread slices
- oz. canned tiny shrimp; drained
- tbsp. mayonnaise
- 2 tbsp. butter; soft

Nutrition: Calories 162 Fat 3g Carbs 12g Protein 4g

DIRECTIONS

1. In a bowl, mix shrimp with cheese, green onion and mayo and stir well.
2. Spread this on part of the bread slices; top with the other bread slices, cut into halves diagonally and spread butter on top.
3. Place sandwiches in your Air Fryer and cook at 350°F, for 5 minutes. Divide shrimp sandwiches on plates and serve them for breakfast.

63. BREAKFAST SOUFFLÉ

PREPARATION: 10 MIN **COOKING:** 18 MIN **SERVINGS:** 4

INGREDIENTS

- eggs; whisked
- tbsp. heavy cream
- 2 tbsp. parsley; chopped.
- 2 tbsp. chives; chopped.
- A pinch of red chili pepper; crushed
- Salt and black pepper to the taste

Nutrition: Calories 300 Fat 7g Carbs 15g Protein 6g

DIRECTIONS

1. Mix the eggs with salt, pepper, heavy cream, red pepper, parsley, and chives. Mix well and divide into 4 soufflé plates.
2. Place the dishes in your deep fryer and cook the soufflé at 350°F for 8 minutes. Serve hot.

64. FRIED TOMATO QUICHE

PREPARATION: 10 MIN **COOKING:** 40 MIN **SERVINGS:** 1

INGREDIENTS

- 1 tbsp. yellow onion; chopped.
- 1/2 cup gouda cheese; shredded
- 1/4 cup tomatoes; chopped.
- 2 eggs
- 1/4 cup milk
- Salt and black pepper to the taste
- Cooking spray

Nutrition: Calories 241 Fat 6g Carbs 14g Protein 6g

DIRECTIONS

1. Grease a ramekin with cooking spray.
2. Crack eggs, add onion, milk, cheese, tomatoes, salt and pepper and stir. Add this in your Air Fryer's pan and cook at 340°F for 30 minutes.

65. BREAKFAST SPANISH OMELET

PREPARATION: 10 MIN **COOKING:** 20 MIN **SERVINGS:** 4

INGREDIENTS

- Eggs
- 1/2 chorizo; chopped
- 1 tbsp. parsley; chopped.
- 1 tbsp. feta cheese; crumbled
- 1 potato; peeled and cubed
- 1/2 cup corn
- 1 tbsp. olive oil
- Salt and black pepper to the taste

DIRECTIONS

1. Heat up your Air Fryer at 350°F and add oil.
2. Add chorizo and potatoes; stir and brown them for a few seconds.
3. In a bowl; mix eggs with corn, parsley, cheese, salt and pepper and whisk.
4. Pour this over chorizo and potatoes; spread and cook for 5 minutes. Divide omelette on plates and serve for breakfast.

Nutrition: *Calories 300 Fat 6g Carbs 12g Protein 6g*

66. SCRAMBLED PANCAKE HASH

PREPARATION: 10 MIN **COOKING:** 25 MIN **SERVINGS:** 4

INGREDIENTS

- 1 egg
- ¼ cup heavy cream
- tbsp. butter
- 1 cup coconut flour
- 1 tsp. ground ginger
- 1 tsp. salt
- 1 tbsp. apple cider vinegar
- 1 tsp. baking soda

DIRECTIONS

1. Combine the salt, baking soda, ground ginger and flour in a mixing bowl. In a separate bowl crack, the egg into it.
2. Add butter and heavy cream.
3. Mix well using a hand mixer. Combine the liquid and dry mixtures and stir until smooth.
4. Preheat your Air Fryer to 400°F. Pour the pancake mixture into the Air Fryer basket tray.
5. Cook the pancake hash for 4 minutes.
6. After this, scramble the pancake hash well and continue to cook for another 5 minutes more.
7. When dish is cooked, transfer it to serving plates, and serve hot!

Nutrition: *Calories 178 Fat 13.3g Carbs 10.7g Protein 4.4g*

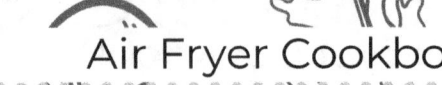

67. ONION FRITTATA

PREPARATION: 20MIN   **COOKING:** 30 MIN   **SERVINGS:** 6

INGREDIENTS

- Eggs; whisked
- 1 tbsp. olive oil
- 1 lb. small potatoes; chopped
- 1 oz. cheddar cheese; grated
- 1/2 cup sour cream
- yellow onions; chopped
- Salt and black pepper to the taste

DIRECTIONS

1. In a large bowl; mix eggs with potatoes, onions, salt, pepper, cheese and sour cream and whisk well.
2. Grease your Air Fryer's pan with the oil, add eggs mix; place in Air Fryer and cook for 20 minutes at 320°F. Slice frittata, divide among plates and serve for breakfast.

Nutrition: *Calories 231 Fat 5g Carbs 8g Protein 4g*

68. PEA TORTILLA

PREPARATION: 10 MIN   **COOKING:** 17 MIN   **SERVINGS:** 8

INGREDIENTS

- 1/2 lb. baby peas
- 1 ½ cup yogurt
- Eggs
- 1/2 cup mint; chopped.
- tbsp. butter
- Salt and black pepper to the taste

DIRECTIONS

1. Heat up a pan that fits your Air Fryer with the butter over medium heat, add peas; mix and cook for a couple of minutes.
2. Meanwhile, in a bowl, mix half of the yogurt with salt, pepper, eggs and mint and whisk well.
3. Pour this over the peas, toss, introduce in your Air Fryer and cook at 350°F, for 7 minutes. Spread the rest of the yogurt over your tortilla; slice and serve.

Nutrition: *Calories 192 Fat 5g Carbs 8g Protein 7g*

69. MUSHROOM QUICHES

PREPARATION: 10 MIN   **COOKING:** 20 MIN   **SERVINGS:** 4

INGREDIENTS

- Button mushrooms; chopped.
- tbsp. ham; chopped
- Eggs
- 1 tbsp. flour
- 1 tbsp. butter; soft
- 9-inch pie dough
- 1/2 tsp. thyme; dried
- 1/4 cup Swiss cheese; grated
- 1 small yellow onion; chopped.
- 1/3 cup heavy cream
- A pinch of nutmeg; ground
- Salt and black pepper to the taste

DIRECTIONS

1. Dust a working surface with the flour and roll the pie dough.
2. Press in on the bottom of the pie pan your Air Fryer has.
3. In a bowl, mix butter with mushrooms, ham, onion, eggs, heavy cream, salt, pepper, thyme and nutmeg and whisk well.
4. Add this over pie crust, spread, sprinkle Swiss cheese all over and place pie pan in your Air Fryer.
5. Cook your quiche at 400°F, for 10 minutes. Slice and serve for breakfast.

Nutrition: *Calories 212 Fat 4g. Carbs 7g Protein 7g*

70. WALNUTS PEAR OATMEAL

PREPARATION: 10 MIN   **COOKING:** 17 MIN   **SERVINGS:** 4

INGREDIENTS

- 1 tbsp. butter; soft
- 1/4 cups brown sugar
- 1 cup water
- 1/2 cup raisins
- 1/2 tsp. cinnamon powder
- 1 cup rolled oats
- 1/2 cup walnuts; chopped.
- 2 cups pear; peeled and chopped.

DIRECTIONS

1. Mix milk with sugar, butter, oats, cinnamon, raisins, pears and walnuts; stir,
2. Introduce in your fryer and cook at 360°F, for 12 minutes.
3. Divide into bowls and serve.

Nutrition: *Calories 230 Fat 6g Carbs 20g Protein 5g*

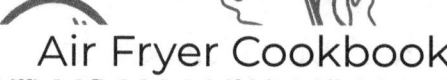 Air Fryer Cookbook

71. BREAKFAST RASPBERRY ROLLS

PREPARATION: 10 MIN **COOKING:** 50 MIN **SERVINGS:** 6

INGREDIENTS

- 1 cup milk
- 1/4 cup sugar
- 1 egg
- tbsp. butter
- ¼ cups flour
- tsp. yeast
- For the filling:
- oz. cream cheese; soft
- oz. raspberries
- 1 tsp. vanilla extract
- tbsp. sugar
- 1 tbsp. cornstarch
- Zest from 1 lemon; grated

DIRECTIONS

1. Mix flour with sugar and yeast and stir.
2. Add milk and egg, stir until you obtain a dough, leave it aside to rise for 30 minutes; transfer dough to a working surface and roll well.
3. Mix cream cheese with sugar, vanilla and lemon zest; stir well and spread over dough.
4. In another bowl, mix raspberries with cornstarch, stir and spread over cream cheese mix.
5. Roll your dough, cut into medium pieces, place them in your Air Fryer; spray them with cooking spray and cook them at 350°F, for 30 minutes. Serve your rolls for breakfast.

Nutrition: *Calories 261 Fat 5g Carbs 9g Protein 6g*

72. BREAD PUDDING

PREPARATION: 10 MIN **COOKING:** 32 MIN **SERVINGS:** 4

INGREDIENTS

- 1/2 lb. white bread; cubed
- 3/4 cup milk
- 3/4 cup water
- tsp. cinnamon powder
- 1 cup flour
- 3/5 cup brown sugar
- tsp. cornstarch
- 1/2 cup apple; peeled; cored and roughly chopped
- 1 tbsp. honey
- 1 tsp. vanilla extract
- oz. soft butter

DIRECTIONS

1. In a bowl, mix bread with apple, milk with water, honey, cinnamon, vanilla and cornstarch and whisk well.
2. Mix flour with sugar and butter and stir until you obtain a crumbled mixture.
3. Press half of the crumble mix on the bottom of your Air Fryer; add bread and apple mix, add the rest of the crumble and cook everything at 350°F, for 22 minutes. Divide bread pudding on plates and serve.

Nutrition: *Calories 261 Fat 7g Carbs 8g Protein 5g*

73. CREAM CHEESE OATS

PREPARATION: 10 MIN **COOKING:** 35 MIN **SERVINGS:** 4

INGREDIENTS

- 1 cup steel oats
- cups milk
- 1 tbsp. butter
- tbsp. white sugar
- oz. cream cheese; soft
- 3/4 cup raisins
- 1 tsp. cinnamon powder
- 1/4 cup brown sugar

DIRECTIONS

1. Heat up a pan that fits your Air Fryer with the butter over medium heat, add oats; stir and toast them for 3 minutes.
2. Add milk and raisins; stir, introduce in your Air Fryer and cook at 350°F, for 20 minutes.
3. Meanwhile; in a bowl, mix cinnamon with brown sugar and stir.
4. In a second bowl, mix white sugar with cream cheese and whisk. Divide oats into bowls and top each with cinnamon and cream cheese.

Nutrition: *Calories 152 Fat 6g Carbs 25g Protein 7g*

74. BREAD ROLLS

PREPARATION: 10 MIN **COOKING:** 22 MIN **SERVINGS:** 4

INGREDIENTS

- potatoes; boiled; peeled and mashed
- 1/2 tsp. turmeric powder
- curry leaf springs
- 1/2 tsp. mustard seeds
- bread slices; white parts only
- 1 coriander bunch; chopped.
- green chilies; chopped
- Small yellow onions; chopped.
- 2 tbsp. olive oil
- Salt and black pepper to the taste

DIRECTIONS

1. Heat up a pan with 1 tsp. oil; add mustard seeds, onions, curry leaves and turmeric, stir and cook for a few seconds.
2. Add mashed potatoes, salt, pepper, coriander and chilies, stir well; take off heat and cool it down.
3. Divide potatoes mix into 8 parts and shape ovals using your wet hands.
4. Wet bread slices with water; press in order to drain excess water and keep one slice in your palm.
5. Add a potato oval over bread slice and wrap it around it.
6. Do the same with the rest of the potato mix and bread.
7. Heat up your Air Fryer at 400°F; add the rest of the oil, add bread rolls; cook them for 12 minutes. Divide bread rolls on plates and serve for breakfast.

Nutrition: *Calories 261 Fat 6g Carbs 12g Protein 7g*

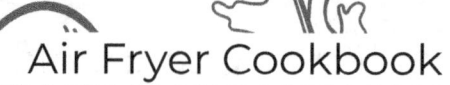

SNACKS

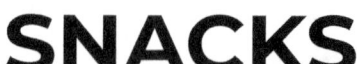

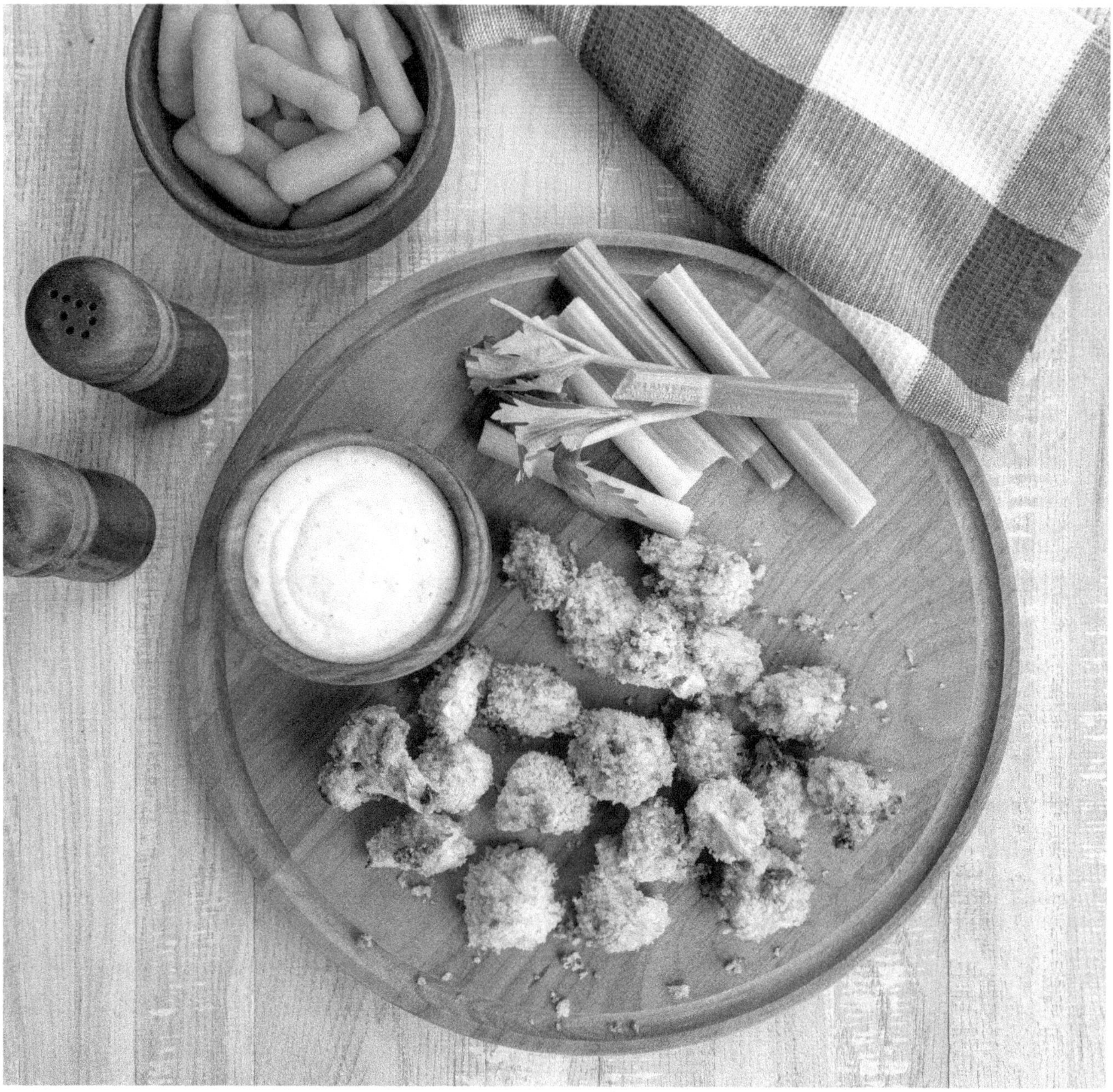

75. ROLLED SALMON SANDWICH

PREPARATION: 5 MIN **COOKING:** 5 MIN **SERVINGS:** 1

INGREDIENTS

- 1 piece of flatbread
- 1 salmon filet
- Pinch of salt
- 1 tbsp. green onion, chopped
- 1/4 tsp. dried sumac
- 1/2 tsp. thyme
- 1/2 tsp. sesame seeds
- 1/4 English cucumber
- 1 tbsp. yogurt

DIRECTIONS

1. Start by peeling and chopping the cucumber. Cut the salmon at a 45-degree angle into 4 slices and lay them flat on the flatbread.
2. Sprinkle salmon with salt to taste. Sprinkle onions, thyme, sumac, and sesame seeds evenly over the salmon.
3. Put the Salmon in the Air Fryer basket and cook at 360°F for at least 3 minutes, but longer if you want a more well-done fish.
4. While you cook your salmon, mix the yogurt and cucumber. Remove your flatbread from the Air Fryer, put it on a plate, and spoon the yogurt mix over the salmon.
5. Fold the flatbread sides in and roll it up for a gourmet lunch that you can take on the go.

Nutrition: *Calories 347 Fat 12.4g Carbs 20.6g Protein 38.9g*

76. BALSAMIC ROASTED CHICKEN

PREPARATION: 10 MIN **COOKING:** 22 MIN **SERVINGS:** 4

INGREDIENTS

- 1/2 cup balsamic vinegar
- 1/4 cup Dijon mustard
- 1/3 cup olive oil
- Juice and zest from 1 lemon
- minced garlic cloves
- 1 tsp. salt
- 1 tsp. pepper
- bone-in, skin-on chicken thighs
- bone-in, skin-on chicken drumsticks
- 1 tbsp. chopped parsley

DIRECTIONS

1. Mix vinegar, lemon juice, mustard, olive oil, garlic, salt, and pepper in a bowl and then pour it into an Air Fryer pan.
2. Roll chicken pieces in the pan, then cover and marinate for at least 2 hours, but up to 24 hours.
3. Preheat the Air Fryer to 360°F and place the chicken on a fresh baking pan, reserving the marinade later.
4. Cook the chicken for 20 minutes.
5. Take the chicken and cover it with foil to keep it warm. Place the marinade in the Air Fryer for about 2 minutes until it simmers down and begins to thicken.
6. Pour marinade over chicken and sprinkle with parsley and lemon zest.

Nutrition: *Calories 1537 Fat 70.5g Carbs 2.4g Protein 210.4g*

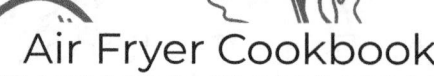
Air Fryer Cookbook

77. CHICKEN CAPERS SANDWICH

PREPARATION: 3 MIN   **COOKING:** 3 MIN   **SERVINGS:** 2

INGREDIENTS

- Leftover chicken breasts or pre-cooked breaded chicken
- 1 large ripe tomato
- oz.' mozzarella cheese slices
- slices of whole-grain bread
- 1/4 cup olive oil
- 1/3 cup fresh basil leaves
- Salt and pepper to taste

Nutrition: *Calories 808 Fat 43.6g Carbs 30.7g Protein 78.4g*

DIRECTIONS

1. Start by slicing tomatoes into thin slices.
2. Layer tomatoes, then cheese over two slices of bread and place on a greased pan that fits the Air Fryer.
3. Grill for about 3 minutes at 370°F
4. Heat chicken while the cheese melts.
5. Remove from Air Fryer, sprinkle with basil, and add chicken.
6. Sprinkle with oil and add salt and pepper.
7. Top with other slices of bread and serve.

78. EASY PROSCIUTTO GRILLED CHEESE

PREPARATION: 5 MIN   **COOKING:** 4 MIN   **SERVINGS:** 1

INGREDIENTS

- slices muenster cheese
- 2 slices white bread
- thinly-shaved pieces of prosciutto
- 1 tbsp. sweet and spicy pickles

Nutrition: *Calories 460 Fat 25.2g Carbs 11.9g Protein 44.2g*

DIRECTIONS

1. Put one slice of cheese on each piece of bread.
2. Put prosciutto on one slice and pickles on the other.
3. Put it in the Air Fryer basket for 4 minutes at 340°F or until the cheese is melted.
4. Combine the sides, cut, and serve.

79. HERB-ROASTED CHICKEN TENDERS

PREPARATION: 5 MIN   **COOKING:** 5 MIN   **SERVINGS:** 2

INGREDIENTS

- 10 oz. chicken tenders
- 1 tbsp. olive oil
- 1/2 tsp. Herbes de Provence
- tbsp. Dijon mustard
- 1 tbsp. honey
- Salt and pepper

Nutrition: *Calories 297 Fat 15.5g Carbs 9.6g Protein 29.8g*

DIRECTIONS

1. Start by preheating the Air Fryer to 345°F.
2. Brush the bottom of the Air Fryer pan with 1/2 tbsp. olive oil.
3. Spice the chicken with herbs, salt, and pepper.
4. Place the chicken in a single flat layer in the pan and drizzle the remaining olive oil over it.
5. Air Fry for about 5 minutes
6. While the chicken is cooking, mix the mustard and honey for a tasty condiment.

80. GROUND BEEF BOWL

PREPARATION: 10 MIN   **COOKING:** 15 MIN   **SERVINGS:** 4

INGREDIENTS

- 2 tbsp. chives
- 1 onion, chopped
- 16 oz ground beef
- 1 tsp. olive oil
- 1 tsp. paprika
- 1 tsp. cumin
- ½ tsp. ground black pepper 1-1/2 lb.' boneless pork loin

Nutrition: *Calories 236 Fat 8.5g Carbs 3.3g Protein 35g*

DIRECTIONS

1. Put the ground beef in the Air Fryer basket.
2. Sprinkle the meat with the cumin, paprika, ground black pepper, and olive oil.
3. Stir it and cook for 7 minutes at 380°F. Stir the meat time to time.
4. After this, add chopped onion and chives.
5. Stir the meat mixture and cook it at 380°F for 8 minutes more or until all the ingredients are cooked.
6. Transfer the ground beef to the bowl and serve!

81. TURMERIC CHICKEN LIVER

PREPARATION: 10 MIN   **COOKING:** 7 MIN   **SERVINGS:** 5

INGREDIENTS

- 17 oz chicken liver
- 2 tbsp. almond flour
- 1 tbsp. coconut oil
- ½ tsp. salt
- ¼ tsp. minced garlic
- ¾ cup chicken stock

Nutrition: *Calories 250, Fat 14.7g, Carbs 3.4g, Protein 26.1g*

DIRECTIONS

1. Place the coconut oil in the Air Fryer basket and preheat it for 20 seconds.
2. Then add chicken liver.
3. Stir it and cook for 2 minutes at 400°F.
4. Then sprinkle the chicken liver with the almond flour, salt, and minced garlic.
5. Add the chicken stock and stir liver and cook it for 5 minutes more or until cooked.
6. Serve the meal immediately!

82. CHICKEN BURGERS

PREPARATION: 15 MIN   **COOKING:** 12 MIN   **SERVINGS:** 3

INGREDIENTS

- ¼ cup fresh parsley, chopped
- 1 garlic clove, chopped
- 1 tbsp. olive oil
- 1 egg
- 10 oz ground chicken
- 1 tsp. paprika
- 1 tsp. almond flour

Nutrition: *Calories 299, Fat 17.9g, Carbs 3.2g, Protein 31.5g*

DIRECTIONS

1. Place the ground chicken in the mixing bowl.
2. Beat the egg into the mixture and sprinkle it with the paprika, almond flour, chopped garlic clove, and chopped parsley.
3. Stir the meat mixture until homogenous. Then make the medium burgers from the mixture.
4. Spray the Air Fryer basket with the olive oil inside and place the chicken burgers there.
5. Cook the meal for 12 minutes at 390°F. Turn the burgers into another side after 6 minutes of cooking.
6. Chill the cooked burgers little and serve!

Air Fryer Cookbook

83. ZUCCHINI CASSEROLE

PREPARATION: 10 MIN **COOKING:** 20 MIN **SERVINGS:** 5

INGREDIENTS

- 1 carrot, sliced
- 1 onion, sliced
- 1 zucchini, sliced
- 1 cup chicken stock
- 1 cup kale, chopped
- 1 tsp. paprika
- 1 tsp. salt
- 3 oz bacon, chopped, cooked
- 1 tbsp. olive oil

DIRECTIONS

1. Combine together the carrot, onion, zucchini, and chopped kale in the mixing bowl. Stir the mixture well. Then add salt and paprika. Stir it.
2. Pour the olive oil into the Air Fryer basket. Add the vegetable mixture and chopped bacon. Stir it well.
3. Then add the chicken stock and cook the casserole for 20 minutes at 375°F. Stir it gently time to time.
4. When the time is over – check if all the ingredients are cooked.
5. Chill the casserole to the room temperature and serve!

Nutrition: *Calories 146, Fat 10.2g, Carbs 6.6g, Protein 7.7g*

84. CHERRY TUSCAN PORK LOIN

PREPARATION: 15 MIN **COOKING:** 40 MIN **SERVINGS:** 5

INGREDIENTS

- 1-lb. pork loin
- ½ lemon
- 1 cup cherry tomatoes
- 1 tsp. chili pepper
- 1 tbsp. olive oil
- 1 onion, chopped
- 1 garlic clove, chopped

DIRECTIONS

1. Pour the olive oil into the air fryer basket.
2. Sprinkle the pork loin with the chili pepper and garlic clove.
3. Place the pork loin in the air fryer basket and cook it for 20 minutes from one side at 360°F.
4. After this, turn the pork loin into another side and cook it for 10 minutes more.
5. Add the cherry tomatoes.
6. Squeeze the lemon juice over the meat and tomatoes and cook the meal for 10 minutes more at 360°F.
7. When the meat is cooked – let it chill for 5 minutes.
8. Enjoy!

Nutrition: *Calories 262g, Fat 15.6g, Carbs 4.3g, Protein 25.5g*

85. MOROCCAN PORK KEBABS

PREPARATION: 40 MIN **COOKING:** 45 MIN **SERVINGS:** 4

INGREDIENTS

- 1/4 cup orange juice
- 1 tbsp. tomato paste
- 1 clove chopped garlic
- 1 tbsp. ground cumin
- 1/8 tsp. ground cinnamon
- tbsp. olive oil
- 1-1/2 tsp.s salt
- 3/4 tsp. black pepper
- 1-1/2 lb. boneless pork loin
- 1 small eggplant
- 1 small red onion
- Pita bread (optional)
- 1/2 small cucumber
- tbsp. chopped fresh mint
- Wooden skewers

Nutrition: *Calories: 465, Fat: 20.8g Carbs: 21.9g, Protein: 48.2g.*

DIRECTIONS

1. Begin by placing wooden skewers in water to soak.
2. Cut pork loin and eggplant into 1- to 1-1/2-inch chunks.
3. Preheat toaster oven to 425°F.
4. Cut cucumber and onions into pieces and chop the mint.
5. Combine the orange juice, tomato paste, garlic, cumin, and cinnamon, 2 tbsp. of oil, 1 tsp. of salt, and 1/2 tsp. of pepper.
6. Add the pork to this mixture and refrigerate for at least 30 minutes, but up to 8 hours.
7. Mix vegetables, remaining oil, and salt and pepper.
8. Skewer the vegetables and bake for 20 minutes.
9. Add the pork to the skewers and bake for an additional 25 minutes.
10. Remove ingredients from skewers and sprinkle with mint; serve with flatbread if using.

86. BANANA CHIPS

PREPARATION: 5 MIN **COOKING:** 15 MIN **SERVINGS:** 8

INGREDIENTS

- ¼ cup peanut butter, soft
- 1 banana, peeled and sliced into 16 pieces
- 1 tbsp. vegetable oil

Nutrition: *Calories 100 Fat 4g Carbs 10g Protein 4g*

DIRECTIONS

1. Put the banana slices in your Air Fryer's basket and drizzle the oil over them.
2. Cook at 360°F for 5 minutes.
3. Transfer to bowls and serve them dipped in peanut butter.

87. LEMONY APPLE BITES

PREPARATION: 5 MIN **COOKING:** 5 MIN **SERVINGS:** 4

INGREDIENTS

- Big apples, cored, peeled and cubed
- 2 tsp.s lemon juice
- ½ cup caramel sauce

Nutrition: *Calories 180 Fat 4g Carbs 10g Protein 3g*

DIRECTIONS

1. In your Air Fryer basket, mix all the ingredients; toss well.
2. Cook at 340°F for 5 minutes.
3. Divide into cups and serve as a snack.

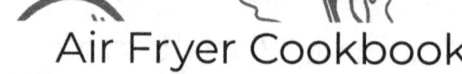

88. BALSAMIC ZUCCHINI SLICES

PREPARATION: 5 MIN **COOKING:** 50 MIN **SERVINGS:** 6

INGREDIENTS

- Zucchinis, thinly sliced
- Salt and black pepper to taste
- Tbsp. avocado oil
- Tbsp. balsamic vinegar

DIRECTIONS

1. Put all of the ingredients into a bowl and mix.
2. Put the zucchini mixture in your Air Fryer's basket and cook at 220°F for 50 minutes.
3. Serve as a snack and enjoy!

Nutrition: *Calories 40 Fat 3g Carbs 3g Protein 7g*

89. TURMERIC CARROT CHIPS

PREPARATION: 5 MIN **COOKING:** 25 MIN **SERVINGS:** 4

INGREDIENTS

- Carrots, thinly sliced
- Salt and black pepper to taste
- ½ tsp. turmeric powder
- ½ tsp. chaat masala
- 1 tsp. olive oil

DIRECTIONS

1. Put all of the ingredients in a bowl and toss well.
2. Put the mixture in your Air Fryer's basket and cook at 370°F for 25 minutes, shaking the fryer from time to time.
3. Serve as a snack.

Nutrition: *Calories 161 Fat 1g Carbs 5g Protein 3g*

90. CHIVES RADISH SNACK

PREPARATION: 5 MIN **COOKING:** 10 MIN **SERVINGS:** 4

INGREDIENTS

- 16 radishes, sliced
- A drizzle of olive oil
- Salt and black pepper to taste
- 1 tbsp. chives, chopped

DIRECTIONS

1. In a bowl, mix the radishes, salt, pepper, and oil; toss well.
2. Place the radishes in your Air Fryer's basket and cook at 350°F for 10 minutes.
3. Divide into bowls and serve with chives sprinkled on top.

Nutrition: *Calories 100 Fat 1g Carbs 4g Protein 1g*

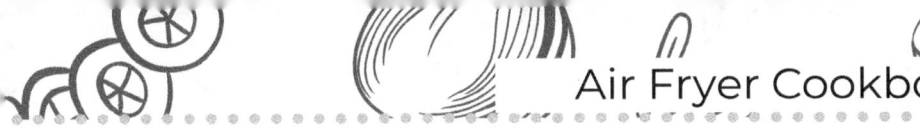

Air Fryer Cookbook

91. LENTILS SNACK

PREPARATION: 5 MIN   **COOKING:** 12 MIN   **SERVINGS:** 4

INGREDIENTS

- 15 oz. canned lentils, drained
- ½ tsp. cumin, ground
- 1 tbsp. olive oil
- 1 tsp. sweet paprika
- Salt and black pepper to taste

DIRECTIONS

1. Place all ingredients in a bowl and blend it well.
2. Transfer the mixture to your Air Fryer and cook at 400°F for 12 minutes.
3. Divide into bowls and serve as a snack -or a side, or appetizer!

Nutrition: *Calories 151 Fat 1g Carbs 10g Protein 6g*

92. AIR FRIED CORN

PREPARATION: 5 MIN   **COOKING:** 10 MIN   **SERVINGS:** 4

INGREDIENTS

- Tbsp. corn kernels
- 2½ tbsp. butter

DIRECTIONS

1. In a saucepan that fits your Air Fryer, mix the corn with the butter.
2. Place the pan inside the Air Fryer and cook at 400°F for 10 minutes.
3. Serve as a snack and enjoy!

Nutrition: *Calories 70 Fat 2g Carbs 7g Protein 3g*

93. BREADED MUSHROOMS

PREPARATION: 10 MIN   **COOKING:** 45 MIN   **SERVINGS:** 4

INGREDIENTS

- 1 lb. small Button mushrooms, cleaned
- 2 cups breadcrumbs
- 6 eggs, beaten
- Salt and pepper to taste
- 2 cups Parmigiano Reggiano cheese, grated

DIRECTIONS

1. Preheat the Air Fryer to 360°F. Pour the breadcrumbs in a bowl, add salt and pepper and mix well. Pour the cheese in a separate bowl and set aside. Dip each mushroom in the eggs, then in the crumbs, and then in the cheese.
2. Slide out the fryer basket and add 6 to 10 mushrooms. Cook them for 20 minutes, in batches, if needed. Serve with cheese dip.

Nutrition: *Calories 487 Carbs 49g Fat 22g Protein 31g*

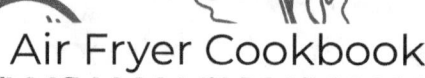

94. CHEESY STICKS WITH SWEET THAI SAUCE

PREPARATION: 2 H **COOKING:** 20 MIN **SERVINGS:** 4

INGREDIENTS

- 12 mozzarella string cheese
- 2 cups breadcrumbs
- 6 eggs
- 1 cup sweet Thai sauce
- tbsp. skimmed milk

DIRECTIONS

1. Pour the crumbs in a medium bowl. Break the eggs into a different bowl and beat with the milk. One after the other, dip each cheese sticks in the egg mixture, in the crumbs, then egg mixture again and then in the crumbs again.
2. Place the coated cheese sticks on a cookie sheet and freeze for 1 to 2 hours. Preheat the Air Fryer to 380°F. Arrange the sticks in the fryer without overcrowding. Cook for 5 minutes, flipping them halfway through cooking to brown evenly. Cook in batches. Serve with a sweet Thai sauce.

Nutrition: *Calories 158 Carbs 14g Fat 7g Protein 9g*

95. BACON WRAPPED AVOCADOS

PREPARATION: 10 MIN **COOKING:** 30 MIN **SERVINGS:** 4

INGREDIENTS

- 12 thick strips bacon
- 2 large avocados, sliced
- ⅓ tsp. salt
- ⅓ tsp. chili powder
- ⅓ tsp. cumin powder

DIRECTIONS

1. Stretch the bacon strips to elongate and use a knife to cut in half to make 24 pieces. Wrap each bacon piece around a slice of avocado from one end to the other end. Tuck the end of bacon into the wrap. Arrange on a flat surface and season with salt, chili and cumin on both sides.
2. Arrange 4 to 8 wrapped pieces in the Air Fryer and cook at 350°F for 8 minutes, or until the bacon is browned and crunchy, flipping halfway through to cook evenly. Remove onto a wire rack and repeat the process for the remaining avocado pieces.

Nutrition: *Calories 193 Carbs 10g Fat 16g Protein 4g*

96. HOT CHICKEN WINGETTES

PREPARATION: 10 MIN **COOKING:** 40 MIN **SERVINGS:** 4

INGREDIENTS

- 15 chicken wingettes
- Salt and pepper to taste
- ⅓ cup hot sauce
- ⅓ cup butter
- ½ tbsp. vinegar

DIRECTIONS

1. Preheat the Air Fryer to 360°F. Season the vignettes with pepper and salt. Add them to the Air Fryer and cook for 35 minutes. Toss every 5 minutes. Once ready, remove them into a bowl. Over low heat, melt the butter in a saucepan. Add the vinegar and hot sauce. Stir and cook for a minute.
2. Turn the heat off. Pour the sauce over the chicken. Toss to coat well. Transfer the chicken to a serving platter. Serve with blue cheese dressing.

Nutrition: *Calories 563 Carbs 2g Fat 28g Protein 35g*

---

97. CARROT CRISPS

PREPARATION: 10 MIN **COOKING:** 10 MIN **SERVINGS:** 4

INGREDIENTS

- 6 large carrots, washed and peeled
- Salt to taste
- Cooking spray

DIRECTIONS

1. Using a mandolin slicer, slice the carrots very thinly height-wise. Put the carrot strips in a bowl and season with salt to taste. Grease the fryer basket lightly with cooking spray, and add the carrot strips. Cook at 350°F for 10 minutes, stirring once halfway through.

Nutrition: *Calories 35 Carbs 8g Fat 3g Protein 1g*

---

98. QUICK CHEESE STICKS

PREPARATION: 5 MIN **COOKING:** 10 MIN **SERVINGS:** 4

INGREDIENTS

- 6 oz bread cheese
- tbsp. butter
- cups panko crumbs

DIRECTIONS

1. Place the butter in a dish and melt it in the microwave, for 2 minutes; set aside. With a knife, cut the cheese into equal-sized sticks. Brush each stick with butter and dip into panko crumbs. Arrange the cheese sticks in a single layer on the fryer basket. Cook at 390°F for 10 minutes. Flip them halfway through, to brown evenly; serve warm.

Nutrition: *Calories 25 Carbs 8g Fat 21g Protein 16g*

99. RADISH CHIPS

PREPARATION: 10 MIN **COOKING:** 20 MIN **SERVINGS:** 4

INGREDIENTS

- Radishes, leaves removed and cleaned
- Salt to season
- Water
- Cooking spray

DIRECTIONS

1. Using a mandolin, slice the radishes thinly. Put them in a pot and pour water on them. Heat the pot on a stovetop, and bring to boil, until the radishes are translucent, for 4 minutes. After 4 minutes, drain the radishes through a sieve; set aside. Grease the fryer basket with cooking spray.
2. Add in the radish slices and cook for 8 minutes, flipping once halfway through. Cook until golden brown, at 400°F. Meanwhile, prepare a paper towel-lined plate. Once the radishes are ready, transfer them to the paper towel-lined plate. Season with salt, and serve with ketchup or garlic mayo.

Nutrition: Calories 25 Carbs 0.2g Fat 2g Protein 0.1g

100. HERBED CROUTONS WITH BRIE CHEESE

PREPARATION: 10 MIN **COOKING:** 10 MIN **SERVINGS:** 4

INGREDIENTS

- tbsp. olive oil
- 1 tbsp. french herbs
- oz brie cheese, chopped
- Sliced bread, halved

Nutrition: Calories 20 Carbs 1.5g Fat 1.3g Protein 0.5g

DIRECTIONS

1. Warm up your Air Fryer to 340° F. Using a bowl, mix oil with herbs. Dip the bread slices in the oil mixture to coat. Place the coated slices on a flat surface. Lay the brie cheese on the slices. Place the slices into your Air Fryer's basket and cook for 7 minutes. Once the bread is ready, cut into cubes.

101. STUFFED JALAPENO

PREPARATION: 10 MIN **COOKING:** 10 MIN **SERVINGS:** 4

INGREDIENTS

- 1 lb. ground pork sausage
- 1 (8 oz.) package cream cheese, softened
- 1 cup shredded Parmesan cheese
- 1 lb. large fresh jalapeno peppers halved lengthwise and seeded
- 1 (8 oz.) bottle Ranch dressing

Nutrition: Calories 168 Protein 9.4g Carbs 12.1g Fat 21.2g

DIRECTIONS

1. Mix pork sausage ground with ranch dressing and cream cheese in a bowl. Cut the jalapeno in half and remove their seeds. Divide the cream cheese mixture into the jalapeno halves. Place the jalapeno pepper in a baking tray that fits the Air Fryer. Set the Baking tray inside the Air Fryer and close the lid. Select the Bake mode at 350°F temperature for 10 minutes. Serve warm.

Air Fryer Cookbook

102. GARLICKY BOK CHOY

PREPARATION: 10 MIN   **COOKING:** 6 MIN   **SERVINGS:** 2

INGREDIENTS

- Bunches baby bok choy
- spray oil
- 1 tsp. garlic powder

Nutrition: *Calories 81 Protein 0.4g Carbs 4.7g Fat 8.3g*

DIRECTIONS

1. Toss bok choy with garlic powder and spread them in the Air Fryer basket. Spray them with cooking oil. Set the Air Fryer basket inside the Air Fryer and close the lid. Select the Air Fry mode at 350°F temperature for 6 minutes. Serve fresh.

103. CHIA SEED CRACKERS

PREPARATION: 15 MIN   **COOKING:** 45 MIN   **SERVINGS:** 48

INGREDIENTS

- 1 Cup raw chia seed
- 3/4 Tsp. salt
- 1/4 Tsp. garlic powder
- 1/4 Tsp. onion powder
- 1 Cup cold water

Nutrition: *Calories 120 Fat 3.9g Carbs 1.9g Protein 1.9g*

DIRECTIONS

1. Put the chia seeds in a bowl. Add salt, garlic powder, and onion powder.
2. Pour into the water. Stir. Cover with plastic wrap. Store in the fridge overnight. Preheat the Air Fryer to 200°F. Cover the baking sheet with a silicone mat or parchment. Transfer the soaked linseed to a prepared baking sheet. Scatter it out with a spatula in a thin, flat rectangle about 1 cm thick. Rate the rectangle in about 32 small rectangles. Bake in the preheated Air Fryer toaster oven up to the chia seeds have darkened and contract slightly, about 3 hours. Let it cool. Break individual cookies.

104. BAKED EGGPLANT CHIPS

PREPARATION: 5 MIN   **COOKING:** 8 MIN   **SERVINGS:** 4

INGREDIENTS

- Medium eggplant, cut into 1/4-inch slices
- 1/2 Cup crushed cornflakes.
- 1/8 Tsp. ground black pepper
- Tbsp. grated goat cheese
- Egg whites

Nutrition: *Calories 92 Fat 2.1g Carbs 13.9g Protein 5.9g*

DIRECTIONS

1. Preheat the Air Fryer to 400°F. Mix the crushed cornflakes, pepper and goat cheese in a small container. Set aside the egg whites in a different container. Dip the eggplant slices in the egg white and cover the crushed cornflakes mixture. Place on a greased baking pan that fits the Air Dryer.
2. Air fry for 3 minutes, then turn and cook bake for another 3 to 5 minutes until golden yellow and crispy.

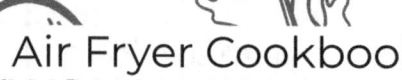
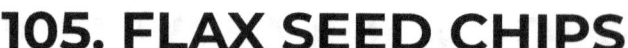

105. FLAX SEED CHIPS

PREPARATION: 8 MIN   **COOKING:** 5 MIN   **SERVINGS:** 4

INGREDIENTS

- 1 Cup almond flour
- 1/2 Cup flax seeds
- 1 1/2 Tsp.s seasoned salt
- 1 Tsp. sea salt
- 1/2 Cup water

DIRECTIONS

1. Preheat the Air Fryer to 300°F. Combine almond flour, flax seeds, 1 1/2 tsp.s seasoned salt and sea salt in a container; Stir in the water up to the dough is completely mixed. Shape the dough into narrow size slices the size of a bite and place them on a pan that fits the Air Dryer. Sprinkle the rounds with seasoned salt. Bake in preheated Air Fryer up to crispy, about 8 minutes. Cool fully and store in an airtight box or in a sealed bag.

Nutrition: *Calories 126.9 Fat 6.1g Carbs 15.9g Protein 2.9g*

106. SALTED HAZELNUTS

PREPARATION: 15 MIN   **COOKING:** 6 MIN   **SERVINGS:** 8

INGREDIENTS

- Cups dry roasted Hazelnuts, no salt added
- Tbsp. coconut oil
- 1 Tsp. garlic powder
- 1 Sprig fresh Thyme, chopped
- 1 1/2 Tsp.s salt

DIRECTIONS

1. Preheat the Air Fryer to 320°F. Mix the Hazelnuts, coconut oil, garlic powder and thyme in a bowl until the nuts are fully covered. Sprinkle with salt. Spread evenly on a baking sheet. Bake in the preheated Air Fryer for 6 minutes.

Nutrition: *Calories 237 Fat 21.3g Carbs 5.9gn Protein 7.4g*

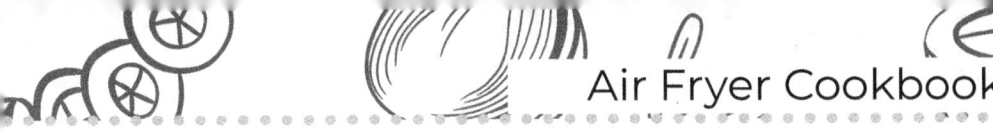

107. BAGUETTE BREAD

PREPARATION: 15 MIN   **COOKING:** 8 MIN   **SERVINGS:** 8

INGREDIENTS

- ¾ cup warm water
- ¾ tsp. quick yeast
- ½ tsp. demerara sugar
- 1 cup bread flour
- ½ cup whole-wheat flour
- ½ cup oat flour
- 1¼ tsp.s salt

Nutrition: *Calories 114 Fat 0.8g Carbs 22.8g Protein 3.8g*

DIRECTIONS

1. In a large bowl, place the water and sprinkle with yeast and sugar. Set aside for 5 minutes or until foamy.
2. Add the bread flour and salt mix until a stiff dough form.
3. Put the dough onto a floured surface and with your hands, knead until smooth and elastic. Shape the dough into a ball.
4. Place the dough into a slightly oiled bowl and turn to coat well.
5. With a plastic wrap, cover the bowl and place in a warm place for about 1 hour or until doubled in size.
6. With your hands, punch down the dough and form into a long slender loaf.
7. Place the loaf onto a lightly greased baking sheet and set aside in warm place, uncovered, for about 30 minutes
8. Heat the Air Fryer 450°F.
9. Carefully, arrange the dough onto the "Wire Rack" and insert in the Air Fryer.
10. Air Fry for 8 minutes.
11. Carefully, invert the bread onto wire rack to cool completely before slicing.
12. Cut the bread into desired-sized slices and serve.

Air Fryer Cookbook

108. YOGURT BREAD

PREPARATION: 20 MIN   **COOKING:** 20 MIN   **SERVINGS:** 10

INGREDIENTS

- 1½ cups warm water, divided
- 1½ tsp.s active dry yeast
- 1 tsp. sugar
- 3 cups all-purpose flour
- 1 cup plain Greek yogurt
- 2 tsp.s kosher salt

Nutrition: *Calories 157 Fat 0.7g Carbs 31g Protein 5.5g*

DIRECTIONS

1. Add ½ cup of the warm water, yeast and sugar in the bowl of a stand mixer, fitted with the dough hook attachment and mix well.
2. Set aside for about 5 minutes
3. Add the flour, yogurt, and salt and mix on medium-low speed until the dough comes together.
4. Then, mix on medium speed for 5 minutes
5. Place the dough into a bowl.
6. With a plastic wrap, cover the bowl and place in a warm place for about 2-3 hours or until doubled in size.
7. Transfer the dough onto a lightly floured surface and shape into a smooth ball.
8. Place the dough onto a greased parchment paper-lined rack.
9. With a kitchen towel, cover the dough and let rest for 15 minutes
10. With a very sharp knife, cut a 4x½-inch deep cut down the center of the dough.
11. Preheat the Air Fryer at 325°F.
12. Carefully, arrange the dough onto the "Wire Rack" and insert in the Air Fryer. Cook for 20 minutes.
13. Carefully, invert the bread onto wire rack to cool completely before slicing.
14. Cut the bread into desired-sized slices and serve.

Air Fryer Cookbook

109. SUNFLOWER SEED BREAD

PREPARATION: 15 MIN   **COOKING:** 18 MIN   **SERVINGS:** 6

INGREDIENTS

- 2/3 cup whole-wheat flour
- 2/3 cup plain flour
- 1/3 cup sunflower seeds
- ½ sachet instant yeast
- 1 tsp. salt
- 2/3-1 cup lukewarm water

DIRECTIONS

1. In a bowl, mix together the flours, sunflower seeds, yeast, and salt.
2. Slowly, add in the water, stirring continuously until a soft dough ball form.
3. Now, move the dough onto a lightly floured surface and knead for about 5 minutes using your hands.
4. Make a ball from the dough and place into a bowl.
5. With a plastic wrap, cover the bowl and place at a warm place for about 30 minutes
6. Grease a cake pan that fits the Air Fryer.
7. Coat the top of dough with water and place into the prepared cake pan.
8. Preheat the Air Fryer at 390°F.
9. Arrange the pan in the Air Fryer basket and insert in the oven. Cook for 18 minutes.
10. Place the pan onto a wire rack to cool for about 10 minutes
11. Carefully, invert the bread onto wire rack to cool completely before slicing.
12. Cut the bread into desired-sized slices and serve.

Nutrition: *Calories 132 Fat 1.7g Carbs 24.4g Protein 4.9g*

110. DATE BREAD

PREPARATION: 15 MIN   **COOKING:** 2 MIN   **SERVINGS:** 10

INGREDIENTS

- 2½ cup dates, pitted and chopped
- ¼ cup butter
- 1 cup hot water
- 1½ cups flour
- ½ cup brown sugar
- 1 tsp. baking powder
- 1 tsp. baking soda
- ½ tsp. salt
- 1 egg

DIRECTIONS

1. In a large bowl, add the dates, butter and top with the hot water.
2. Set aside for about 5 minutes
3. In another bowl, mix together the flour, brown sugar, baking powder, baking soda, and salt.
4. In the same bowl of dates, mix well the flour mixture, and egg.
5. Grease a baking pan.
6. Place the mixture into the prepared pan.
7. Preheat the Air Fryer at 340°F.
8. Arrange the pan in Air Fryer basket and insert in the oven. Cook for about 22 minutes.
9. Place the pan onto a wire rack to cool for about 10 minutes
10. Carefully, invert the bread onto wire rack to cool completely before slicing.
11. Cut the bread into desired-sized slices and serve.

Nutrition: *Calories 269 Fat 5.4g Carbs 55.1g Protein 3.6g*

111. DATE & WALNUT BREAD

PREPARATION: 15 MIN　　**COOKING:** 35 MIN　　**SERVINGS:** 5

INGREDIENTS

- 1 cup dates, pitted and sliced
- ¾ cup walnuts, chopped
- 1 tbsp. instant coffee powder
- 1 tbsp. hot water
- 1¼ cups plain flour
- ¼ tsp. salt
- ½ tsp. baking powder
- ½ tsp. baking soda
- ½ cup condensed milk
- ½ cup butter, softened
- ½ tsp. vanilla essence

Nutrition: *Calories 593 Fat 32.6g Carbs 69.4g Protein 11.2g*

DIRECTIONS

1. In a large bowl, add the dates, butter and top with the hot water.
2. Set aside for about 30 minutes
3. Dry out well and set aside.
4. In a small bowl, add the coffee powder and hot water and mix well.
5. In a large bowl, mix together the flour, baking powder, baking soda and salt.
6. In another large bowl, add the condensed milk and butter and beat until smooth.
7. Add the flour mixture, coffee mixture and vanilla essence and mix until well combined.
8. Fold in dates and ½ cup of walnut.
9. Line a baking pan with a lightly greased parchment paper.
10. Place the mixture into the prepared pan and sprinkle with the remaining walnuts.
11. Preheat the Air Fryer at 320°F.
12. Arrange the pan in Air Fryer basket and insert in the oven. Cook for 35 minutes.
13. Place the pan onto a wire rack to cool for about 10 minutes
14. Carefully, invert the bread onto wire rack to cool completely before slicing.
15. Cut the bread into desired-sized slices and serve.

112. BROWN SUGAR BANANA BREAD

PREPARATION: 15 MIN　　**COOKING:** 30 MIN　　**SERVINGS:** 4

INGREDIENTS

- 1 egg
- 1 ripe banana, peeled and mashed
- ¼ cup milk
- 2 tbsp. canola oil
- 2 tbsp. brown sugar
- ¾ cup plain flour
- ½ tsp. baking soda

Nutrition: *Calories 214 Fat 8.7g Carbs 29.9g Protein 4.6g*

DIRECTIONS

1. Line a very small baking pan with a greased parchment paper.
2. In a small bowl, add the egg and banana and beat well.
3. Add the milk, oil and sugar and beat until well combined.
4. Add the flour and baking soda and mix until just combined.
5. Place the mixture into prepared pan.
6. Preheat the Air Fryer at 320°F.
7. Arrange the pan in Air Fryer basket and insert in the oven. Cook for 30 minutes.
8. Place the pan onto a wire rack to cool for about 10 minutes
9. Carefully, invert the bread onto wire rack to cool completely before slicing.
10. Cut the bread into desired-sized slices and serve.

113. CINNAMON BANANA BREAD

PREPARATION: 15 MIN   **COOKING:** 20 MIN   **SERVINGS:** 8

INGREDIENTS

- 1 1/3 cups flour
- 2/3 cup sugar
- 1 tsp. baking soda
- 1 tsp. baking powder
- 1 tsp. ground cinnamon
- 1 tsp. salt
- ½ cup milk
- ½ cup olive oil
- 3 bananas, peeled and sliced

DIRECTIONS

1. In the bowl of a stand mixer, add all the ingredients and mix well.
2. Grease a loaf pan.
3. Place the mixture into the prepared pan.
4. Preheat the Air Fryer at 320°F.
5. Arrange the pan in Air Fryer basket and insert in the oven. Cook for 20 minutes.
6. Place the pan onto a wire rack to cool for about 10 minutes
7. Carefully, invert the bread onto wire rack to cool completely before slicing.
8. Cut the bread into desired-sized slices and serve.

Nutrition: *Calories 295 Fat 13.3g Carbs 44g Protein 3.1g*

114. BANANA & WALNUT BREAD

PREPARATION: 15 MIN   **COOKING:** 25 MIN   **SERVINGS:** 6

INGREDIENTS

- 1½ cups self-rising flour
- ¼ tsp. bicarbonate of soda
- 5 tbsp. plus 1 tsp. butter
- 2/3 cup plus ½ tbsp. caster sugar
- 2 medium eggs
- 3½ oz. walnuts, chopped
- 2 cups bananas, peeled and mashed

DIRECTIONS

1. In a bowl, mix together the flour and bicarbonate of soda.
2. In another bowl, add the butter, and sugar and beat until pale and fluffy.
3. Add the eggs, one at a time along with a little flour and mix well.
4. Stir in the remaining flour and walnuts. Add the bananas and mix until well combined.
5. Grease a loaf pan. Place the mixture into the prepared pan.
6. Preheat the Air Fryer at 350°F.
7. Arrange the pan in Air Fryer basket and insert in the oven. Cook for 10 minutes.
8. After 10 minutes of cooking, set the temperature at 320°F for 15 minutes
9. Place the pan onto a wire rack to cool for about 10 minutes
10. Carefully, invert the bread onto wire rack to cool completely before slicing.
11. Cut the bread into desired-sized slices and serve.

Nutrition: *Calories 270 Fat 12.8g Carbs 35.5g Protein 5.8g*

115. BANANA & RAISIN BREAD

PREPARATION: 15 MIN **COOKING:** 40 MIN **SERVINGS:** 6

INGREDIENTS

- 1½ cups cake flour
- 1 tsp. baking soda
- ½ tsp. ground cinnamon
- Salt, to taste
- ½ cup vegetable oil
- 2 eggs
- ½ cup sugar
- ½ tsp. vanilla extract
- 3 medium bananas, peeled and mashed
- ½ cup raisins, chopped finely

DIRECTIONS

1. In a large bowl, mix together the flour, baking soda, cinnamon, and salt.
2. In another bowl, beat well eggs and oil.
3. Add the sugar, vanilla extract, and bananas and beat until well combined.
4. Add the flour mixture and stir until just combined.
5. Place the mixture into a lightly greased baking pan and sprinkle with raisins.
6. With a piece of foil, cover the pan loosely.
7. Preheat the Air Fryer at 300°F.
8. Arrange the pan in Air Fryer basket and insert in the oven. Cook for 30 minutes.
9. After 30 minutes of cooking, set the temperature to 285°F for 10 minutes
10. Place the pan onto a wire rack to cool for about 10 minutes
11. Carefully, invert the bread onto wire rack to cool completely before slicing.
12. Cut the bread into desired-sized slices and serve.

Nutrition: *Calories 448 Fat 20.2 Carbs 63.9g Protein 6.1g*

116. 3-INGREDIENTS BANANA BREAD

PREPARATION: 10 MIN **COOKING:** 20 MIN **SERVINGS:** 6

INGREDIENTS

- 2 (6.4-oz.) banana muffin mix
- 1 cup water
- 1 ripe banana, peeled and mashed

DIRECTIONS

1. In a bowl, add all the ingredients and with a whisk, mix until well combined.
2. Place the mixture into a lightly greased loaf pan.
3. Preheat the Air Fryer at 360°F.
4. Arrange the pan in Air Fryer basket and insert in the oven. Cook for 20 minutes.
5. Place the pan onto a wire rack to cool for about 10 minutes
6. Carefully, invert the bread onto wire rack to cool completely before slicing.
7. Cut the bread into desired-sized slices and serve.

Nutrition: *Calories 144 Fat 3.8g Carbs 25.5g Protein 1.9g*

117. YOGURT BANANA BREAD

PREPARATION: 15 MIN **COOKING:** 28 MIN **SERVINGS:** 5

INGREDIENTS

- 1 medium very ripe banana, peeled and mashed
- 1 large egg
- 1 tbsp. canola oil
- 1 tbsp. plain Greek yogurt
- ¼ tsp. pure vanilla extract
- ½ cup all-purpose flour
- ¼ cup granulated white sugar
- ¼ tsp. ground cinnamon
- ¼ tsp. baking soda
- 1/8 tsp. sea salt

DIRECTIONS

1. In a bowl, add the mashed banana, egg, oil, yogurt and vanilla and beat until well combined.
2. Add the flour, sugar, baking soda, cinnamon and salt and mix until just combined.
3. Place the mixture into a lightly greased mini loaf pan.
4. Preheat the Air Fryer at 350°F.
5. Arrange the pan in Air Fryer basket and insert in the oven. Cook for 28 minutes.
6. Place the pan onto a wire rack to cool for about 10 minutes
7. Carefully, invert the bread onto wire rack to cool completely before slicing.
8. Cut the bread into desired-sized slices and serve.

Nutrition: *Calories 145 Fat 4g Carbs 25g Protein 3g*

118. SOUR CREAM BANANA BREAD

PREPARATION: 15 MIN **COOKING:** 37 MIN **SERVINGS:** 8

INGREDIENTS

- ¾ cup all-purpose flour
- ¼ tsp. baking soda
- ¼ tsp. salt
- 2 ripe bananas, peeled and mashed
- ½ cup granulated sugar
- ¼ cup sour cream
- ¼ cup vegetable oil
- 1 large egg
- ½ tsp. pure vanilla extract

DIRECTIONS

1. In a large bowl, mix together the flour, baking soda and salt.
2. In another bowl, add the bananas, egg, sugar, sour cream, oil and vanilla and beat until well combined.
3. Add the flour mixture and mix until just combined.
4. Preheat the Air Fryer at 310°F.
5. Arrange the pan in Air Fryer basket and insert in the oven. Cook for 37 minutes.
6. Place the pan onto a wire rack to cool for about 10 minutes
7. Carefully, invert the bread onto wire rack to cool completely before slicing.
8. Cut the bread into desired-sized slices and serve.

Nutrition: *Calories 201 Fat 9.2g Carbs 28.6g Protein 2.6g*

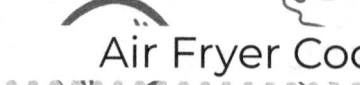
Air Fryer Cookbook

119. PEANUT BUTTER BANANA BREAD

PREPARATION: 15 MIN **COOKING:** 40 MIN **SERVINGS:** 6

INGREDIENTS

- 1 cup plus 1 tbsp. all-purpose flour
- ¼ tsp. baking soda
- 1 tsp. baking powder
- ¼ tsp. salt
- 1 large egg
- 1/3 cup granulated sugar
- ¼ cup canola oil
- 2 tbsp. creamy peanut butter
- 2 tbsp. sour cream
- 1 tsp. vanilla extract
- 2 medium ripe bananas, peeled and mashed
- ¾ cup walnuts, roughly chopped

DIRECTIONS

1. In a bowl and mix the flour, baking powder, baking soda, and salt together.
2. In another large bowl, add the egg, sugar, oil, peanut butter, sour cream, and vanilla extract and beat until well combined.
3. Add the bananas and beat until well combined. Add the flour mixture and mix until just combined.
4. Gently, fold in the walnuts. Place the mixture into a lightly greased pan.
5. Preheat the Air Fryer at 330°F.
6. Arrange the pan in Air Fryer basket and insert in the oven. Cook for 40 minutes.
7. Place the pan onto a wire rack to cool for about 10 minutes
8. Carefully, invert the bread onto wire rack to cool completely before slicing.
9. Cut the bread into desired-sized slices and serve.

Nutrition: Calories 384 Fat 23g Carbs 39.3g Protein 8.9g

120. CHOCOLATE BANANA BREAD

PREPARATION: 15 MIN **COOKING:** 20 MIN **SERVINGS:** 8

INGREDIENTS

- 2 cups flour
- ½ tsp. baking soda
- ½ tsp. baking powder
- ½ tsp. salt
- ¾ cup sugar
- 1/3 cup butter, softened
- 3 eggs
- 1 tbsp. vanilla extract
- 1 cup milk
- ½ cup bananas, peeled and mashed
- 1 cup chocolate chips

DIRECTIONS

1. In a bowl, mix together the flour, baking soda, baking powder, and salt.
2. In another large bowl, add the butter, and sugar and beat until light and fluffy.
3. Add the eggs, and vanilla extract and whisk until well combined.
4. Add the flour mixture and mix until well combined.
5. Add the milk, and mashed bananas and mix well.
6. Gently, fold in the chocolate chips. Place the mixture into a lightly greased loaf pan.
7. Preheat the Air Fryer at 360°F.
8. Arrange the pan in Air Fryer basket and insert in the oven. Cook for 20 minutes.
9. Place the pan onto a wire rack to cool for about 10 minutes Carefully, invert the bread onto wire rack to cool completely before slicing.
10. Cut the bread into desired-sized slices and serve.

Nutrition: Calories 416 Fat 16.5g Carbs 59.2g Protein 8.1g

121. ALLSPICE CHICKEN WINGS

PREPARATION: 0 MIN **COOKING:** 45 MIN **SERVINGS:** 8

INGREDIENTS

- ½ tsp. celery salt
- ½ tsp. bay leaf powder
- ½ tsp. ground black pepper
- ½ tsp. paprika
- ¼ tsp. dry mustard
- ¼ tsp. cayenne pepper
- ¼ tsp. allspice
- 2 lb. chicken wings

DIRECTIONS

1. Grease the Air Fryer basket and preheat to 340°F. In a bowl, mix celery salt, bay leaf powder, black pepper, paprika, dry mustard, cayenne pepper, and allspice. Coat the wings thoroughly in this mixture.
2. Arrange the wings in an even layer in the basket of the Air Fryer. Cook the chicken until it's no longer pinks around the bone, for 30 minutes then, increase the temperature to 380°F and cook for 6 minutes more, until crispy on the outside.

Nutrition: *Calories 332 Fat 10.1g Carbs 31.3g Protein 12g*

122. FRIDAY NIGHT PINEAPPLE STICKY RIBS

PREPARATION: 10 MIN **COOKING:** 20 MIN **SERVINGS:** 4

INGREDIENTS

- 2 lb. cut spareribs
- 7 oz salad dressing
- 1 (5-oz) can pineapple juice
- 2 cups water
- Garlic salt to taste
- Salt and black pepper

DIRECTIONS

1. Sprinkle the ribs with salt and pepper, and place them in a saucepan. Pour water and cook the ribs for 12 minutes on high heat.
2. Dry out the ribs and arrange them in the fryer; sprinkle with garlic salt. Cook it for 15minutes at 390°F.
3. Prepare the sauce by combining the salad dressing and the pineapple juice. Serve the ribs drizzled with the sauce.

Nutrition: *Calories 316 Fat 3.1g Carbs 1.9g Protein 5g*

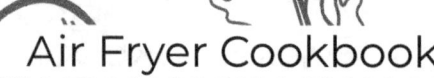

123. EGG ROLL WRAPPED WITH CABBAGE AND PRAWNS

PREPARATION: 10 MIN   **COOKING:** 40 MIN   **SERVINGS:** 4

INGREDIENTS

- 2 tbsp. vegetable oil
- 1-inch piece fresh ginger, grated
- 1 tbsp. minced garlic
- 1 carrot, cut into strips
- ¼ cup chicken broth
- 2 tbsp. reduced-sodium soy sauce
- 1 tbsp. sugar
- 1 cup shredded Napa cabbage
- 1 tbsp. sesame oil
- 8 cooked prawns, minced
- 1 egg
- 8 egg roll wrappers

DIRECTIONS

1. In a skillet over high heat, heat vegetable oil, and cook ginger and garlic for 40 seconds, until fragrant. Stir in carrot and cook for another 2 minutes. Pour in chicken broth, soy sauce, and sugar and bring to a boil.
2. Add cabbage and let simmer until softened, for 4 minutes. Remove skillet from the heat and stir in sesame oil. Let cool for 15 minutes. Strain cabbage mixture, and fold in minced prawns. Whisk an egg in a small bowl. Fill each egg roll wrapper with prawn mixture, arranging the mixture just below the center of the wrapper.
3. Fold the bottom part over the filling and tuck under. Fold in both sides and tightly roll up. Use the whisked egg to seal the wrapper. Repeat until all egg rolls are ready. Place the rolls into a greased Air Fryer basket, spray them with oil and cook for 12 minutes at 370°F, turning once halfway through.

Nutrition: *Calories 215 Fat 7.9g Carbs 6.7g Protein 8g*

124. SESAME GARLIC CHICKEN WINGS

PREPARATION: 10 MIN   **COOKING:** 40 MIN   **SERVINGS:** 4

INGREDIENTS

- 1-lb. chicken wings
- 1 cup soy sauce, divided
- ½ cup brown sugar
- ½ cup apple cider vinegar
- 2 tbsp. fresh ginger, minced
- 2 tbsp. fresh garlic, minced
- 1 tsp. finely ground black pepper
- 2 tbsp. cornstarch
- 2 tbsp. cold water
- 1 tsp. sesame seeds

DIRECTIONS

1. In a bowl, add chicken wings, and pour in half cup soy sauce. Refrigerate for 20 minutes; Dry out and pat dry. Arrange the wings in the Air Fryer and cook for 30 minutes at 380°F, turning once halfway through. Make sure you check them towards the end to avoid overcooking.
2. In a skillet and over medium heat, stir sugar, half cup soy sauce, vinegar, ginger, garlic, and black pepper. Cook until sauce has reduced slightly, about 4 to 6 minutes
3. Dissolve 2 tbsp. of cornstarch in cold water, in a bowl, and stir in the slurry into the sauce, until it thickens, for 2 minutes. Pour the sauce over wings and sprinkle with sesame seeds.

Nutrition: *Calories 413 Fat 8.3g Carbs 7g Protein 8.3g*

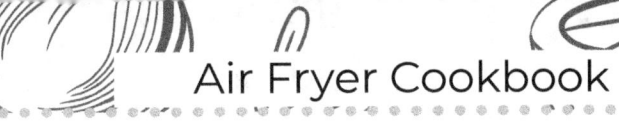

125. SAVORY CHICKEN NUGGETS WITH PARMESAN CHEESE

PREPARATION: 5 MIN **COOKING:** 20 MIN **SERVINGS:** 4

INGREDIENTS

- 1 lb. chicken breast, boneless, skinless, cubed
- ½ tsp. ground black pepper
- ¼ tsp. kosher salt
- ¼ tsp. seasoned salt
- 2 tbsp. olive oil
- 5 tbsp. plain breadcrumbs
- 2 tbsp. panko breadcrumbs
- 2 tbsp. grated Parmesan cheese

DIRECTIONS

1. Preheat the Air Fryer to 380°F and grease. Season the chicken with pepper, kosher salt, and seasoned salt; set aside. In a bowl, pour olive oil. In a separate bowl, add crumb, and Parmesan cheese.
2. Place the chicken pieces in the oil to coat, then dip into breadcrumb mixture, and transfer to the Air Fryer. Work in batches if needed. Lightly spray chicken with cooking spray.
3. Cook the chicken for 10 minutes, flipping once halfway through. Cook until golden brown on the outside and no pinker on the inside.

Nutrition: *Calories 312 Fat 8.9g Carbs 7g Protein 10g*

126. BUTTERNUT SQUASH WITH THYME

PREPARATION: 5 MIN **COOKING:** 20 MIN **SERVINGS:** 4

INGREDIENTS

- 2 cups peeled, butternut squash, cubed
- 1 tbsp. olive oil
- ¼ tsp. salt
- ¼ tsp. black pepper
- ¼ tsp. dried thyme
- 1 tbsp. finely chopped fresh parsley

DIRECTIONS

1. In a bowl, add squash, oil, salt, pepper, and thyme, and toss until squash is well-coated.
2. Place squash in the Air Fryer and cook for 14 minutes at 360°F.
3. When ready, sprinkle with freshly chopped parsley and serve chilled.

Nutrition: *Calories 219 Fat 4.3g Carbs 9.4g Protein 7.8*

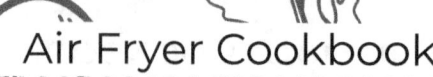 Air Fryer Cookbook

127. CHICKEN BREASTS IN GOLDEN CRUMB

PREPARATION: 10 MIN **COOKING** 25 MIN **SERVINGS:** 4

INGREDIENTS

- 1 ½ lb. chicken breasts, boneless, cut into strips
- 1 egg, lightly beaten
- 1 cup seasoned breadcrumbs
- Salt and black pepper to taste
- ½ tsp. dried oregano

DIRECTIONS

1. Preheat the Air Fryer to 390°F. Season the chicken with oregano, salt, and black pepper. In a small bowl, whisk in some salt and pepper to the beaten egg. In a separate bowl, add the crumbs. Dip chicken tenders in the egg wash, then in the crumbs.
2. Roll the strips in the breadcrumbs and press firmly, so the breadcrumbs stick well. Spray the chicken tenders with cooking spray and arrange them in the Air Fryer. Cook for 14 minutes, until no longer pink in the center, and nice and crispy on the outside.

Nutrition: *Calories 223 Fat 3.2g Carbs 4.3 Protein 5g*

128. YOGURT CHICKEN TACOS

PREPARATION: 5 MIN **COOKING:** 20 MIN **SERVINGS:** 4

INGREDIENTS

- 1 cup cooked chicken, shredded
- 1 cup shredded mozzarella cheese
- ¼ cup salsa
- ¼ cup Greek yogurt
- Salt and ground black pepper
- 8 flour tortillas

DIRECTIONS

1. In a bowl, mix chicken, cheese, salsa, and yogurt, and season with salt and pepper. Spray one side of the tortilla with cooking spray. Lay 2 tbsp. of the chicken mixture at the center of the non-oiled side of each tortilla.
2. Roll tightly around the mixture. Arrange taquitos into your Air Fryer basket, without overcrowding. Cook in batches if needed. Place the seam side down, or it will unravel during cooking crisps.
3. Cook it for 12 to 14 minutes, or until crispy, at 380°F.

Nutrition: *Calories 312 Fat 3g Carbs 6.5g Protein 6.2g*

129. FLAWLESS KALE CHIPS

PREPARATION: 5 MIN   **COOKING:** 20 MIN   **SERVINGS:** 4

INGREDIENTS

- 4 cups chopped kale leaves; stems removed
- 2 tbsp. olive oil
- 1 tsp. garlic powder
- ½ tsp. salt
- ¼ tsp. onion powder
- ¼ tsp. black pepper

DIRECTIONS

1. In a bowl, mix kale and oil together, until well-coated. Add in garlic, salt, onion, and pepper and toss until well-coated. Arrange half the kale leaves to Air Fryer, in a single layer.
2. Cook for 8 minutes at 350°F, shaking once halfway through. Remove chips to a sheet to cool; do not touch.

Nutrition: *Calories 312 Fat 5.3g Carbs 5g Protein 7g*

130. VERMICELLI NOODLES & VEGETABLES ROLLS

PREPARATION: 5 MIN   **COOKING:** 25 MIN   **SERVINGS:** 8

INGREDIENTS

- 8 spring roll wrappers
- 1 cup cooked and cooled vermicelli noodles
- 2 garlic cloves, finely chopped
- 1 tbsp. minced fresh ginger
- 2 tbsp. soy sauce
- 1 tsp. sesame oil
- 1 red bell pepper, seeds removed, chopped
- 1 cup finely chopped mushrooms
- 1 cup finely chopped carrot
- ½ cup finely chopped scallions

DIRECTIONS

1. In a saucepan, add garlic, ginger, soy sauce, pepper, mushroom, carrot and scallions, and stir-fry over high heat for a few minutes, until soft. Add in vermicelli noodles; remove from the heat.
2. Place the spring roll wrappers onto a working board. Spoon the dollops of veggie and noodle mixture at the center of each spring roll wrapper. Roll the spring rolls and tuck the corners and edges in to create neat and secure rolls.
3. Spray with oil and transfer them to the Air Fryer. Cook for 12 minutes at 340°F, turning once halfway through. Cook until golden and crispy. Serve with soy or sweet chili sauce.

Nutrition: *Calories 312 Fat 5g Carbs 5.4g Protein 3g*

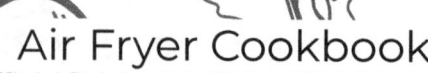
Air Fryer Cookbook

131. CHEESE FISH BALLS

PREPARATION: 5 MIN **COOKING:** 40 MIN **SERVINGS:** 6

INGREDIENTS

- 1 cup smoked fish, flaked
- 2 cups cooked rice
- 2 eggs, lightly beaten
- 1 cup grated Grana Padano cheese
- ¼ cup finely chopped thyme
- Salt and black pepper to taste
- 1 cup panko crumbs

DIRECTIONS

1. In a bowl, add fish, rice, eggs, Parmesan cheese, thyme, salt and pepper into a bowl; stir to combine. Shape the mixture into 12 even-sized balls. Roll the balls in the crumbs then spray with oil.
2. Arrange the balls into the fryer and cook for 16 minutes at 400°F, until crispy.

Nutrition: *Calories 234 Fat 5.2g Carbs 4.3g Protein 6.2g*

132. BEEF BALLS WITH MIXED HERBS

PREPARATION: 5 MIN **COOKING:** 25 MIN **SERVINGS:** 4

INGREDIENTS

- 1 lb. ground beef
- 1 onion, finely chopped
- 3 garlic cloves, finely chopped
- 2 eggs
- 1 cup breadcrumbs
- ½ cup fresh mixed herbs
- 1 tbsp. mustard
- Salt and black pepper to taste
- Olive oil

DIRECTIONS

1. In a bowl, add beef, onion, garlic, eggs, crumbs, herbs, mustard, salt, and pepper and mix with hands to combine.
2. Shape into balls and arrange them in the Air Fryer's basket. Drizzle with oil and cook for 16 minutes at 380°F, turning once halfway through.

Nutrition: *Calories 315 Fat 5g Carbs 9g Protein 8g*

133. ROASTED PUMPKIN SEEDS

PREPARATION: 10 MIN **COOKING:** 40 MIN **SERVINGS:** 4

INGREDIENTS

- 1 cup pumpkin seeds, pulp removed, rinsed
- 1 tbsp. butter, melted
- 1 tbsp. brown sugar
- 1 tsp. orange zest
- ½ tsp. cardamom
- ½ tsp. salt

DIRECTIONS

1. Cook the seeds for 4 minutes at 320°F, in your Air Fryer, to avoid moisture. In a bowl, whisk melted butter, sugar, zest, cardamom and salt.
2. Add the seeds to the bowl and toss to coat thoroughly.
3. Transfer the seeds to the Air Fryer and cook for 35 minutes at 300°F, shaking the basket every 10-12 minutes Cook until lightly browned.

Nutrition: *Calories 536 Fat 13g Carbs 5g Protein 7g*

134. BUTTERY PARMESAN BROCCOLI FLORETS

PREPARATION: 5 MIN   **COOKING:** 20 MIN   **SERVINGS:** 2

INGREDIENTS

- 2 tbsp. butter, melted
- 1 egg white
- 1 garlic clove, grated
- ¼ tsp. salt
- A pinch of black pepper
- ½ lb. broccoli florets
- ⅓ cup grated Parmesan cheese

DIRECTIONS

1. In a bowl, whisk together the butter, egg, garlic, salt, and black pepper.
2. Toss in broccoli to coat well.
3. Top with Parmesan cheese and; toss to coat.
4. Arrange broccoli in a single layer in the Air Fryer, without overcrowding.
5. Cook it in batches for 10 minutes at 360°F.
6. Remove to a serving plate and sprinkle with Parmesan cheese.

Nutrition: *Calories 350 Fat 27g Carbs 20g Protein 15 g*

135. SPICY CHICKPEAS

PREPARATION: 5 MIN   **COOKING:** 10 MIN   **SERVINGS:** 4

INGREDIENTS

- 1 (15-oz.) can chickpeas rinsed and Dry-out
- 1 tbsp. olive oil
- ½ tsp. ground cumin
- ½ tsp. cayenne pepper
- ½ tsp. smoked paprika
- Salt, as required

DIRECTIONS

1. In a bowl, add all the ingredients and toss to coat well.
2. Preheat the Air Fryer at 390°F.
3. Arrange the chickpeas in Air Fryer basket and insert in the Air Fryer. Cook for 10 minutes.
4. Serve warm.

Nutrition: *Calories 146 Fat 4.5g Carbs 18.8g Protein 6.3g*

136. ROASTED PEANUTS

PREPARATION: 5 MIN   **COOKING:** 14 MIN   **SERVINGS:** 6

INGREDIENTS

- 1½ cups raw peanuts
- Nonstick cooking spray

DIRECTIONS

1. Preheat the Air Fryer at 320°F.
2. Arrange the peanuts in Air Fryer basket and insert in the Air Fryer. Cook for 14 minutes.
3. Toss the peanuts twice.
4. After 9 minutes of cooking, spray the peanuts with cooking spray.
5. Serve warm.

Nutrition: *Calories 207 Fat 18g Carbs 5.9g Protein 9.4g*

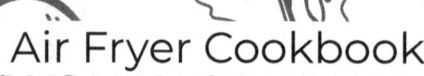
Air Fryer Cookbook

137. ROASTED CASHEWS

PREPARATION: 5 MIN **COOKING:** 5 MIN **SERVINGS:** 6

INGREDIENTS

- 1½ cups raw cashew nuts
- 1 tsp. butter, melted
- Salt and freshly ground black pepper, as needed

DIRECTIONS

1. In a bowl, mix together all the ingredients.
2. Preheat the Air Fryer at 355°F.
3. Arrange the cashew in Air Fryer basket and insert in the Air Fryer. Cook for 5 minutes.
4. Shake the cashews once halfway through.

Nutrition: *Calories 202 Fat 16.5g Carbs 11.2g Protein 5.3g*

138. FRENCH FRIES

PREPARATION: 15 MIN **COOKING:** 30 MIN **SERVINGS:** 4

INGREDIENTS

- 1 lb. potatoes, peeled and cut into strips
- 3 tbsp. olive oil
- ½ tsp. onion powder
- ½ tsp. garlic powder
- 1 tsp. paprika

DIRECTIONS

1. In a large bowl of water, soak the potato strips for about 1 hour.
2. Dry out the potato strips well and pat them dry with the paper towels.
3. In a large bowl, add the potato strips and the remaining ingredients and toss to coat well.
4. Preheat the Air Fryer at 370°F.
5. Arrange the potatoe fries in Air Fryer basket and insert in the Air Fryer. Cook for 30 minutes.
6. Serve warm.

Nutrition: *Calories 172 Fat 10.7g Carbs 18.6g Protein 2.1g*

139. ZUCCHINI FRIES

PREPARATION: 10 MIN **COOKING:** 12 MIN **SERVINGS:** 4

INGREDIENTS

- 1 lb. zucchini, sliced into 2½-inch sticks
- Salt, as required
- 2 tbsp. olive oil
- ¾ cup panko breadcrumbs

DIRECTIONS

1. In a colander, add the zucchini and sprinkle with salt. Set aside for about 10 minutes. Gently pat dry the zucchini sticks with the paper towels and coat with oil.
2. In a shallow dish, add the breadcrumbs. Coat the zucchini sticks with breadcrumbs evenly.
3. Preheat the Air Fryer at 400°F.
4. Arrange the pan in Air Fryer basket and insert in the oven. Cook for 12 minutes.
5. Serve warm.

Nutrition: *Calories 151 Fat 8.6g Carbs 6.9g Protein 1.9g*

140. SPICY CARROT FRIES

PREPARATION: 10 MIN **COOKING:** 12 MIN **SERVINGS:** 2

INGREDIENTS

- 1 large carrot, peeled and cut into sticks
- 1 tbsp. fresh rosemary, chopped finely
- 1 tbsp. olive oil
- ¼ tsp. cayenne pepper
- Salt and ground black pepper, as required

DIRECTIONS

1. In a bowl, add all the ingredients and mix well.
2. Preheat the Air Fryer at 390°F.
3. Arrange the pan in Air Fryer basket and insert in the oven. Cook for 12 minutes.
4. Serve warm.

Nutrition: *Calories 81 Fat 8.3g Carbs 4.7g Protein 0.4g*

141. CINNAMON CARROT FRIES

PREPARATION: 10 MIN **COOKING:** 12 MIN **SERVINGS:** 6

INGREDIENTS

- 1 lb. carrots, peeled and cut into sticks
- 1 tsp. maple syrup
- 1 tsp. olive oil
- ½ tsp. ground cinnamon
- Salt, to taste

DIRECTIONS

1. In a bowl, add all the ingredients and mix well.
2. Preheat the Air Fryer at 400°F.
3. Arrange the pan in Air Fryer basket and insert in the oven. Cook for 12 minutes.
4. Serve warm.

Nutrition: *Calories 41 Fat 0.8g Carbs 8.3g Protein 0.6g*

142. SQUASH FRIES

PREPARATION: 10 MIN **COOKING:** 35 MIN **SERVINGS:** 2

INGREDIENTS

- 14 oz. butternut squash, peeled, seeded and cut into strips
- 2 tsp.s olive oil
- ½ tsp. ground cinnamon
- ½ tsp. red chili powder
- ¼ tsp. garlic salt
- Salt and freshly ground black pepper, as needed

DIRECTIONS

1. In a bowl, add all the ingredients and toss to coat well.
2. Preheat the Air Fryer at 400°F.
3. Arrange the pan in Air Fryer basket and insert in the oven. Cook for 30 minutes.
4. Serve warm.

Nutrition: *Calories 134 Fat 5g Carbs 24.3g Protein 2.1g*

Air Fryer Cookbook

143. AVOCADO FRIES

PREPARATION: 15 MIN   **COOKING:** 7 MIN   **SERVINGS:** 2

INGREDIENTS

- ¼ cup all-purpose flour
- Salt and freshly ground black pepper, as needed
- 1 egg 1 tsp. water
- ½ cup panko breadcrumbs
- 1 avocado, peeled, pitted and sliced into 8 pieces
- Non-stick cooking spray

DIRECTIONS

1. In a shallow bowl, mix together the flour, salt, and black pepper.
2. In a second bowl, mix well egg and water.
3. In a third bowl, put the breadcrumbs.
4. Coat the avocado slices with flour mixture, then dip into egg mixture and finally, coat evenly with the breadcrumbs.
5. Now, spray the avocado slices evenly with cooking spray.
6. Preheat the Air Fryer at 400°F.
7. Arrange the pan in Air Fryer basket and insert in the oven. Cook for 7 minutes.
8. Serve warm.

Nutrition: *Calories 340 Fat 14g Carbs 30g Protein 23g*

144. DILL PICKLE FRIES

PREPARATION: 15 MIN   **COOKING:** 15 MIN   **SERVINGS:** 8

INGREDIENTS

- 1 (16-oz.) jar spicy dill pickle spears Dry out and pat dried
- ¾ cup all-purpose flour
- ½ tsp. paprika
- 1 egg, beaten
- ¼ cup milk
- 1 cup panko breadcrumbs
- Nonstick cooking spray

DIRECTIONS

1. In a shallow dish, mix together the flour, and paprika.
2. In a second dish, place the milk and egg and mix well.
3. In a third dish, put the breadcrumbs.
4. Coat the pickle spears with flour mixture, then dip into egg mixture and finally, coat evenly with the breadcrumbs.
5. Now, spray the pickle spears evenly with cooking spray.
6. Preheat the Air Fryer at 400°F.
7. Arrange the pan in Air Fryer basket and insert in the oven. Cook for 15 minutes.
8. Serve warm.
9. Flip the fries once halfway through.
10. Serve warm.

Nutrition: *Calories 110 Fat 1.9g Carbs 12.8g Protein 2.7g*

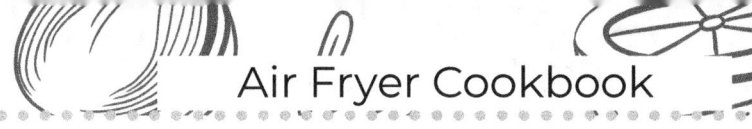

145. MOZZARELLA STICKS

PREPARATION: 15 MIN **COOKING:** 12 MIN **SERVINGS:** 3

INGREDIENTS

- ¼ cup white flour
- 2 eggs
- 3 tbsp. nonfat milk
- 1 cup plain breadcrumbs
- 1 lb. Mozzarella cheese block cut into 3x½-inch sticks

DIRECTIONS

1. In a shallow dish, add the flour.
2. In a second shallow dish, mix together the eggs, and milk.
3. In a third shallow dish, place the breadcrumbs.
4. Coat the Mozzarella sticks with flour, then dip into egg mixture and finally, coat evenly with the breadcrumbs.
5. Preheat the Air Fryer at 400°F.
6. Arrange the pan in Air Fryer basket and insert in the oven. Cook for 12 minutes.
7. Serve warm

Nutrition: *Calories 254 Fat 6.6g Carbs 35.2g Protein 12.8g*

146. TORTILLA CHIPS

PREPARATION: 10 MIN **COOKING:** 3 MIN **SERVINGS:** 3

INGREDIENTS

- 4 corn tortillas cut into triangles
- 1 tbsp. olive oil
- Salt, to taste

DIRECTIONS

1. Coat the tortilla chips with oi and then, sprinkle each side of the tortillas with salt.
2. Preheat the Air Fryer at 390°F.
3. Arrange the pan in Air Fryer basket and insert in the oven. Cook for 3 minutes.
4. Serve warm.

Nutrition: *Calories 110 Fat 5.6g Carbs 14.3g Protein 1.8g*

SIDE DISHES

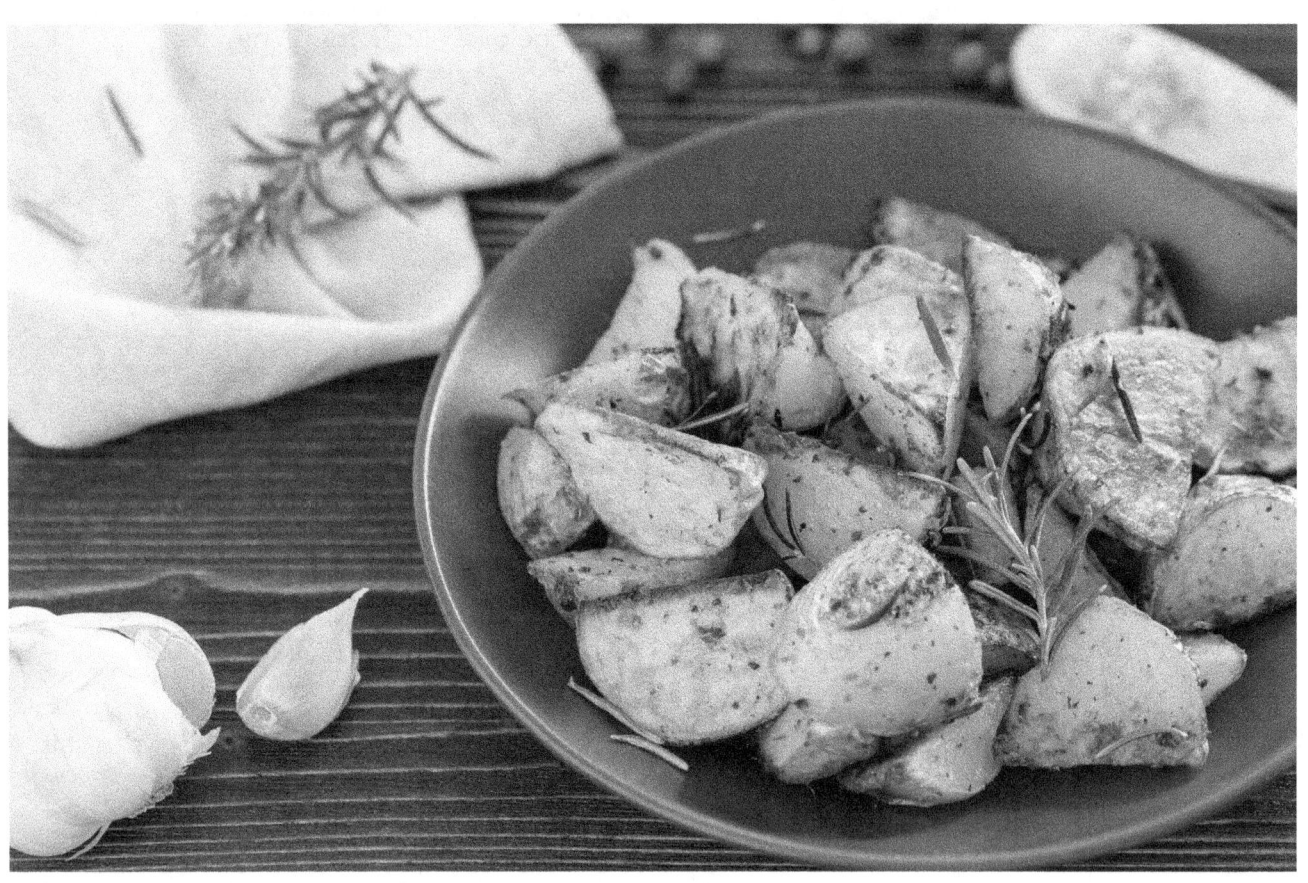

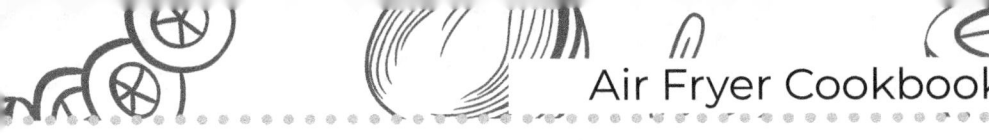

147. SKY-HIGH ROASTED CORN

PREPARATION: 5 MIN   **COOKING:** 10 MIN   **SERVINGS:** 4

INGREDIENTS

- 4 ears of husk-less corn
- 1 tbsp. of olive oil
- 1 tsp. of salt
- 1 tsp. of black pepper

DIRECTIONS

1. Heat up your Air Fryer to 400°F.
2. Sprinkle the ears of corn with the olive oil, salt and black pepper.
3. Place it inside your Air Fryer and cook it for 10 minutes at 400°F.
4. Serve and enjoy!

Nutrition: *Calories 100 Fat 1g Carbs 22g Protein 3g*

148. RAVISHING AIR-FRIED CARROTS WITH HONEY GLAZE

PREPARATION: 5 MIN   **COOKING:** 10 MIN   **SERVINGS:** 1

INGREDIENTS

- 3 cups of chopped into ½-inch pieces carrots
- 1 tbsp. of olive oil
- 2 tbsp. of honey
- 1 tbsp. of brown sugar
- salt and black pepper

DIRECTIONS

1. Heat up your Air Fryer to 390°F.
2. Using a bowl, add and toss the carrot pieces, olive oil, honey, brown sugar, salt, and the black pepper until it is properly covered.
3. Place it inside your Air Fryer and add the seasoned glazed carrots.
4. Cook it for 12 minutes at a 390°F, and then shake after 6 minutes. Serve and enjoy!

Nutrition: *Calories 90 Fat 3.5g Carbs 13g Protein 1g*

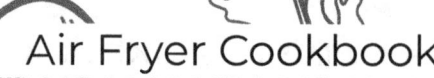

149. FLAMING BUFFALO CAULIFLOWER BITES

PREPARATION: 5 MIN **COOKING:** 20 MIN **SERVINGS:** 4

INGREDIENTS

- 1 large chopped into florets cauliflower head
- 3 beaten eggs
- 2/3 cup of cornstarch
- 2 tbsp. of melted butter
- ¼ cup of hot sauce

DIRECTIONS

1. Heat up your Air Fryer to 360°F.
2. Using a large mixing bowl, add and mix the eggs and the cornstarch properly.
3. Add the cauliflower, gently toss it until it is properly covered with the batter, shake it off in case of any excess batter and set it aside.
4. Grease your Air Fryer basket with a nonstick cooking spray and add the cauliflower bites which will require you to work in batches.
5. Cook the cauliflower bites for 15 to 20 minutes or until it has a golden-brown color and a crispy texture, while still shaking occasionally.
6. Then, using a small mixing bowl, add and mix the melted butter and hot sauce properly.
7. Once the cauliflower bites are done, remove it from your Air Fryer and place it into a large bowl. Pour the buffalo sauce over the cauliflower bites and toss it until it is properly covered.
8. Serve and enjoy!

Nutrition: *Calories 240 Fat 5.5g Carbs 37g Protein 8.8g*

150. PLEASANT AIR-FRIED EGGPLANT

PREPARATION: 5 MIN **COOKING:** 20 MIN **SERVINGS:** 4

INGREDIENTS

- 2 thinly sliced or chopped into chunks eggplants
- 1 tsp. of salt
- 1 tsp. of black pepper
- 1 cup of rice flour
- 1 cup of white wine

DIRECTIONS

1. Using a bowl, add the rice flour, white wine and mix properly until it gets smooth.
2. Add the salt, black pepper and stir again.
3. Dredge the eggplant slices or chunks into the batter and remove any excess batter.
4. Heat up your Air Fryer to 390°F.
5. Grease your Air Fryer basket with a nonstick cooking spray.
6. Add the eggplant slices or chunks into your Air Fryer and cook it for 15 to 20 minutes or until it has a golden brown and crispy texture, while still shaking it occasionally.
7. Carefully remove it from your Air Fryer and allow it to cool off. Serve and enjoy!

Nutrition: *Calories 380 Fat 15g Carbs 51g Protein 13g*

151. CAULIFLOWER HASH

PREPARATION: 10 MIN **COOKING:** 15 MIN **SERVINGS:** 6

INGREDIENTS

- 9 oz. asparagus
- 1 tsp. almond flour
- 1 tbsp. almond flakes
- ¼ tsp. salt
- 1 tsp. olive oil

DIRECTIONS

1. Combine the almond flour and almond flakes; stir the mixture well.
2. Sprinkle the asparagus with the olive oil and salt.
3. Shake it gently and coat in the almond flour mixture.
4. Place the asparagus in the Air Fryer basket and cook at 400°F for 5 minutes, stirring halfway through.
5. Then cool a little and serve.

Nutrition: *Calories 143 Fat 11g Carbs 8.6g Protein 6.4g*

152. ASPARAGUS WITH ALMONDS

PREPARATION: 10 MIN **COOKING:** 5 MIN **SERVINGS:** 2

INGREDIENTS

- 1 cup egg whites
- 1/4 cup mushrooms; chopped
- 2 tbsp. chives; chopped
- 1/4 cup tomato; chopped
- 2 tbsp. skim milk
- Salt and black pepper to the taste

DIRECTIONS

1. In a bowl, mix egg whites with tomato, milk, mushrooms, chives, salt and pepper;
2. Whisk well and pour into your Air Fryer's pan. Cook at 320°F, for 15 minutes;
3. Cool omelet down, slice, divide among plates and serve.

Nutrition: *Calories 100 Fat 3g Carbs 7g Carbs 4g*

Air Fryer Cookbook

153. ZUCCHINI CUBES

PREPARATION: 7 MIN   **COOKING:** 8 MIN   **SERVINGS:** 2

INGREDIENTS

- 1 zucchini
- ½ tsp. ground black pepper
- 1 tsp. oregano
- 2 tbsp. chicken stock
- ½ tsp. coconut oil

DIRECTIONS

1. Chop the zucchini into cubes.
2. Combine the ground black pepper, and oregano; stir the mixture.
3. Sprinkle the zucchini cubes with the spice mixture and stir well.
4. After this, sprinkle the vegetables with the chicken stock.
5. Place the coconut oil in the Air Fryer basket and preheat it to 360°F for 20 seconds.
6. Then add the zucchini cubes and cook the vegetables for 8 minutes at 390°F, stirring halfway through.
7. Transfer to serving plates and enjoy!

Nutrition: *Calories 30 Fat 1.5g Carbs 4.3g Protein 1.4g*

154. SWEET POTATO & ONION MIX

PREPARATION: 10 MIN   **COOKING:** 15 MIN   **SERVINGS:** 4

INGREDIENTS

- 2 sweet potatoes, peeled
- 1 red onion, peeled
- 1 white onion, peeled
- 1 tsp. olive oil
- ¼ cup almond milk

DIRECTIONS

1. Chop the sweet potatoes and the onions into cubes.
2. Sprinkle the sweet potatoes with olive oil.
3. Place the sweet potatoes in the Air Fryer basket and cook for 5 minutes at 400°F.
4. Then stir the sweet potatoes and add the chopped onions.
5. Pour in the almond milk and stir gently.
6. Cook the mix for 10 minutes more at 400°F.
7. When the mix is cooked, let it cool a little and serve.

Nutrition: *Calories 56 Fat 4.8g Carbs 3.5g Protein 0.6g*

155. SPICY EGGPLANT CUBES

PREPARATION: 10 MIN   **COOKING:** 20 MIN   **SERVINGS:** 2

INGREDIENTS

- 12 oz. eggplants
- ½ tsp. cayenne pepper
- ½ tsp. ground black pepper
- ½ tsp. cilantro
- ½ tsp. ground paprika

Nutrition: *Calories 67 Fat 2.8g Carbs 10.9g Protein 1.9g*

DIRECTIONS

1. Rinse the eggplants and slice them into cubes.
2. Sprinkle the eggplant cubes with the cayenne pepper and ground black pepper.
3. Add the cilantro and ground paprika.
4. Stir the mixture well and let it rest for 10 minutes.
5. After this, sprinkle the eggplants with olive oil and place in the Air Fryer basket.
6. Cook the eggplants for 20 minutes at 380°F, stirring halfway through.
7. When the eggplant cubes are done, serve them right away!

156. ROASTED GARLIC HEAD

PREPARATION: 5 MIN   **COOKING:** 10 MIN   **SERVINGS:** 4

INGREDIENTS

- 1-lb. garlic head
- 1 tbsp. olive oil
- 1 tsp. thyme

Nutrition: *Calories 200 Fat 4.1g Carbs 37.7g Protein 7.2g*

DIRECTIONS

1. Cut the ends of the garlic head and place it in the Air Fryer basket.
2. Then sprinkle the garlic head with the olive oil and thyme.
3. Cook the garlic head for 10 minutes at 400°F.
4. When the garlic head is cooked, it should be soft and aromatic.
5. Serve immediately.

157. WRAPPED ASPARAGUS

PREPARATION: 10 MIN   **COOKING:** 5 MIN   **SERVINGS:** 4

INGREDIENTS

- 12 oz. asparagus
- ½ tsp. ground black pepper
- 3 oz. turkey fillet, sliced
- ¼ tsp. chili flakes

Nutrition: *Calories 133 Fat 9g Carbs 3.8g Protein 9.8g*

DIRECTIONS

1. Sprinkle the asparagus with the ground black pepper and chili flakes.
2. Stir carefully.
3. Wrap the asparagus in the sliced turkey fillet and place in the Air Fryer basket.
4. Cook the asparagus at 400°F for 5 minutes, turning halfway through cooking.
5. Let the wrapped asparagus cool for 2 minutes before serving.

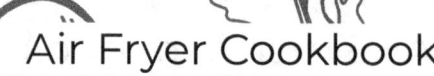
Air Fryer Cookbook

158. BAKED YAMS WITH DILL

PREPARATION: 10 MIN   **COOKING:** 8 MIN   **SERVINGS:** 2

INGREDIENTS

- 2 yams
- 1 tbsp. fresh dill
- 1 tsp. coconut oil
- ½ tsp. minced garlic

Nutrition: Calories 25 Fat 2.3g Carbs 1.2g Protein 0.4g

DIRECTIONS

1. Wash the yams carefully and cut them into halves.
2. Sprinkle the yam halves with the coconut oil and then rub with the minced garlic.
3. Place the yams in the Air Fryer basket and cook for 8 minutes at 400°F.
4. After this, mash the yams gently with a fork and then sprinkle with the fresh dill.
5. Serve the yams immediately.

159. HONEY ONIONS

PREPARATION: 10 MIN   **COOKING:** 20 MIN   **SERVINGS:** 2

INGREDIENTS

- 2 large white onions
- 1 tbsp. raw honey
- 1 tsp. water
- 1 tbsp. paprika

Nutrition: Calories 102 Fat 0.6g Carbs 24.6g Protein 2.2g

DIRECTIONS

1. Peel the onions and using a knife, make cuts in the shape of a cross.
2. Then combine the raw honey and water; stir.
3. Add the paprika and stir the mixture until smooth.
4. Place the onions in the Air Fryer basket and sprinkle them with the honey mixture.
5. Cook the onions for 16 minutes at 380°F.
6. When the onions are cooked, they should be soft.
7. Transfer the cooked onions to serving plates and serve.

160. DELIGHTFUL ROASTED GARLIC SLICES

PREPARATION: 10 MIN   **COOKING:** 8 MIN   **SERVINGS:** 4

INGREDIENTS

- 1 tsp. coconut oil
- ½ tsp. dried cilantro
- ¼ tsp. cayenne pepper
- 12 oz. garlic cloves, peeled

Nutrition: Calories 137 Fat 1.6g Carbs 28.2g Protein 5.4g

DIRECTIONS

1. Sprinkle the garlic cloves with the cayenne pepper and dried cilantro.
2. Mix the garlic up with the spices, and then transfer to the Air Fryer basket.
3. Add the coconut oil and cook the garlic for 8 minutes at 400°F, stirring halfway through.
4. When the garlic cloves are done, transfer them to serving plates and serve.

161. COCONUT OIL ARTICHOKES

PREPARATION: 10 MIN **COOKING:** 13 MIN **SERVINGS:** 4

INGREDIENTS

- 1 lb. artichokes
- 1 tbsp. coconut oil
- 1 tbsp. water
- ½ tsp. minced garlic
- ¼ tsp. cayenne pepper

Nutrition: Calories 83 Fat 3.6g Carbs 12.1g Protein 3.7g

DIRECTIONS

1. Trim the ends of the artichokes, sprinkle them with the water, and rub them with the minced garlic.
2. Sprinkle with the cayenne pepper and the coconut oil.
3. After this, wrap the artichokes in foil and place in the Air Fryer basket.
4. Cook for 10 minutes at 370°F.
5. Then remove the artichokes from the foil and cook them for 3 minutes more at 400°F.
6. Transfer the cooked artichokes to serving plates and allow to cool a little. Serve!

162. ROASTED MUSHROOMS

PREPARATION: 10 MIN **COOKING:** 5 MIN **SERVINGS:** 2

INGREDIENTS

- 12 oz. mushroom hats
- ¼ cup fresh dill, chopped
- ¼ tsp. onion, chopped
- 1 tsp. olive oil
- ¼ tsp. turmeric

Nutrition: Calories 73 Fat 3.1g Carbs 9.2g Protein 6.6g

DIRECTIONS

1. Combine the chopped dill and onion.
2. Add the turmeric and stir the mixture.
3. After this, add the olive oil and mix until homogenous.
4. Then fill the mushroom hats with the dill mixture and place them in the Air Fryer basket.
5. Cook the mushrooms for 5 minutes at 400°F.
6. When the vegetables are cooked, let them cool to room temperature before serving.

163. MASHED YAMS

PREPARATION: 10 MIN **COOKING:** 10 MIN **SERVINGS:** 5

INGREDIENTS

- 1 lb. yams
- 1 tsp. olive oil
- 1 tbsp. almond milk
- ¾ tsp. salt
- 1 tsp. dried parsley

Nutrition: Calories 120 Fat 1.8g Carbs 25.1g Protein 1.4g

DIRECTIONS

1. Peel the yams and chop.
2. Place the chopped yams in the Air Fryer basket and sprinkle with the salt and dried parsley.
3. Add the olive oil and stir the mixture.
4. Cook the yams at 400°F for 10 minutes, stirring twice during cooking.
5. When the yams are done, blend them well with a hand blender until smooth.
6. Add the almond milk and stir carefully.
7. Serve, and enjoy!

164. CAULIFLOWER RICE

PREPARATION: 10 MIN   **COOKING:** 12 MIN   **SERVINGS:** 4

INGREDIENTS

- 14 oz. cauliflower heads
- 1 tbsp. coconut oil
- 2 tbsp. fresh parsley, chopped

DIRECTIONS

1. Wash the cauliflower heads carefully and chop them into small pieces of rice.
2. Place the cauliflower in the Air Fryer and add coconut oil.
3. Stir carefully and cook for 10 minutes at 370°F.
4. Then add the fresh parsley and stir well.
5. Cook the cauliflower rice for 2 minutes more at 400°F.
6. After this, gently toss the cauliflower rice and serve immediately.

Nutrition: *Calories 55 Fat 3.5g Carbs 5.4g Protein 2g*

165. SHREDDED CABBAGE

PREPARATION: 15 MIN   **COOKING:** 15 MIN   **SERVINGS:** 4

INGREDIENTS

- 15 oz. cabbage
- ¼ tsp. salt
- ¼ cup chicken stock
- ½ tsp. paprika

DIRECTIONS

1. Shred the cabbage and sprinkle it with the salt and paprika.
2. Stir the cabbage and let it sit for 10 minutes.
3. Then transfer the cabbage to the Air Fryer basket and add the chicken stock.
4. Cook the cabbage for 15 minutes at 250°F, stirring halfway through.
5. When the cabbage is soft, it is done. Serve immediately, while still hot

Nutrition: *Calories 132 Fat 2.1g Carbs 32.1g Protein 1.78g*

166. FRIED LEEKS RECIPE

PREPARATION: 5 MIN   **COOKING:** 10 MIN   **SERVINGS:** 4

INGREDIENTS

- 4 leeks; ends cut off and halved
- 1 tbsp. butter; melted
- 1 tbsp. lemon juice
- Salt and black pepper to the taste

DIRECTIONS

1. Coat leeks with melted butter, flavor with salt and pepper, put in your Air Fryer and cook at 350°F, for 7 minutes.
2. Arrange on a platter, drizzle lemon juice all over and serve

Nutrition: *Calories 100 Fat 4g Carbs 6g Protein 2g*

167. BRUSSELS SPROUTS AND TOMATOES MIX RECIPE

PREPARATION: 5 MIN   **COOKING:** 10 MIN   **SERVINGS:** 4

INGREDIENTS

- 1 lb. Brussels sprouts; trimmed
- 6 cherry tomatoes; halved
- 1/4 cup green onions; chopped.
- 1 tbsp. olive oil
- Salt and black pepper to the taste

DIRECTIONS

1. Season Brussels sprouts with salt and pepper, put them in your Air Fryer and cook at 350°F, for 10 minutes
2. Transfer them to a bowl, add salt, pepper, cherry tomatoes, green onions and olive oil, toss well and serve.

Nutrition: *Calories 121 Fat 4g Carbs 11g Protein 4g*

168. RADISH HASH RECIPE

PREPARATION: 5 MIN   **COOKING:** 15 MIN   **SERVINGS:** 4

INGREDIENTS

- 1/2 tsp. onion powder
- 1/3 cup parmesan; grated
- 4 eggs
- 1 lb. radishes; sliced
- Salt and black pepper to the taste

DIRECTIONS

1. In a bowl; mix radishes with salt, pepper, onion, eggs and parmesan and stir well
2. Transfer radishes to a pan that fits your Air Fryer and cook at 350°F, for 7 minutes
3. Divide hash on plates and serve.

Nutrition: *Calories 80 Fat 5g Carbs 5g Protein 7g*

169. BROCCOLI SALAD RECIPE

PREPARATION: 5 MIN   **COOKING:** 20 MIN   **SERVINGS:** 4

INGREDIENTS

- 1 broccoli head; florets separated
- 1 tbsp. Chinese rice wine vinegar
- 1 tbsp. peanut oil
- 6 garlic cloves; minced
- Salt and black pepper to the taste

DIRECTIONS

1. In a bowl; mix broccoli with salt, pepper and half of the oil, toss, transfer to your Air Fryer and cook at 350°F, for 8 minutes; shaking the fryer halfway
2. Transfer broccoli to a salad bowl, add the rest of the peanut oil, garlic and rice vinegar, toss really well and serve.

Nutrition: *Calories 121 Fat 3g Carbs 4g Protein 4g*

170. CHILI BROCCOLI

PREPARATION: 5 MIN **COOKING:** 15 MIN **SERVINGS:** 4

INGREDIENTS

- 1-lb. broccoli florets
- 2 tbsp. olive oil
- 2 tbsp. chili sauce
- Juice of 1 lime
- A pinch of salt and black pepper

DIRECTIONS

1. Combine all of the ingredients in a bowl, and toss well.
2. Put the broccoli in your Air Fryer's basket and cook at 400°F for 15 minutes.
3. Divide between plates and serve.

Nutrition: *Calories 173 Fat 6g Carbs 6g Protein 8g*

171. PARMESAN BROCCOLI AND ASPARAGUS

PREPARATION: 5 MIN **COOKING:** 15 MIN **SERVINGS:** 4

INGREDIENTS

- 1 broccoli head, florets separated
- ½ lb. asparagus, trimmed
- Juice of 1 lime
- Salt and black pepper to the taste
- 2 tbsp. olive oil
- 3 tbsp. parmesan, grated

DIRECTIONS

1. In a small bowl, combine the asparagus with the broccoli and all the other ingredients except the parmesan, toss, transfer to your Air Fryer's basket and cook at 400°F for 15 minutes.
2. Divide between plates, sprinkle the parmesan on top and serve.

Nutrition: *Calories 172 Fat 5g Carbs 4g Protein 9g*

172. BUTTER BROCCOLI MIX

PREPARATION: 5 MIN **COOKING:** 15 MIN **SERVINGS:** 4

INGREDIENTS

- 1-lb. broccoli florets
- A pinch of salt and black pepper
- 1 tsp. sweet paprika
- ½ tbsp. butter, melted

DIRECTIONS

1. In a small bowl, combine the broccoli with the rest of the ingredients, and toss.
2. Put the broccoli in your Air Fryer's basket, cook at 350°F for 15 minutes, divide between plates and serve.

Nutrition: *Calories 130 Fat 3g Carbs 4g Protein 8g*

173. BALSAMIC KALE

PREPARATION: 2 MIN **COOKING:** 12 MIN **SERVINGS:** 6

INGREDIENTS

- 2 tbsp. olive oil
- 3 garlic cloves, minced
- 2 and ½ lb. kale leaves
- Salt and black pepper to the taste
- 2 tbsp. balsamic vinegar

DIRECTIONS

1. In a pan that fits the Air Fryer, combine all the ingredients and toss.
2. Put the pan in your Air Fryer and cook at 300°F for 12 minutes.
3. Divide between plates and serve.

Nutrition: *Calories 122 Fat 4g Carbs 4g Protein 5g*

174. KALE AND OLIVES

PREPARATION: 5 MIN **COOKING:** 15 MIN **SERVINGS:** 4

INGREDIENTS

- 1 an ½ lb. kale, torn
- 2 tbsp. olive oil
- Salt and black pepper to the taste
- 1 tbsp. hot paprika
- 2 tbsp. black olives, pitted and sliced

DIRECTIONS

1. In a pan that fits the Air Fryer, combine all the ingredients and toss.
2. Put the pan in your Air Fryer, cook at 370°F for 15 minutes, divide between plates and serve.

Nutrition: *Calories 154 Fat 3g Carbs 4g Protein 6g*

175. KALE AND MUSHROOMS MIX

PREPARATION: 5 MIN **COOKING:** 15 MIN **SERVINGS:** 4

INGREDIENTS

- 1 lb. brown mushrooms, sliced
- 1-lb. kale, torn
- Salt and black pepper to the taste
- 2 tbsp. olive oil
- 14 oz. coconut milk

DIRECTIONS

1. In a pot that fits your Air Fryer, mix the kale with the rest of the ingredients and toss.
2. Put the pan in the fryer, cook at 380°F for 15 minutes, divide between plates and serve.

Nutrition: *Calories 162 Fat 4g Carbs 3g Protein 5g*

176. OREGANO KALE

PREPARATION: 5 MIN   **COOKING:** 10 MIN   **SERVINGS:** 4

INGREDIENTS

- 1-lb. kale, torn
- 1 tbsp. olive oil
- A pinch of salt and black pepper
- 2 tbsp. oregano, chopped

DIRECTIONS

1. In a pan that fits the Air Fryer, combine all the ingredients and toss.
2. Put the pan in the Air Fryer and cook at 380°F for 10 minutes.
3. Divide between plates and serve.

Nutrition: *Calories 140 Fat 3g Carbs 3g Protein 5g*

177. KALE AND BRUSSELS SPROUTS

PREPARATION: 5 MIN   **COOKING:** 15 MIN   **SERVINGS:** 8

INGREDIENTS

- 1-lb. Brussels sprouts, trimmed
- 2 cups kale, torn
- 1 tbsp. olive oil
- Salt and black pepper to the taste
- 3 oz. mozzarella, shredded

DIRECTIONS

1. In a pan that fits the Air Fryer, combine all the ingredients except the mozzarella and toss.
2. Put the pan in the Air Fryer and cook at 380°F for 15 minutes.
3. Divide between plates, sprinkle the cheese on top and serve.

Nutrition: *Calories 170 Fat 5g Carbs 4g Protein 7g*

178. SPICY OLIVES AND AVOCADO MIX

PREPARATION: 5 MIN   **COOKING:** 15 MIN   **SERVINGS:** 4

INGREDIENTS

- 2 cups kalamata olives, pitted
- 2 small avocados, pitted, peeled and sliced
- ¼ cup cherry tomatoes, halved
- Juice of 1 lime
- 1 tbsp. coconut oil, melted

DIRECTIONS

1. In a pan that fits the Air Fryer, combine the olives with the other ingredients, toss, put the pan in your Air Fryer and cook at 370°F for 15 minutes.
2. Divide the mix between plates and serve.

Nutrition: *Calories 153 Fat 3g Carbs 4g Protein 6g*

179. OLIVES, GREEN BEANS AND BACON

PREPARATION: 5 MIN   **COOKING:** 15 MIN   **SERVINGS:** 4

INGREDIENTS

- ½ lb. green beans, trimmed and halved
- 1 cup black olives, pitted and halved
- ¼ cup bacon, cooked and crumbled
- 1 tbsp. olive oil
- ¼ cup tomato sauce

DIRECTIONS

1. In a pan that fits the Air Fryer, combine all the ingredients, toss, put the pan in the Air Fryer and cook at 380°F for 15 minutes.
2. Divide between plates and serve.

Nutrition: *Calories 160 Fat 4g Carbs 5g Protein 4g*

180. CAJUN OLIVES AND PEPPERS

PREPARATION: 4 MIN   **COOKING:** 12 MIN   **SERVINGS:** 4

INGREDIENTS

- 1 tbsp. olive oil
- ½ lb. mixed bell peppers, sliced
- 1 cup black olives, pitted and halved
- ½ tbsp. Cajun seasoning

DIRECTIONS

1. In a pan that fits the Air Fryer, combine all the ingredients.
2. Put the pan it in your Air Fryer and cook at 390°F for 12 minutes.
3. Divide the mix between plates and serve.

Nutrition: *Calories 151 Fat 3g Carbs 4g Protein 5g*

181. CRISP KALE

PREPARATION: 5 MIN   **COOKING:** 8 MIN   **SERVINGS:** -

INGREDIENTS

- •4 Handfuls Kale, Washed & Stemless
- •1 Tbsp. Olive Oil
- •Pinch Sea Salt

DIRECTIONS

1. Start by heating it to 360°F, and then combine your ingredients together making sure your kale is coated evenly.
2. Place the kale in your fryer and cook for eight minutes.

Nutrition: *Calories 121 Fat 4g Carbs 5g Protein 8g*

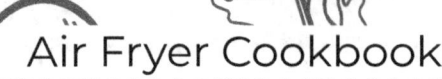

182. IMPLE BASIL POTATOES

PREPARATION: 15 MIN **COOKING:** 40 MIN **SERVINGS:** -

INGREDIENTS

- 18 Medium Potatoes
- 5 Tbsp. Olive Oil
- 4 Tsp.s Basil, Dried
- 1 ½ Tsp.s Garlic Powder
- Salt & Pepper to Taste
- Oz. Butter

DIRECTIONS

1. Turn on your Air Fryer to 390°F.
2. Cut your potatoes lengthwise, and make sure to cut them thin.
3. Lightly coat your potatoes with both your butter and oil.
4. Add in salt and pepper, and then cook for 40 minutes.

Nutrition: *Calories 140 Fat 5g Carbs 8g Protein 9g*

183. SWEET POTATO FRIES

PREPARATION: 10 MIN **COOKING:** 12-15 MIN **SERVINGS:** -

INGREDIENTS

- 3 Large Sweet Potatoes, Peeled
- 1 Tbsp. Olive Oil
- A Pinch Tsp. Sea Salt

DIRECTIONS

1. Turn on your Air Fryer to 390°F.
2. Start by cutting your sweet potatoes in quarters, cutting them lengthwise to make fries.
3. Combine the uncooked fries with a tbsp. of sea salt and olive oil. Make sure all of your fries are coated well.
4. Place your sweet potato pieces in your basket, cooking for 12 minutes.
5. Cook for two to three minutes more if you want it to be crispier.
6. Add more salt to taste, and serve when cooled.

Nutrition: *Calories 150 Fat 6g Carbs 8g Protein 9g*

184. CRISP & SPICY CABBAGE

PREPARATION: 5 MIN **COOKING:** 10 MIN **SERVINGS:** -

INGREDIENTS

- 1/2 Head White Cabbage, Chopped & Washed
- 1 Tbsp. Coconut Oil, Melted
- ¼ Tsp. Cayenne Pepper
- ¼ Tsp. Chili Powder
- ¼ Tsp. Garlic Powder

DIRECTIONS

1. Turn on your Air Fryer to 390°F.
2. Mix your cabbage, spices and coconut oil together in a bowl, making sure your cabbage is coated well.
3. Place it in the fryer and cook for ten minutes.

Nutrition: *Calories 100 Fat 2g Carbs 3g Protein 5g*

185. ROSEMARY POTATOES

PREPARATION: 5 MIN **COOKING:** 12-15 MIN **SERVINGS:** -

INGREDIENTS

- Three Large Red Potatoes, Cubed & Not Peeled
- 1 Tbsp. of Olive Oil
- Pinch Sea Salt
- ½ Tsp. Rosemary, Dried

DIRECTIONS

1. Start by preheating your fryer to 390°F.
2. Combine your potatoes with olive oil, salt and rosemary. Make sure your potatoes are coated properly.
3. Cook for 12 minutes, and then check them. If you'd like them to be crispier than you can cook them for another two to three minutes.
4. You can serve them on their own or with sour cream.

Nutrition: *Calories 150 Fat 5g Carbs 9g Protein 9g*

186. SIMPLE GARLIC POTATOES

PREPARATION: 10 MIN **COOKING:** 15 MIN **SERVINGS:** -

INGREDIENTS

- 3 Baking Potatoes, Large
- 2 Tbsp. Olive Oil
- 2 Tbsp. Garlic, Minced
- 1 Tbsp. Salt
- ½ Tbsp. Onion Powder

DIRECTIONS

1. Turn on your Air Fryer to 390°F.
2. Create holes in your potato, and then sprinkle it with oil and salt.
3. Mix your garlic and onion powder together, and then rub it on the potatoes evenly.
4. Put it into your Air Fryer basket, and then bake for thirty-five to forty minutes.

Nutrition: *Calories 160 Fat 6g Carbs 9g Protein 9g*

187. CRISPY BRUSSELS SPROUTS

PREPARATION: 5 MIN **COOKING:** 10 MIN **SERVINGS:** 2

INGREDIENTS

- ½ lb. brussels sprouts, cut in half
- ½ tbsp. oil
- ½ tbsp. unsalted butter, melted

DIRECTIONS

1. Rub sprouts with oil.
2. Place into the Air Fryer basket. Cook at 400°F for 10 minutes. Stir once at the halfway mark.
3. Remove the Air Fryer basket and drizzle with melted butter. Serve.

Nutrition: *Calories 90 Fat 6.1g Carb: 4g Protein 2.9g*

188. FLATBREAD

PREPARATION: 5 MIN   **COOKING:** 7 MIN   **SERVINGS:** 2

INGREDIENTS

- 1 cup shredded mozzarella cheese
- ¼ cup almond flour
- 1 oz. full-fat cream cheese softened

DIRECTIONS

1. Melt mozzarella in the microwave for 30 seconds. Stir in almond flour until smooth.
2. Add cream cheese. Continue mixing until dough forms. Knead with wet hands if necessary.
3. Divide the dough into two pieces and roll out to ¼-inch thickness between two pieces of parchment.
4. Cover the Air Fryer basket with parchment and place the flatbreads into the Air Fryer basket. Work in batches if necessary.
5. Cook at 320°F for 7 minutes. Flip once at the halfway mark.
6. Serve.

Nutrition: *Calories 296 Fat 22.6g Carb: 3.3g Protein 16.3g*

189. CREAMY CABBAGE

PREPARATION: 10 MIN   **COOKING:** 20 MIN   **SERVINGS:** 2

INGREDIENTS

- ½ green cabbage head, chopped
- ½ yellow onion, chopped
- Salt and black pepper, to taste
- ½ cup whipped cream
- 1 tbsp. cornstarch

DIRECTIONS

1. Put cabbage and onion in the Air Fryer.
2. In a bowl, mix cornstarch with cream, salt, and pepper. Stir and pour over cabbage.
3. Toss and cook at 400°F for 20 minutes.
4. Serve.

Nutrition: *Calories 208 Fat 10g Carb: 16g Protein 5g*

190. VEGETABLE EGG ROLLS

PREPARATION: 15 MIN **COOKING:** 10 MIN **SERVINGS:** 8

INGREDIENTS

- ½ cup chopped mushrooms
- ½ cup grated carrots
- ½ cup chopped zucchini
- green onions, chopped
- tbsp. low-sodium soy sauce
- egg roll wrappers
- 1 tbsp. cornstarch
- 1 egg, beaten

DIRECTIONS

1. In a medium bowl, combine the mushrooms, carrots, zucchini, green onions, and soy sauce, and stir together.
2. Place the egg roll wrappers on a work surface. Top each with about 3 tbsp. of the vegetable mixture.
3. In a small bowl, combine the cornstarch and egg and mix well. Brush some of this mixture on the edges of the egg roll wrappers. Roll up the wrappers, enclosing the vegetable filling. Brush some of the egg mixture on the outside of the egg rolls to seal.
4. Air fry at 380°F for 7 to 10 minutes or until the egg rolls are brown and crunchy.

Nutrition: *Calories 112 Fat 1g Carbs 21g Protein 4g*

191. VEGGIES ON TOAST

PREPARATION: 12 MIN **COOKING:** 11 MIN **SERVINGS:** 4

INGREDIENTS

- 1 red bell pepper, cut into ½-inch strips
- 1 cup sliced button or cremini mushrooms
- 1 small yellow squash, sliced
- green onions, cut into ½-inch slices
- Extra light olive oil for misting
- to 6 pieces sliced French or Italian bread
- tbsp. softened butter
- ½ cup soft goat cheese

DIRECTIONS

1. Combine the red pepper, mushrooms, squash, and green onions in the Air Fryer and mist with oil. Roast at 375°F for 7 to 9 minutes or until the vegetables are tender, shaking the basket once during cooking time.
2. Remove the vegetables from the basket and set aside.
3. Spread the bread with butter and place in the Air Fryer, butter-side up. Toast for 2 to 4 minutes or until golden brown.
4. Spread the goat cheese on the toasted bread and top with the vegetables; serve warm.
5. Variation tip: To add even more flavor, drizzle the finished toasts with extra-virgin olive oil and balsamic vinegar.

Nutrition: *Calories 162 Fat 11g Carbs 9g Protein 7g*

192. JUMBO STUFFED MUSHROOMS

PREPARATION: 10 MIN **COOKING:** 20 MIN **SERVINGS:** 4

INGREDIENTS

- Jumbo portobello mushrooms
- 1 tbsp. olive oil
- ¼ cup ricotta cheese
- tbsp. Parmesan cheese, divided
- 1 cup frozen chopped spinach, thawed and drained
- ⅓ cup bread crumbs
- ¼ tsp. minced fresh rosemary

DIRECTIONS

1. Wipe the mushrooms with a damp cloth. Remove the stems and discard. Using a spoon, gently scrape out most of the gills.
2. Rub the mushrooms with the olive oil. Put in the Air Fryer basket, hollow side up, and bake for 3 minutes. Carefully remove the mushroom caps, because they will contain liquid. Drain the liquid out of the caps.
3. In a medium bowl, combine the ricotta, 3 tbsp. of Parmesan cheese, spinach, bread crumbs, and rosemary, and mix well.
4. Stuff this mixture into the drained mushroom caps. Sprinkle with the remaining 2 tbsp. of Parmesan cheese. Put the mushroom caps back into the basket.
5. Bake at 375°F for 4 to 6 minutes or until the filling is hot and the mushroom caps are tender.

Nutrition: *Calories 117 Fat 7g Carbs 8g Protein 7g*

193. MUSHROOM PITA PIZZAS

PREPARATION: 10 MIN **COOKING:** 5 MIN **SERVINGS:** 4

INGREDIENTS

- (3-inch) pitas
- 1 tbsp. olive oil
- ¾ cup pizza sauce
- 1 (4 oz.) jar sliced mushrooms, drained
- ½ tsp. dried basil
- green onions, minced
- 1 cup grated mozzarella or provolone cheese
- 1 cup sliced grape tomatoes

DIRECTIONS

1. Brush each piece of pita with oil and top with the pizza sauce.
2. Add the mushrooms and sprinkle with basil and green onions. Top with the grated cheese.
3. Bake 370°F for 3 to 6 minutes or until the cheese is melted and starts to brown. Top with the grape tomatoes and serve immediately.

Nutrition: *Calories 231 Fat 9g Carbs 25g Protein 13g*

194. SPINACH QUICHE

PREPARATION: 10 MIN **COOKING:** 20 MIN **SERVINGS:** 3

INGREDIENTS

- Eggs
- 1 cup frozen chopped spinach, thawed and drained
- ⅓ cup heavy cream
- Tbsp. honey mustard
- ½ cup grated Swiss or Havarti cheese
- ½ tsp. dried thyme
- Pinch of salt
- Freshly ground black pepper
- Nonstick baking spray with flour

DIRECTIONS

1. In a medium bowl, beat the eggs until blended. Stir in the spinach, cream, honey mustard, cheese, thyme, salt, and pepper.
2. Spray a 6-by-6-by-2-inch pan baking pan with nonstick spray. Pour the egg mixture into the pan.
3. Bake at 360°F for 18 to 22 minutes or until the egg mixture is puffed, light golden brown, and set.
4. Let cool for 5 minutes, then cut into wedges to serve.

Nutrition: *Calories 203 Fat 15g Carbs 6g Protein 11g*

195. YELLOW SQUASH FRITTERS

PREPARATION: 15 MIN **COOKING:** 7 MIN **SERVINGS:** 4

INGREDIENTS

- 1 (3 oz.) package cream cheese, softened
- 1 egg, beaten
- ½ tsp. dried oregano
- Pinch of salt
- Freshly ground black pepper
- 1 medium yellow summer squash, grated
- ⅓ cup grated carrot
- ⅔ cup bread crumbs
- tbsp. olive oil

DIRECTIONS

1. In a medium bowl, combine the cream cheese, egg, oregano, and salt and pepper. Add the squash and carrot, and mix well. Stir in the breadcrumbs.
2. Form about 2 tbsp. of this mixture into a patty about ½ inch thick. Repeat with remaining mixture. Brush the fritters with olive oil.
3. Air-fry at 390°F until crisp and golden, about 7 to 9 minutes.

Nutrition: *Calories 234 Fat 17g Carbs 16g Protein 6g*

196. PESTO GNOCCHI

PREPARATION: 5 MIN **COOKING:** 20 MIN **SERVINGS:** 4

INGREDIENTS

- 1 tbsp. olive oil
- 1 onion, finely chopped
- cloves garlic, sliced
- 1 (16 oz.) package shelf-stable gnocchi
- 1 (8 oz.) jar pesto
- ⅓ cup grated Parmesan cheese

DIRECTIONS

1. Combine the oil, onion, garlic, and gnocchi in a 6-by-6-by-2-inch pan and put into the Air Fryer.
2. Bake at 365°F for 10 minutes, then remove the pan and stir.
3. Return the pan to the Air Fryer and cook for 8 to 13 minutes or until the gnocchi are lightly browned and crisp.
4. Remove the pan from the Air Fryer. Stir in the pesto and Parmesan cheese, and serve immediately.

Nutrition: *Calories 646 Fat 32g Carbs 69g Protein 22g*

197. ENGLISH MUFFIN TUNA SANDWICHES

PREPARATION: 8 MIN **COOKING:** 5 MIN **SERVINGS:** 4

INGREDIENTS

- 1 (6 oz.) can chunk light tuna, drained
- ¼ cup mayonnaise
- tbsp. mustard
- 1 tbsp. lemon juice
- green onions, minced
- English muffins, split with a fork
- tbsp. softened butter
- thin slices provolone or Muenster cheese

DIRECTIONS

1. In a small bowl, combine the tuna, mayonnaise, mustard, lemon juice, and green onions.
2. Butter the cut side of the English muffins. Grill butter-side up in the Air Fryer at 375°F for 2 to 4 minutes or until light golden brown. Remove the muffins from the Air Fryer basket.
3. Top each muffin with one slice of cheese and return to the Air Fryer. Grill for 2 to 4 minutes or until the cheese melts and starts to brown.
4. Remove the muffins from the Air Fryer, top with the tuna mixture, and serve.

Nutrition: *Calories 389 Fat 23g Carbs 25g Protein 21g*

198. TUNA ZUCCHINI MELTS

PREPARATION: 15 MIN **COOKING:** 10 MIN **SERVINGS:** 4

INGREDIENTS

- Corn tortillas
- Tbsp. softened butter
- 1 (6 oz.) can chunk light tuna, drained
- 1 cup shredded zucchini, drained by squeezing in a kitchen towel
- ⅓ cup mayonnaise
- Tbsp. mustard
- 1 cup shredded Cheddar or Colby cheese

DIRECTIONS

1. Spread the tortillas with the softened butter. Place in the Air Fryer basket and grill at 350°F for 2 to 3 minutes or until the tortillas are crisp. Remove from basket and set aside.
2. In a medium bowl, combine the tuna, zucchini, mayonnaise, and mustard, and mix well.
3. Divide the tuna mixture among the toasted tortillas. Top each with some of the shredded cheese.
4. Grill in the Air Fryer for 2 to 4 minutes or until the tuna mixture is hot, and the cheese melts and starts to brown. Serve.

Nutrition: *Calories 428 Fat 30g Carbs 19g Protein 22g*

199. SHRIMP AND GRILLED CHEESE SANDWICHES

PREPARATION: 10 MIN **COOKING:** 5 MIN **SERVINGS:** 4

INGREDIENTS

- 1¼ cups shredded Colby, Cheddar, or Havarti cheese
- 1 (6 oz.) can tiny shrimp, drained
- tbsp. mayonnaise
- tbsp. minced green onion
- slices whole grain or whole-wheat bread
- tbsp. softened butter

DIRECTIONS

1. In a medium bowl, combine the cheese, shrimp, mayonnaise, and green onion, and mix well.
2. Spread this mixture on two of the slices of bread. Top with the other slices of bread to make two sandwiches. Spread the sandwiches lightly with butter.
3. Grill in the Air Fryer at 380°F for 5 to 7 minutes or until the bread is browned and crisp and the cheese is melted. Cut in half and serve warm.

Nutrition: *Calories 276 Fat 14g Carbs 16g Protein 22g*

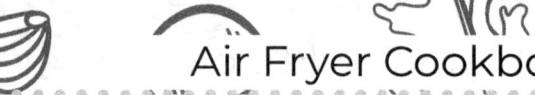

200. SHRIMP CROQUETTES

PREPARATION: 12 MIN   **COOKING:** 8 MIN   **SERVINGS:** 3-4

INGREDIENTS

- ⅔ lb. cooked shrimp, shelled and deveined
- 1½ cups bread crumbs, divided
- 1 egg, beaten
- 1 tbsp. lemon juice
- Green onions, finely chopped
- ½ tsp. dried basil
- Pinch of salt
- Freshly ground black pepper
- 2 tbsp. olive oil

DIRECTIONS

1. Finely chop the shrimp. Take about 1 tbsp. of the finely chopped shrimp and chop it further until it's almost a paste. Set aside.
2. In a medium bowl, combine ½ cup of the bread crumbs with the egg and lemon juice. Let stand for 5 minutes.
3. Stir the shrimp, green onions, basil, salt, and pepper into the bread crumb mixture.
4. Combine the remaining 1 cup of bread crumbs with the olive oil on a shallow plate; mix well.
5. Form the shrimp mixture into 1½-inch round balls and press firmly with your hands. Roll in the bread crumb mixture to coat.
6. Air fry at 380°F the little croquettes in batches for 6 to 8 minutes or until they are brown and crisp. Serve with cocktail sauce for dipping, if desired.

Nutrition: *Calories 330 Fat 12g Carbs 31g Protein 24g*

POULTRY

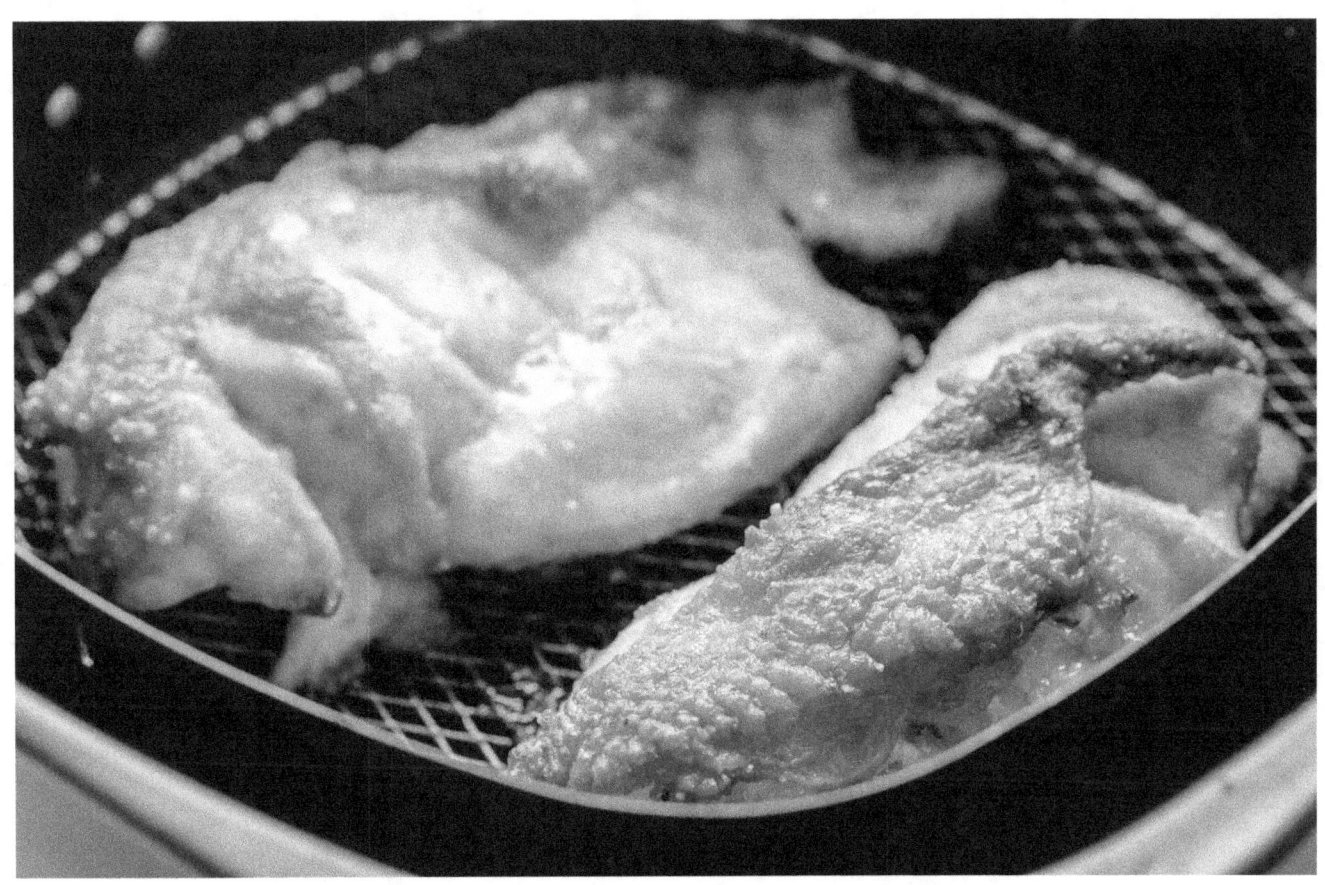

201. TURKEY BREASTS

PREPARATION: 5 MIN **COOKING:** 1 H **SERVINGS:** 4

INGREDIENTS

- 3 lbs. Boneless turkey breast
- ¼ cup Mayonnaise
- 2 tsps. Poultry seasoning
- Salt and pepper to taste
- ½ tsp. Garlic powder

DIRECTIONS

1. Preheat the Air Fryer to 360°F. Season the turkey with mayonnaise, seasoning, salt, garlic powder, and black pepper. Cook the turkey in the Air Fryer for 1 hour at 360°F.
2. Turn after every 15 minutes. The turkey is done when it reaches 165°F.

Nutrition: *Calories 558 Fat 18g Carbs 1g Protein 98g*

202. BBQ CHICKEN BREASTS

PREPARATION: 5 MIN **COOKING:** 15 MIN **SERVINGS:** 4

INGREDIENTS

- 4, about 6 oz. each Boneless, skinless chicken breast
- 2 tbsps. BBQ seasoning
- Cooking spray

DIRECTIONS

1. Rub the chicken with BBQ seasoning and marinate in the refrigerator for 45 minutes. Preheat the Air Fryer at 400°F. Grease the basket with oil and place the chicken.
2. Then spray oil on top. Cook for 13 to 14 minutes, flipping at the halfway mark. Serve.

Nutrition: *Calories 131 Fat 3g Carbs 2g Protein 24g*

203. ROTISSERIE CHICKEN

PREPARATION: 5 MIN **COOKING:** 1 H **SERVINGS:** 4

INGREDIENTS

- 1 Whole chicken, cleaned and patted dry
- 2 tbsps Olive oiL
- 1 tbsp. Seasoned salt

DIRECTIONS

1. Remove the giblet packet from the cavity. Rub the chicken with oil and salt. Place in the Air Fryer basket, breast-side down. Cook at 350°F for 30 minutes.
2. Then flip and cook another 30 minutes. Chicken is done when it reaches 165°F.

Nutrition: *Calories 534 Fat 36g Carbs 0g Protein 35g*

204. HONEY-MUSTARD CHICKEN BREASTS

PREPARATION: 5 MIN **COOKING:** 25 MIN **SERVINGS:** 6

INGREDIENTS

- 6 (6-oz, each) Boneless, skinless chicken breasts
- 2 tbsps. minced Fresh rosemary
- 3 tbsps. honey
- 1 tbsp. dijon mustard
- Salt and pepper to taste

DIRECTIONS

1. Combine the mustard, honey, pepper, rosemary and salt in a bowl. Rub the chicken with this mixture.
2. Grease the Air Fryer basket with oil. Air fry the chicken at 350°F for 20 to 24 minutes or until the chicken reaches 165°F. Serve.

Nutrition: *Calories 236 Fat 5g Carbs 9.8g Protein 38g*

---

205. CHICKEN PARMESAN WINGS

PREPARATION: 5 MIN **COOKING:** 15 MIN **SERVINGS:** 4

INGREDIENTS

- Chicken wings – 2 lbs. cut into drumettes, pat dried
- Parmesan – ½ cup, plus 6 tbsps. grated
- 1 tsp. herbs de Provence
- 1 tsp. paprika
- Salt to taste

DIRECTIONS

1. Combine the parmesan, herbs, paprika, and salt in a bowl and rub the chicken with this mixture. Preheat the Air Fryer at 350°F.
2. Grease the basket with cooking spray. Cook for 15 minutes. Flip once at the halfway mark. Garnish with parmesan and serve.

Nutrition: *Calories 490 Fat 22g Carbs 1g Protein 72g*

---

206. AIR FRYER CHICKEN

PREPARATION: 5 MIN **COOKING:** 30 MIN **SERVINGS:** 4

INGREDIENTS

- 2 lbs. chicken wings
- Salt and pepper to taste
- Cooking spray

DIRECTIONS

1. Flavor the chicken wings with salt and pepper. Grease the Air Fryer basket with cooking spray. Add chicken wings and cook at 400°F for 35 minutes.
2. Flip 3 times during cooking for even cooking. Serve.

Nutrition: *Calories 277 Fat 8g Carbs 1g Protein 50g*

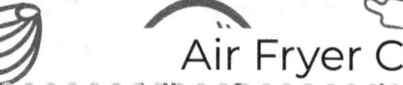
Air Fryer Cookbook

207. WHOLE CHICKEN

PREPARATION: 5 MIN **COOKING:** 40 MIN **SERVINGS:** 6

INGREDIENTS

- Whole chicken – 1 (2 ½ lb.) washed and pat dried
- 2 tbsps. dry rub –
- 1 tsp. salt
- Cooking spray

DIRECTIONS

1. Preheat the Air Fryer at 350°F. Rub the dry rub on the chicken. Then rub with salt. Cook it at 350°F for 45 minutes. After 30 minutes, flip the chicken and finish cooking.
2. Chicken is done when it reaches 165°F.

Nutrition: *Calories 412 Fat 28g Carbs 1g Protein 35g*

208. HONEY DUCK BREASTS

PREPARATION: 5 MIN **COOKING:** 25 MIN **SERVINGS:** 2

INGREDIENTS

- Smoked duck breast – 1, halved
- Honey – 1 tsp.
- Tomato paste – 1 tsp.
- Mustard – 1 tbsp.
- Apple vinegar – ½ tsp.

DIRECTIONS

1. Mix tomato paste, honey, mustard, and vinegar in a bowl. Whisk well. Add duck breast pieces and coat well. Cook in the Air Fryer at 370°F for 15 minutes.
2. Remove the duck breast from the Air Fryer and add to the honey mixture. Coat again. Cook again at 370°F for 6 minutes. Serve.

Nutrition: *Calories 274 Fat 11g Carbs 22g Protein 13g*

209. CREAMY COCONUT CHICKEN

PREPARATION: 5 MIN **COOKING:** 20 MIN **SERVINGS:** 4

INGREDIENTS

- 4 big chicken legs
- Turmeric powder – 5 tsps.
- Ginger – 2 tbsps. grated
- Salt and black pepper to taste
- Coconut cream – 4 tbsps.

DIRECTIONS

1. In a bowl, mix salt, pepper, ginger, turmeric, and cream. Whisk. Add chicken pieces, coat and marinate for 2 hours.
2. Transfer chicken to the preheated Air Fryer and cook at 370°F for 25 minutes. Serve.

Nutrition: *Calories 300 Fat 4g Carbs 22g Protein 20g*

210. BUFFALO CHICKEN TENDERS

PREPARATION: 5 MIN **COOKING:** 20 MIN **SERVINGS:** 4

INGREDIENTS

- 1 lb. boneless, skinless chicken tenders
- ¼ cup Hot sauce
- Pork rinds – 1 ½ oz., finely ground
- Chili powder – 1 tsp.
- Garlic powder – 1 tsp.

DIRECTIONS

1. Put the chicken breasts in a bowl and pour hot sauce over them. Toss to coat. Mix ground pork rinds, chili powder and garlic powder in another bowl.
2. Place each tender in the ground pork rinds, and coat well. With wet hands, press down the pork rinds into the chicken. Place the tender in a single layer into the Air Fryer basket. Cook at 375°F for 20 minutes. Flip once. Serve.

Nutrition: *Calories 160 Fat 4.4g Carbs 0.6g Protein 27.3g*

211. TERIYAKI WINGS

PREPARATION: 5 MIN **COOKING:** 20 MIN **SERVINGS:** 4

INGREDIENTS

- Chicken wings – 2 lb.
- Teriyaki sauce – ½ cup
- Minced garlic – 2 tsp.
- Ground ginger - ¼ tsp.
- Baking powder – 2 tsp.

DIRECTIONS

1. Except for the baking powder, place all ingredients in a bowl and marinate for 1 hour in the refrigerator. Place wings into the Air Fryer basket and sprinkle with baking powder.
2. Gently rub into wings. Cook at 400°F for 25 minutes. Shake the basket two or three times during cooking. Serve.

Nutrition: *Calories 446 Fat 29.8g Carbs 3.1g Protein 41.8g*

212. LEMONY DRUMSTICKS

PREPARATION: 5 MIN **COOKING:** 20 MIN **SERVINGS:** 2

INGREDIENTS

- Baking powder – 2 tsps.
- Garlic powder – ½ tsp.
- Chicken drumsticks – 8
- Salted butter – 4 tbsps. melted
- Lemon pepper seasoning – 1 tbsp.

DIRECTIONS

1. Sprinkle garlic powder and baking powder over drumsticks and rub into chicken skin. Place drumsticks into the Air Fryer basket. Cook at 375°F for 25 minutes. Flip the drumsticks once halfway through the Cooking Time.
2. Remove when cooked. Mix seasoning and butter in a bowl. Add drumsticks to the bowl and toss to coat. Serve.

Nutrition: *Calories 532 Carbs 1.2g Fat 32.3g Protein 48.3g*

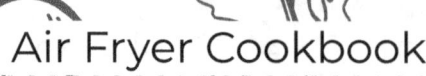

213. PARMESAN CHICKEN TENDERS

PREPARATION: 5 MIN   **COOKING:** 10 MIN   **SERVINGS:** 4

INGREDIENTS

- 1 lb. chicken tenderloins
- 3 large egg whites
- ½ cup Italian-style bread crumbs
- ¼ cup grated Parmesan cheese

DIRECTIONS

1. Spray the Air Fryer basket with olive oil. Trim off any white fat from the chicken tenders. In a bowl, whisk the egg whites until frothy. In a separate small mixing bowl, combine the bread crumbs and Parmesan cheese. Mix well.
2. Dip the chicken tenders into the egg mixture, then into the Parmesan and bread crumbs. Shake off any excess breading. Place the chicken tenders in the greased Air Fryer basket in a single layer. Generously spray the chicken with olive oil to avoid powdery, uncooked breading.
3. Set the temperature of your Air Fryer to 370°F. Set the timer and bake for 4 minutes. Using tongs, flip the chicken tenders and bake for 4 minutes more. Check that the chicken has reached an internal temperature of 165°F. Add Cooking Time if needed. Once the chicken is fully cooked, plate, serve, and enjoy.

Nutrition: Calories 210 Fat 4g Carbs 10g Protein 33g

214 EASY LEMON CHICKEN THIGHS

PREPARATION: 5 MIN   **COOKING:** 10 MIN   **SERVINGS:** 4

INGREDIENTS

- Salt and black pepper to taste
- 2 tbsp. olive oil
- 2 tbsp. Italian seasoning
- 2 tbsp. freshly squeezed lemon juice
- 1 lemon, sliced

DIRECTIONS

1. Place the chicken thighs in a medium mixing bowl and season them with the salt and pepper. Add the olive oil, Italian seasoning, and lemon juice and toss until the chicken thighs are thoroughly coated with oil. Add the sliced lemons. Place the chicken thighs into the Air Fryer basket in a single layer.
2. Set the temperature of your Air Fryer to 350°F. Set the timer and cook for 10 minutes. Using tongs, flip the chicken. Reset the timer and cook for 10 minutes more. Check that the chicken has reached an internal temperature of 165°F. Add Cooking Time if needed. Once the chicken is fully cooked, plate, serve, and enjoy.

Nutrition: Calories 325 Carbs 1g Fat 26g Protein 20g

Air Fryer Cookbook

215. AIR FRYER GRILLED CHICKEN BREASTS

PREPARATION: 5 MIN   **COOKING:** 14 MIN   **SERVINGS:** 4

INGREDIENTS

- ½ tsp. garlic powder
- salt and black pepper to taste
- 1 tsp. dried parsley
- 2 tbsp. olive oil, divided
- 3 boneless, skinless chicken breasts

Nutrition: *Calories 182 Carbs 0g Fat 9g Protein 26g*

DIRECTIONS

1. In a small bowl, combine together the garlic powder, salt, pepper, and parsley. Using 1 tbsp. of olive oil and half of the seasoning mix, rub each chicken breast with oil and seasonings. Place the chicken breast in the Air Fryer basket.
2. Set the temperature of your Air Fryer to 370°F. Set the timer and grill for 7 minutes.
3. Using tongs, flip the chicken and brush the remaining olive oil and spices onto the chicken. Reset the timer and grill for 7 minutes more. Check that the chicken has reached an internal temperature of 165°F. Add Cooking Time if needed.
4. When the chicken is cooked, transfer it to a platter and serve.

216. CRISPY AIR FRYER BUTTER CHICKEN

PREPARATION: 5 MIN   **COOKING:** 15 MIN   **SERVINGS:** 4

INGREDIENTS

- 2 (8 oz.) boneless, skinless chicken breasts
- 1 sleeve Ritz crackers
- 4 tbsp. (½ stick) cold unsalted butter, cut into 1-tbsp. slices

Nutrition: *Calories 750 Fat 40g Carbs 38g Protein 57g*

DIRECTIONS

1. 1. Spray the Air Fryer basket with olive oil, or spray an Air Fryer–size baking sheet with olive oil or cooking spray.
2. 2. Dip the chicken breasts in water. Put the crackers in a resealable plastic bag. Using a mallet or your hands, crush the crackers. Place the chicken breasts inside the bag one at a time and coat them with the cracker crumbs.
3. 3. Place the chicken in the greased Air Fryer basket, or on the greased baking sheet set into the Air Fryer basket. Put 1 to 2 dabs of butter onto each piece of chicken.
4. 4. Set the temperature of your Air Fryer to 370°F. Set the timer and bake for 7 minutes.
5. 5. Using tongs, flip the chicken. Spray the chicken generously with olive oil to avoid uncooked breading. Reset the timer and bake for 7 minutes more.
6. 6. Check that the chicken has reached an internal temperature of 165°F. Add Cooking Time if needed. Using tongs, remove the chicken from the Air Fryer and serve.

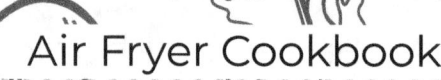

217. LIGHT AND AIRY BREADED CHICKEN BREASTS

PREPARATION: 5 MIN   **COOKING:** 15 MIN   **SERVINGS:** 2

INGREDIENTS

- 2 large eggs
- 1 cup bread crumbs or panko bread crumbs
- 1 tsp. Italian seasoning
- 4 to 5 tbsp. vegetable oil
- 2 boneless, skinless, chicken breasts

Nutrition: *Calories 833 Fat 46g Carbs 40g Protein 65g*

DIRECTIONS

1. Preheat the Air Fryer to 370°F. Spray the Air Fryer basket with olive oil or cooking spray. In a small bowl, whisk the eggs until frothy. In a separate small mixing bowl, mix together the bread crumbs, Italian seasoning, and oil. Dip the chicken in the egg mixture, then in the bread crumb mixture. Place the chicken directly into the greased Air Fryer basket, or on the greased baking sheet set into the basket.
2. Spray the chicken generously and thoroughly with olive oil to avoid powdery, uncooked breading. Set the timer and fry for 7 minutes. Using tongs, flip the chicken and generously spray it with olive oil. Reset the timer and fry for 7 minutes more. Check that the chicken has reached an internal temperature of 165°F. Add Cooking Time if needed. Once the chicken is fully cooked, use tongs to remove it from the Air Fryer and serve.

218. CHICKEN FILLETS, BRIE & HAM

PREPARATION: 5 MIN   **COOKING:** 15 MIN   **SERVINGS:** 4

INGREDIENTS

- 2 Large Chicken Fillets
- Freshly Ground Black Pepper
- 4 Small Slices of Brie (Or your cheese of choice)
- 1 Tbsp. Freshly Chopped Chives
- 4 Slices Cured Ham

Nutrition: *Calories 850 Fat 50g Carbs 43g Protein 76g*

DIRECTIONS

1. Slice the fillets into four and make incisions as you would for a hamburger bun. Leave a little "hinge" uncut at the back. Season the inside and pop some brie and chives in there. Close them, and wrap them each in a slice of ham. Brush with oil and pop them into the basket.
2. Heat your fryer to 350°F. Roast the little parcels until they look tasty (15 min)

219. AIR FRYER CORNISH HEN

PREPARATION: 5 MIN   **COOKING:** 30 MIN   **SERVINGS:** 2

INGREDIENTS

- 2 tbsp. Montreal chicken seasoning
- 1 (1½- to 2-lb.) Cornish hen

Nutrition: *Calories 520 Fat 36g Carbs 0g Protein 45g*

DIRECTIONS

1. Preheat the Air Fryer to 390°F. Rub the seasoning over the chicken, coating it thoroughly.
2. Put the chicken in the basket. Set the timer and roast for 15 minutes.
3. Flip the chicken and cook for another 15 minutes. Check that the chicken has reached an internal temperature of 165°F. Add Cooking Time if needed.

220. AIR FRIED TURKEY WINGS

PREPARATION: 5 MIN **COOKING:** 26 MIN **SERVINGS:** 4

INGREDIENTS

- 2 lb. turkey wings
- 3 tbsp. olive oil or sesame oil
- 3 to 4 tbsp. chicken rub

DIRECTIONS

1. Put the turkey wings in a large mixing bowl. Pour the olive oil into the bowl and add the rub. Using your hands, rub the oil mixture over the turkey wings. Place the turkey wings in the Air Fryer basket.
2. Fix the temperature of your Air Fryer to 380°F. Set the timer and roast for 13 minutes.
3. Using tongs, flip the wings. Reset the timer and roast for 13 minutes more. Remove the turkey wings from the Air Fryer, plate, and serve.

Nutrition: Calories 521 Fat 34g Carbs 4g Protein 52g

221. CHICKEN-FRIED STEAK SUPREME

PREPARATION: 10 MIN **COOKING:** 30 MIN **SERVINGS:** 8

INGREDIENTS

- ½ lb. beef-bottom round, sliced into strips
- 1 cup of breadcrumbs
- 2 medium-sized eggs
- Pinch of salt and pepper
- ½ tbsp. of ground thyme

DIRECTIONS

1. Cover the basket of the Air Fryer with a layer of tin foil, leaving the edges open to allow air to flow through the basket. Preheat the Air Fryer to 350°F. In a bowl, whisk the eggs until fluffy and until the yolks and whites are fully combined, and set aside. In a separate bowl, mix the breadcrumbs, thyme, salt and pepper, and set aside. One by one, dip each piece of raw steak into the bowl with dry ingredients, coating all sides; then submerge into the bowl with wet ingredients, then dip again into the dry ingredients. This double coating will ensure an extra crisp air fry. Lay the coated steak pieces on the foil covering the Air Fryer basket, in a single flat layer.
2. Set the Air Fryer timer for 15 minutes. After 15 minutes, the Air Fryer will turn off and the steak should be mid-way cooked and the breaded coating starting to brown. Using tongs, turn each piece of steak over to ensure a full all-over fry. Reset the Air Fryer to 320°F for 15 minutes. After 15 minutes, when the Air Fryer shuts off, remove the fried steak strips using tongs and set on a serving plate. Eat once cool enough to handle and enjoy.

Nutrition: Calories 421 Fat 26g Carbs 8g Protein 46g

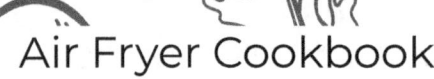

222. CAESAR MARINATED GRILLED CHICKEN

PREPARATION: 10 MIN **COOKING:** 25 MIN **SERVINGS:** 4

INGREDIENTS

- ¼ cup crouton
- 1 tsp. lemon zest. Form into ovals, skewer and grill.
- 1/2 cup Parmesan
- 1/4 cup breadcrumbs
- 1-lb. ground chicken
- 2 tbsp. Caesar dressing and more for drizzling
- 2-4 romaine leaves

DIRECTIONS

1. In a shallow dish, mix well chicken, 2 tbsp. Caesar dressing, parmesan, and breadcrumbs. Mix well with hands. Form into 1-inch oval patties. Thread chicken pieces in skewers. Place on skewer rack in Air Fryer.
2. For 12 minutes, cook on 360°F. Halfway through Cooking Time, turnover skewers. If needed, cook in batches. Serve on a bed of lettuce and sprinkle with croutons and extra dressing.

Nutrition: *Calories 342 Fat 12g Carbs 8g Protein 36g*

223. CHEESY CHICKEN TENDERS

PREPARATION: 10 MIN **COOKING:** 30 MIN **SERVINGS:** 4

INGREDIENTS

- 1 large white meat chicken breast
- 1 cup of breadcrumbs
- 2 medium-sized eggs
- Pinch of salt and pepper
- 1 tbsp. of grated or powdered parmesan cheese

DIRECTIONS

1. Cover the basket of the Air Fryer with a layer of tin foil, leaving the edges open to allow air to flow through the basket. Preheat the Air Fryer to 350°F. In a bowl, whisk the eggs until fluffy and until the yolks and whites are fully combined, and set aside. In a separate bowl, mix the breadcrumbs, parmesan, salt and pepper, and set aside. One by one, dip each piece of raw chicken into the bowl with dry ingredients, coating all sides; then submerge into the bowl with wet ingredients, then dip again into the dry ingredients. Put the coated chicken pieces on the foil covering the Air Fryer basket, in a single flat layer.
2. Set the Air Fryer timer for 15 minutes. After 15 minutes, the Air Fryer will turn off and the chicken should be mid-way cooked and the breaded coating starting to brown. Flip each piece of chicken over to ensure a full all over fry. Reset the Air Fryer to 320°F or another 15 minutes. After 15 minutes, when the Air Fryer shuts off, remove the fried chicken strips using tongs and set on a serving plate. Eat once cool enough to handle, and enjoy.

Nutrition: *Calories 278 Fat 15g Carbs 7g Protein 29g*

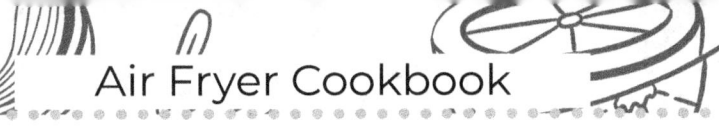

224. MINTY CHICKEN-FRIED PORK CHOPS

PREPARATION: 10 MIN **COOKING:** 30 MIN **SERVINGS:** 4

INGREDIENTS

- 4 medium-sized pork chops
- 1 cup of breadcrumbs
- 2 medium-sized eggs
- Pinch of salt and pepper
- ½ tbsp. of mint, either dried and ground; or fresh, rinsed, and finely chopped

DIRECTIONS

1. Cover the basket of the Air Fryer with a layer of tin foil, leaving the edges open to allow air to flow through the basket. Preheat the Air Fryer to 350°F. In a mixing bowl, whisk the eggs until fluffy and until the yolks and whites are fully combined, and set aside. In a separate bowl, mix the breadcrumbs, mint, salt and pepper, and set aside. One by one, dip each raw pork chop into the bowl with dry ingredients, coating all sides; then submerge into the bowl with wet ingredients, then dip again into the dry ingredients. Lay the coated pork chops on the foil covering the Air Fryer basket, in a single flat layer.
2. Set the Air Fryer timer for 15 minutes. After 15 minutes, the Air Fryer will turn off and the pork should be mid-way cooked and the breaded coating starting to brown. Using tongs, turn each piece of steak over to ensure a full all-over fry. Reset the Air Fryer to 320° for 15 minutes. After 15 minutes remove the fried pork chops using tongs and set on a serving plate.

Nutrition: *Calories 262 Fat 17g Carbs 7g Protein 32g*

225. BACON LOVERS' STUFFED CHICKEN

PREPARATION: 10 MIN **COOKING:** 20 MIN **SERVINGS:** 4

INGREDIENTS

- 4 (5 oz.) boneless, skinless chicken breasts, sliced into ¼ inch thick
- 2 packages Boursin cheese
- 8 slices thin-cut bacon or beef bacon
- Sprig of fresh cilantro, for garnish

DIRECTIONS

1. Spray the Air Fryer basket with avocado oil. Preheat the Air Fryer to 400°F. Put one of the chicken breasts on a cutting board. With a sharp knife held parallel to the cutting board, make a 1-inch-wide incision at the top of the breast. Carefully cut into the breast to form a large pocket, leaving a ½-inch border along the sides and bottom. Repeat with the other 3 chicken breasts. Snip the corner of a large resealable plastic bag to form a ¾-inch hole. Place the Boursin cheese in the bag and pipe the cheese into the pockets in the chicken breasts, dividing the cheese evenly among them. Wrap 2 slices of bacon around each chicken breast and secure the ends with toothpicks.
2. Place the bacon-wrapped chicken in the Air Fryer basket and cook until the bacon is crisp and the chicken's internal temperature reaches 165°F, about 18 to 20 minutes, flipping after 10 minutes. Garnish with a sprig of cilantro before serving, if desired.

Nutrition: *Calories 446 Fat 17g Carbs 13g Protein 36g*

226. AIR FRYER TURKEY BREAST

PREPARATION: 5 MIN   **COOKING:** 60 MIN   **SERVINGS:** 6

INGREDIENTS

- Pepper and salt
- 1 oven-ready turkey breast
- Turkey seasonings of choice

Nutrition: *Calories 212 Fat 12g Carbs 6g Protein 24g*

DIRECTIONS

1. Preheat the Air Fryer to 350°F.
2. Season turkey with pepper, salt, and other desired seasonings.
3. Place turkey in Air Fryer basket.
4. Set temperature to 350°F, and set time to 60 minutes. Cook 60 minutes. The meat should be at 165°F when done. Allow to rest 10-15 minutes before slicing. Enjoy.

227. MUSTARD CHICKEN TENDERS

PREPARATION: 5 MIN   **COOKING:** 20 MIN   **SERVINGS:** 4

INGREDIENTS

- ½ C. coconut flour
- 1 tbsp. spicy brown mustard
- 2 beaten eggs
- 1 lb. of chicken tenders

Nutrition: *Calories 346 Fat 10g Carbs 12g Protein 31g*

DIRECTIONS

1. Season tenders with pepper and salt.
2. Place a thin layer of mustard onto tenders and then dredge in flour and dip in egg.
3. Add to the Air Fryer, set temperature to 390°F, and set time to 20 minutes.

228. CHICKEN MEATBALLS

PREPARATION: 5 MIN   **COOKING:** 15 MIN   **SERVINGS:** 2

INGREDIENTS

- ½ lb. chicken breast
- 1 tbsp. of garlic
- 1 tbsp. of onion
- ½ chicken broth
- 1 tbsp. of oatmeal, whole wheat flour or of your choice

Nutrition: *Calories 45 Fat 1.57g Carbs 1.94g Protein 5.43g*

DIRECTIONS

1. Place all of the ingredients in a food processor and beat well until well mixed and ground.
2. If you don't have a food processor, ask the butcher to grind it and then add the other ingredients, mixing well.
3. Make balls and place them in the Air Fryer basket.
4. Program the Air Fryer for 15 minutes at 400°F.
5. Half the time shake the basket so that the meatballs loosen and fry evenly.

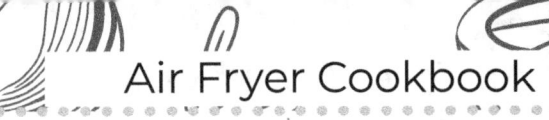

229. HOMEMADE BREADED NUGGET IN DORITOS

PREPARATION: 10 MIN **COOKING:** 15 MIN **SERVINGS:** 4

INGREDIENTS

- ½ lb. boneless, skinless chicken breast
- ¼ lb. Doritos snack
- 1 cup of wheat flour
- 1 egg
- Salt, garlic and black pepper to taste.

DIRECTIONS

1. Cut the chicken breast in the width direction, 1 to 1.5 cm thick, so that it is already shaped like pips.
2. Season with salt, garlic, black pepper to taste and some other seasonings if desired.
3. You can also season with those seasonings or powdered onion soup.
4. Put the Doritos snack in a food processor or blender and beat until everything is crumbled, but don't beat too much, you don't want flour.
5. Now bread, passing the pieces of chicken breast first in the wheat flour, then in the beaten eggs and finally in the Doritos, without leaving the excess flour, eggs or Doritos.
6. Place the seeds in the Air Fryer basket and program for 15 minutes at 400°F, and half the time they brown evenly.

Nutrition: *Calories 42 Fat 1.44g Carbs 1.65g Protein 5.29g*

230. CHICKEN BREAST

PREPARATION: 30 MIN **COOKING:** 25 MIN **SERVINGS:** 6

INGREDIENTS

- 1 lb. diced clean chicken breast
- ½ lemon
- Smoked paprika to taste
- Black pepper or chili powder, to taste
- Salt to taste

DIRECTIONS

1. Flavor the chicken with salt, paprika and pepper and marinate.
2. Store in Air Fryer and turn on for 15 minutes at 350°F.
3. Turn the chicken over and raise the temperature to 200°C, and turn the Air Fryer on for another 5 minutes or until golden.
4. Serve immediately.

Nutrition: *Calories 124 Fat 1.4g Carbs 0g Protein 26.1g*

231. BREADED CHICKEN WITHOUT FLOUR

PREPARATION: 10 MIN   **COOKING:** 15 MIN   **SERVINGS:** 6

INGREDIENTS

- 1 1/6 oz. of grated parmesan cheese
- 1 unit of egg
- 1 lb. of chicken (breast)
- Salt and black pepper to taste

Nutrition: Calories 114 Fat 5.9g Carbs 13g Protein 2.3g

DIRECTIONS

1. Cut the chicken breast into 6 fillets and season with a little salt and pepper.
2. Beat the egg in a bowl.
3. Pass the chicken breast in the egg and then in the grated cheese, sprinkling the fillets.
4. Non-stick and put in the Air Fryer at 400°F for about 30 minutes or until golden brown.

232. BARBECUE WITH CHORIZO AND CHICKEN

PREPARATION: 5 MIN   **COOKING:** 35 MIN   **SERVINGS:** 4

INGREDIENTS

- 4 chicken thighs
- 2 Tuscan sausages
- 4 small onions

Nutrition: Calories 135 Fat 5g Carbs 0g Protein 6g

DIRECTIONS

1. Preheat the fryer to 400°F for 5 minutes. Season the meat the same way you would if you were going to use the barbecue.
2. Put in the fryer, lower the temperature to 320°F and set for 30 minutes.
3. After 20 minutes, check if any of the meat has reached the point of your preference. If so, take whichever is ready and return to the fryer with the others for another 10 minutes, now at 400°F. If not, return them to Air Fryer for the last 10 minutes at 400°F.

233. ROASTED THIGH

PREPARATION: 5 MIN   **COOKING:** 30 MIN   **SERVINGS:** 1

INGREDIENTS

- 3 chicken thighs and thighs
- 2 red seasonal bags
- 1 clove garlic
- ½ tsp. of salt
- 1 pinch of black pepper

Nutrition: Calories 278 Fat 18g Carbs 0.1g Protein 31g

DIRECTIONS

1. Season chicken with red season, minced garlic, salt, and pepper. Leave to act for 5-10 minutes to obtain the flavor.
2. Put the chicken in the basket of the Air Fryer and bake at 390°F for 20 minutes.
3. After that time, remove the Air Fryer basket and check the chicken spot. If it is still raw or not golden enough, turn it over and leave it for another 10 minutes at 350°F.
4. After the previous step, your chicken will be ready on the Air Fryer! Serve with doré potatoes and leaf salad.

234. COXINHA FIT

PREPARATION: 10 MIN **COOKING:** 10-15 MIN **SERVINGS:** 4

INGREDIENTS

- ½ lb. seasoned and minced chicken
- 1 cup light cottage cheese
- 1 egg
- Condiments to taste
- Flaxseed or oatmeal

DIRECTIONS

1. In a bowl, mix all of the ingredients together except flour.
2. Knead well with your hands and mold into coxinha format.
3. If you prefer you can fill it, add chicken or cheese.
4. Repeat the process until all the dough is gone.
5. Pass the drumsticks in the flour and put them in the fryer.
6. Bake for 10 to 15 minutes at 390°F or until golden.

Nutrition: Calories 220 Fat 18g Carbs 40g Protein 100g

235. ROLLED TURKEY BREAST

PREPARATION: 5 MIN **COOKING:** 10 MIN **SERVINGS:** 4

INGREDIENTS

- 1 box of cherry tomatoes
- ¼ lb. turkey blanket

Nutrition: Calories 172 Fat 2g Carbs 3g Protein 34g

DIRECTIONS

1. Wrap the turkey and blanket in the tomatoes, close with the help of toothpicks.
2. Take to Air Fryer for 10 minutes at 390°F.
3. You can increase the filling with ricotta and other preferred light ingredients.

236. CHICKEN IN BEER

PREPARATION: 5 MIN **COOKING:** 10 MIN **SERVINGS:** 4

INGREDIENTS

- 2 ¼ lbs chicken thigh and thigh
- ½ can of beer
- 4 cloves of garlic
- 1 large onion
- Pepper and salt to taste

DIRECTIONS

1. Wash the chicken pieces and, if desired, remove the skin to be healthier.
2. Place on an ovenproof plate.
3. In the blender, beat the other ingredients: beer, onion, garlic, and add salt and pepper, all together.
4. Cover the chicken with this mixture; it has to stay like swimming in the beer.
5. Take to the preheated Air Fryer at 390°F for 45 minutes.
6. It will roast when it has a brown cone on top and the beer has dried a bit.

Nutrition: Calories 674 Fat 41.94g Carbs 5.47g Protein 61.94g

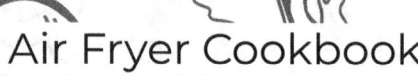

237. CHICKEN FILLET

PREPARATION: 5 MIN   **COOKING:** 10 MIN   **SERVINGS:** 4

INGREDIENTS

- 4 chicken fillets
- salt to taste
- 1 garlic clove, crushed
- thyme to taste
- black pepper to taste

Nutrition: *Calories 90 Fat 1g Carbs 1g Protein 17g*

DIRECTIONS

1. Add seasoning to fillets, wrapping well for flavor. Heat up the Air Fryer for 5 minutes at 350°F. Place the fillets in the basket, program for 20 minutes at 350°F.
2. With 5 minutes remaining, turn the fillets and raise the temperature to 390°F. Serve!

238. CHICKEN WITH LEMON AND BAHIAN SEASONING

PREPARATION: 2 H   **COOKING:** 20 MIN   **SERVINGS:** 4

INGREDIENTS

- 5 pieces of chicken to bird;
- 2 garlic cloves, crushed;
- 4 tbsp. of lemon juice;
- 1 coffee spoon of Bahian spices;
- salt and black pepper to taste.

Nutrition: *Calories 316.2 Fat 15.3g Carbs 4.9g Protein 32.8g*

DIRECTIONS

1. Place the chicken pieces in a covered bowl and add the spices. Add the lemon juice. Cover the container and let the chicken marinate for 2 hours.
2. Place each piece of chicken in the basket of the Air Fryer, without overlapping the pieces. Set the fryer for 20 minutes at 390°F. In half the time, brown evenly. Serve!

239. BASIC BBQ CHICKEN

PREPARATION: 5 MIN   **COOKING:** 20 MIN   **SERVINGS:** 4

INGREDIENTS

- 2 tbsp. Worcestershire Sauce
- 1 tbsp. honey
- ¾ cup ketchup
- 2 tsp.s chipotle chili powder
- 6 chicken drumsticks

Nutrition: *Calories 145 Fat 2.6g Carbs 4.5g Protein 13g*

DIRECTIONS

1. Heat up the Air Fryer to 370°F for 5 minutes.
2. Use a big bowl to mix the Worcestershire sauce, honey, ketchup and chili powder. Whisk it up well.
3. Drop in the drumsticks and turn them so they are all coated with the mixture.
4. Grease the basket of the Air Fryer with nonstick spray and place 3 chicken drumsticks in.
5. Cook for 17 minutes for large drumsticks 15 minutes for smaller ones, flipping when it reaches half the time.
6. Repeat with the other three drumsticks.

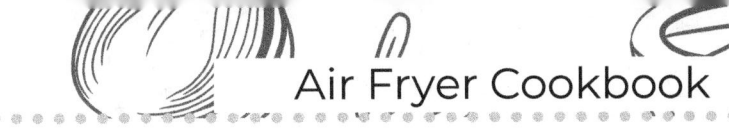

Air Fryer Cookbook

240. BASIC NO FRILLS TURKEY BREAST

PREPARATION: 5 MIN   **COOKING:** 50 MIN   **SERVINGS:** 4

INGREDIENTS

- 1 bone in turkey breast (about 8 lb.)
- 2 tbsp. olive oil
- 2 tbsp. sea salt
- 1 tbsp. black pepper

DIRECTIONS

1. Warm up the Air Fryer to 360°F for about 8 minutes.
2. Rub the washed turkey breast with the olive oil both on the skin and on the inside of the cavity.
3. Sprinkle on the sea salt and black pepper.
4. Remove the basket from the Air Fryer and spray with butter or olive oil flavored nonstick spray.
5. Put the turkey in with the breast side down.
6. Cook 20 minutes and carefully turn the breast over.
7. Spray with cooking oil and cook another 20 minutes.
8. When done test with thermometer and it should read 165°F. If not, put it back in for a few minutes.
9. Let the breast rest at least 15 minutes before cutting and serving.

Nutrition: *Calories 375 Fat 6.8g Carbs 8.2g Protein 15g*

241. FAIRE-WORTHY TURKEY LEGS

PREPARATION: 5 MIN   **COOKING:** 10 MIN   **SERVINGS:** 4

INGREDIENTS

- 1 turkey leg
- 1 tsp. olive oil
- 1 tsp. poultry seasoning
- 1 tsp. garlic powder
- salt and black pepper to taste

DIRECTIONS

1. Warm up the Air Fryer to 350°F for about 4 minutes.
2. Coat the leg with the olive oil. Just use your hands and rub it in.
3. In a small bowl, mix the poultry seasoning, garlic powder, salt and pepper. Rub it on the turkey leg.
4. Coat the inside of the Air Fryer basket with nonstick spray and place the turkey leg in.
5. Cook for 27 minutes, turning at 14 minutes. Be sure the leg is done by inserting a meat thermometer in the fleshy part of the leg and it should read 165°F

Nutrition: *Calories 325 Fat 10g Carbs 8.3g Protein 18g*

242. HERB AIR FRIED CHICKEN THIGHS

PREPARATION: 5 MIN   **COOKING:** 50 MIN   **SERVINGS:** 4

INGREDIENTS

- 2 lb. deboned chicken thighs
- 1 tsp. rosemary
- 1 tsp. thyme
- 1 tsp. garlic powder
- 1 large lemon

Nutrition: Calories 534 Fat 27.8g Carbs 2.5g Protein 66.2g

DIRECTIONS

1. Trim fat from thighs and salt and pepper all sides.
2. In a bowl, combine the rosemary, thyme, and garlic powder. Sprinkle over the chicken thighs and press the mixture in putting them on a baking sheet.
3. Cut the lemon and squeeze the juice over all the chicken thighs. Cover with plastic wrap and put in the refrigerator for 30 minutes.
4. Warm up the Air Fryer to 360°F for 6 minutes and spray with butter flavored cooking spray.
5. Place the thighs in the Air Fryer basket, as many will fit in one layer.
6. Cook for 15 minutes, turning after 7 minutes. Check internal temperature to make sure it is at 180°F before serving.

243. QUICK & EASY LEMON PEPPER CHICKEN

PREPARATION: 10 MIN   **COOKING:** 30 MIN   **SERVINGS:** 4

INGREDIENTS

- 2 chicken breasts, boneless & skinless
- 1 1/2 tsp. granulated garlic
- 1 tbsp. lemon pepper seasoning
- 1 tsp. salt

Nutrition: Calories 285 Fat 10.9g Carbs 1.8g Protein 42.6g

DIRECTIONS

1. Preheat the Air Fryer to 360°F.
2. Season chicken breasts with lemon pepper seasoning, granulated garlic, and salt.
3. Place chicken into the Air Fryer basket and cook for 30 minutes. Turn chicken halfway through.
4. Serve and enjoy.

244. SPICY JALAPENO HASSEL BACK CHICKEN

PREPARATION: 10 MIN   **COOKING:** 15 MIN   **SERVINGS:** 2

INGREDIENTS

- 2 chicken breasts, boneless and skinless
- 1/2 cup cheddar cheese, shredded
- tbsp. pickled jalapenos, chopped
- 2 oz cream cheese, softened
- bacon slices, cooked and crumbled

Nutrition: Calories 736 Fat 49g Carbs 3.7g Protein 65.5g

DIRECTIONS

1. In a bowl, mix together 1/2 cheddar cheese, pickled jalapenos, cream cheese, and bacon.
2. Stuff cheddar cheese mixture into the slits.
3. Place chicken into the Air Fryer basket and cook at 350°F for 14 minutes.
4. Sprinkle remaining cheese on top of the chicken and air fry for 1 minute more.
5. Serve and enjoy.

245. TASTY HASSEL BACK CHICKEN

PREPARATION: 10MIN **COOKING:** 18 MIN **SERVINGS:** 2

INGREDIENTS

- 2 chicken breasts, boneless and skinless
- 1/2 cup sauerkraut, squeezed and remove excess liquid
- thin Swiss cheese slices, tear into pieces
- thin deli corned beef slices, tear into pieces
- Salt and Pepper\

Nutrition: Calories 724 Fat 39.9g Carbs 3.6g Protein 83.6g

DIRECTIONS

1. Make five slits on top of chicken breasts. Season chicken with pepper and salt.
2. Stuff each slit with beef, sauerkraut, and cheese.
3. Spray chicken with cooking spray and place in the Air Fryer basket.
4. Cook chicken at 350°F for 18 minutes.
5. Serve and enjoy.

246. WESTERN TURKEY BREAST

PREPARATION: 10 MIN **COOKING:** 60 MIN **SERVINGS:** 8

INGREDIENTS

- 2 lbs. turkey breast, boneless
- 1 tbsp. olive oil
- 1 1/2 tsp. paprika
- 1 1/2 tsp. garlic powder
- Salt and pepper

Nutrition: Calories 254 Fat 5.6g Carbs 10.4g Protein 38.9g

DIRECTIONS

1. Preheat the Air Fryer to 350°F.
2. In a bowl, mix paprika, garlic powder, pepper, and salt together.
3. Rub oil and spice mixture all over turkey breast.
4. Place turkey breast skin side down in the Air Fryer basket and cook for 25 minutes.
5. Turn turkey breast and cover with foil and cook for 35-45 minutes more or until the internal temperature of the turkey reaches 160°F.
6. Remove turkey breast from the Air Fryer and allow it to cool for 10 minutes.
7. Slice and serve.

247. LEMON PEPPER TURKEY BREAST

PREPARATION: 10 MIN **COOKING:** 60 MIN **SERVINGS:** 6

INGREDIENTS

- 2 lbs turkey breast, de-boned
- 1 tsp. lemon pepper seasoning
- 1 tbsp. Worcestershire sauce
- tbsp. olive oil
- 1/2 tsp. salt

Nutrition: Calories 279 Fat 8.4g Carbs 10.3g Protein 38.8g

DIRECTIONS

1. Add olive oil, Worcestershire sauce, lemon pepper seasoning, and salt into the zip-lock bag. Add turkey breast to the marinade and coat well and marinate for 1-2 hours.
2. Remove turkey breast from marinade and place it into the Air Fryer basket.
3. Cook at 350°F for 25 minutes. Turn turkey breast and cook for 35 minutes more or until the internal temperature of turkey breast reaches 165°F.
4. Slice and serve.

Air Fryer Cookbook

248. TENDER TURKEY LEGS

PREPARATION: 10 MIN   **COOKING:** 27 MIN   **SERVINGS:** 4

INGREDIENTS

- turkey legs
- 1/4 tsp. oregano
- 1/4 tsp. rosemary
- 1 tbsp. butter
- Salt and Pepper

Nutrition: *Calories 182 Fat 9.9g Carbs 1.9g Protein 20.2g*

DIRECTIONS

1. Season turkey legs with pepper and salt.
2. In a small bowl, mix together butter, oregano, and rosemary.
3. Rub the butter mixture all over turkey legs.
4. Preheat the Air Fryer to 350°F.
5. Place turkey legs into the Air Fryer basket and cook for 27 minutes.
6. Serve and enjoy.

249. PERFECT CHICKEN BREASTS

PREPARATION: 10 MIN   **COOKING:** 15 MIN   **SERVINGS:** 4

INGREDIENTS

- 1 lb. chicken breasts, skinless and boneless
- 1 tsp. poultry seasoning
- tsp. olive oil
- 1 tsp. salt

Nutrition: *Calories 237 Fat 10.8g Carbs 0.3g Protein 32.9g*

DIRECTIONS

1. Drizzle oil on the chicken breasts and season with poultry seasoning and salt.
2. Place chicken breasts into the Air Fryer basket and cook at 360°F for 10 minutes. Flip chicken and cook for 5 minutes more.
3. Serve and enjoy.

250. RANCH GARLIC CHICKEN WINGS

PREPARATION: 10 MIN   **COOKING:** 25 MIN   **SERVINGS:** 4

INGREDIENTS

- 1 lb. chicken wings
- garlic cloves, minced
- 1/4 cup butter, melted
- tbsp. ranch seasoning mix

Nutrition: *Calories 552 Fat 28.3g Carbs 1.3g Protein 66g*

DIRECTIONS

1. Add chicken wings into a zip-lock bag.
2. Mix together butter, garlic, and ranch seasoning and pour over chicken wings. Seal bag shakes well and places in the refrigerator overnight.
3. Place marinated chicken wings into the Air Fryer basket and cook at 360°F for 20 minutes. Shake Air Fryer basket twice.
4. Turn temperature to 390°F and cook chicken wings for 5 minutes more.
5. Serve and enjoy.

251. RANCH CHICKEN THIGHS

PREPARATION: 10 MIN **COOKING:** 23 MIN **SERVINGS:** 4

INGREDIENTS

- Chicken thighs, bone-in & skin-on
- 1/2 tbsp. ranch dressing mix

DIRECTIONS

1. Add chicken thighs into the mixing bowl and sprinkle with ranch dressing mix. Toss well to coat.
2. Spray chicken thighs with cooking spray and place into the Air Fryer basket.
3. Cook at 380°F for 23 minutes. Turn chicken halfway through.
4. Serve and enjoy.

Nutrition: Calories 558 Fat 21.7g Carbs 0.5g Protein 84.6g

252. TACO RANCH CHICKEN WINGS

PREPARATION: 10 MIN **COOKING:** 30 MIN **SERVINGS:** 4

INGREDIENTS

- 2 lbs. chicken wings
- 1 tsp. ranch seasoning
- 1 1/2 tsp. taco seasoning
- 1 tsp. olive oil

DIRECTIONS

1. Preheat the Air Fryer to 400°F.
2. In a mixing bowl, add chicken wings, ranch seasoning, taco seasoning, and oil and toss well to coat.
3. Place chicken wings into the Air Fryer basket and cook for 15 minutes.
4. Turn chicken wings to another side and cook for 15 minutes more.
5. Serve and enjoy.

Nutrition: Calories 444 Fat 18g Carbs 0g Protein 65.6g

253. SIMPLE CAJUN CHICKEN WINGS

PREPARATION: 10 MIN **COOKING:** 25 MIN **SERVINGS:** 4

INGREDIENTS

- 2 lbs. chicken wings
- 1/3 cup ranch dressing
- 1 tbsp. + 1/2 tsp. Cajun seasoning

DIRECTIONS

1. Rub 1 tbsp. Cajun seasoning all over chicken wings.
2. Place chicken wings into the Air Fryer basket and cook at 400°F for 25 minutes. Turn chicken wings halfway through.
3. Meanwhile, in a small bowl, mix together ranch dressing and 1 tsp. Cajun seasoning.
4. Serve chicken wings with Cajun ranch dressing.

Nutrition: Calories 437 Fat 16.9g Carbs 1.1g Protein 65.9g

Air Fryer Cookbook

254. SIMPLE AIR FRIED CHICKEN

PREPARATION: 10 MIN **COOKING:** 10 MIN **SERVINGS:** 4

INGREDIENTS

- oz chicken, skinless and boneless
- 1/2 tsp. black pepper
- 1/2 tsp. salt
- 1/2 cup almond meal
- 1 egg, beaten

Nutrition: Calories 285 Fat 12.8g Carbs 3.7g Protein 38.1g

DIRECTIONS

1. Preheat the Air Fryer at 330°F.
2. Add egg in a bowl and whisk until frothy and season with pepper and salt.
3. In a shallow dish, mix together almond meal and salt.
4. Dip chicken into the egg mixture then coats with almond meal.
5. Place coated chicken into the Air Fryer basket and cook for 10 minutes.
6. Serve and enjoy.

255. BUFFALO WINGS

PREPARATION: 5 MIN **COOKING:** 15 MIN **SERVINGS:** 4

INGREDIENTS

- 32 oz chicken wings
- 1/4 cup hot sauce
- tbsp. grass-fed butter, melted
- Salt

Nutrition: Calories 678 Fat 34 g Carbs 0.4 g Protein 87.7 g

DIRECTIONS

1. Add chicken wings into the bowl. Pour hot sauce and butter over chicken wings and toss well.
2. Place marinated chicken wings into the refrigerator for 1-2 hours.
3. Preheat the Air Fryer at 400°F for 3 minutes
4. Place marinated chicken wings into the Air Fryer basket and cook for 12 minutes. shake basket halfway through.
5. Serve and enjoy.

256. HONEY LIME CHICKEN WINGS

PREPARATION: 10 MIN **COOKING:** 50 MIN **SERVINGS:** 66

INGREDIENTS

- 2 lbs chicken wings
- tbsp. fresh lime juice
- salt and black pepper
- 1/4 tsp. white pepper powder
- tbsp. honey

Nutrition: Calories 311 Fat 11.2g Carbs 6.1g Protein 43.8g

DIRECTIONS

1. In a bowl, place all the ingredients and coat well.
2. Place marinated chicken wings into the refrigerator for 1-2 hours.
3. Preheat the Air Fryer to 360°F.
4. Place marinated chicken wings into the Air Fryer basket and cook for 12 minutes. Shake Air Fryer basket halfway through.
5. Turn temperature to 400°F and cook for 3 minutes more. Serve and enjoy.

257. SIMPLE CHICKEN DRUMSTICKS

PREPARATION: 10 MIN   **COOKING:** 16 MIN   **SERVINGS:** 4

INGREDIENTS

- 1 1/2 lbs chicken drumsticks
- tbsp. chicken seasoning
- 1 tsp. black pepper
- 1 tbsp. olive oil
- 1 tsp. salt

DIRECTIONS

1. In a small bowl, mix together chicken seasoning, olive oil, pepper, and salt.
2. Rub seasoning mixture all over the chicken.
3. Place seasoned chicken into the Air Fryer basket and cook for 10 minutes. Flip halfway through.
4. Turn temperature to 300°F and cook for 6 minutes more. Serve and enjoy.

Nutrition: Calories 319 Fat 13.2g Carbs 0.3g Protein 46.8g

258. HEALTHY CHICKEN WINGS

PREPARATION: 10 MIN   **COOKING:** 25 MIN   **SERVINGS:** 4

INGREDIENTS

- lbs. chicken wings
- 1 tbsp. pepper
- 1 tbsp. garlic powder
- tbsp. seasoning salt

DIRECTIONS

1. In a bowl, mix all of the ingredients except for the chicken wings.
2. Add chicken wings in a bowl and toss until well coated.
3. Preheat the Air Fryer at 370°F for 5 minutes.
4. Put the chicken wings into the basket of the Air Fryer and cook for 20 minutes. Shake basket halfway through.
5. Serve and enjoy.

Nutrition: Calories 442 Fat 16.9g Carbs 2.6g Protein 66.1g

259. THAI CHICKEN THIGHS

PREPARATION: 10MIN   **COOKING:** 20 MIN   **SERVINGS:** 4

INGREDIENTS

- 1 lb. chicken thighs, boneless and skinless
- tsp. ginger, minced
- garlic cloves, chopped
- 1/2 cup coconut milk
- tbsp. curry paste

DIRECTIONS

1. Add all ingredients into the zip-lock bag and shake well and place bag in the refrigerator for overnight.
2. Add marinated chicken and the sauce in a pie dish.
3. Place dish in Air Fryer and cook for 20 minutes at 165°F. Serve and enjoy.

Nutrition: Calories 341 Fat 20g Carbs 5.2g Protein 34.1g

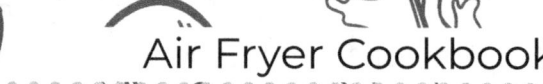
Air Fryer Cookbook

260. CHICKEN PATTIES

PREPARATION: 10 MIN **COOKING:** 13 MIN **SERVINGS:** 8

INGREDIENTS

- lbs ground chicken
- 1 cup homemade salsa
- 1/2 small onion, chopped
- 1 1/2 cups egg whites
- Salt and Pepper

DIRECTIONS

1. Add egg whites, salsa, and onion into the blender and blend until combined.
2. Add ground chicken and egg mixture into the large mixing bowl. Season with pepper and salt and mix until well combined.
3. Make small patties from meat mixture.
4. Spray Air Fryer basket with cooking spray.
5. Place chicken patties in Air Fryer and cook for 12-13 minutes at 345°F. Cook in batches. Serve and enjoy.

Nutrition: Calories 357 Fat 12.7g Carbs 2.8g Protein 54.7g

261. CAJUN SEASONED CHICKEN DRUMSTICKS

PREPARATION: 5 MIN **COOKING:** 15 MIN **SERVINGS:** 2

INGREDIENTS

- chicken drumsticks, skinless
- 1 tbsp. Cajun seasoning
- tsp. olive oil

DIRECTIONS

1. Add all ingredients to the zip-lock bag. Shake bag well and place in refrigerator for half hour.
2. Place marinated chicken drumsticks in Air Fryer basket and cook for 15 minutes at 400°F.
3. Serve and enjoy.

Nutrition: Calories 118 Fat 7.3g Carbs 0g Protein 12.7g

262. HONEY GARLIC CHICKEN

PREPARATION: 10 MIN **COOKING:** 15 MIN **SERVINGS:** 2

INGREDIENTS

- Chicken drumsticks, skinless
- 1/2 tsp. garlic, minced
- tsp. honey
- tsp. olive oil

DIRECTIONS

1. Put all of the ingredients to a bowl and mix until well coated.
2. Place chicken in refrigerator for half hour.
3. Place marinated chicken into the Air Fryer and cook for 15 minutes at 400°F.
4. Serve and enjoy.

Nutrition: Calories 140 Fat 7.3g Carbs 6g Protein 12.7g

263. SRIRACHA CHICKEN WINGS

PREPARATION: 10 MIN   **COOKING:** 35 MIN   **SERVINGS:** 2

INGREDIENTS

- 1 lb. chicken wings
- 1/2 lime juice
- 1 tbsp. grass-fed butter
- tbsp. sriracha sauce
- 1/4 cup honey

Nutrition: Calories 711 Fat 32.6g Carbs 35.9g Protein 65.8g

DIRECTIONS

1. Preheat the Air Fryer to 360°F.
2. Add chicken wings in Air Fryer basket and cook for 30 minutes.
3. Meanwhile, in a pan, add all remaining ingredients and bring to boil for 3 minutes.
4. Once chicken wings are done then toss with sauce and serve.

264. SWEET & SPICY CHICKEN WINGS

PREPARATION: 10 MIN   **COOKING:** 20 MIN   **SERVINGS:** 8

INGREDIENTS

- lbs. chicken wings
- tbsp. honey
- 1/2 cup buffalo sauce
- tbsp. grass-fed butter, melted
- Salt and Pepper

Nutrition: Calories 262 Fat 11.7g Carbs 4.6g Protein 32.9g

DIRECTIONS

1. Put the chicken wings into the basket of the Air Fryer and cook for 20 minutes at 400°F. Shake Air Fryer basket 2 times during the cooking.
2. In a large bowl, combine together honey, buffalo sauce, butter, pepper, and salt.
3. Add cooked chicken wings into the bowl and toss until well coated with sauce.
4. Serve and enjoy.

265. GINGER GARLIC CHICKEN

PREPARATION: 10 MIN   **COOKING:** 30 MIN   **SERVINGS:** 2

INGREDIENTS

- chicken thighs, skinless and boneless
- 1/2 tsp. ground ginger
- 1 garlic clove, minced
- tbsp. ketchup
- 1/2 cup honey

Nutrition: Calories 554 Fat 16.3g Carbs 37.2g Protein 63.7g

DIRECTIONS

1. Cut chicken thighs into the small pieces and place them into the Air Fryer basket and cook for 25 minutes at 390°F.
2. Meanwhile, in a pan heat together honey, ketchup, garlic, and ground ginger for 4-5 minutes.
3. Once the chicken is cooked then transfer into the mixing bowl.
4. Pour honey mixture over the chicken and toss until well coated.
5. Serve and enjoy.

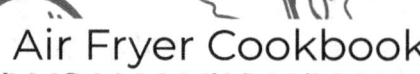
Air Fryer Cookbook

266. SALT AND PEPPER WINGS

PREPARATION: 5 MIN **COOKING:** 10 MIN **SERVINGS:** 4

INGREDIENTS

- 2 tsp.s salt
- 2 tsp.s fresh ground pepper
- 2 lb. chicken wings

Nutrition: Calories 342 Fat 14.8g Carbs 1g Protein 49.2g

DIRECTIONS

1. In a bowl, mix the salt and pepper.
2. Add the wings to the bowl and mix with your hands to coat every last one.
3. Put 8 to 10 wings in the Air Fryer basket that has been sprayed with nonstick cooking spray. Set for 350°F (there is no need to preheat) and cook about 15 minutes, turning once at 7 minutes.
4. Repeat with rest of wings and serve hot.

267. PARMESAN CHICKEN WINGS

PREPARATION: 10 MIN **COOKING:** 25 MIN **SERVINGS:** 4

INGREDIENTS

- 1 1/2 lbs. chicken wings
- 3/4 tbsp. garlic powder
- 1/4 cup parmesan cheese, grated
- 2 tbsp. arrowroot powder
- Salt and Pepper

Nutrition: Calories 386 Fat 15.3g Carbs 5.6g Protein 53.5g

DIRECTIONS

1. Preheat the Air Fryer to 380°F.
2. In a bowl, mix the garlic powder, parmesan cheese, arrowroot powder, pepper, and salt together. Add chicken wings and toss until well coated.
3. Put the chicken wings into the Air Fryer basket. Spray top of chicken wings with cooking spray.
4. Select chicken and press start. Shake Air Fryer basket halfway through. Serve and enjoy.

268. WESTERN CHICKEN WINGS

PREPARATION: 10 MIN **COOKING:** 15 MIN **SERVINGS:** 4

INGREDIENTS

- 2 lbs. chicken wings
- 1 tsp. Herb de Provence
- 1 tsp. paprika
- 1/2 cup parmesan cheese, grated
- Salt and Pepper

Nutrition: Calories 473 Fat 19.6g Carbs 0.8g Protein 69.7g

DIRECTIONS

1. Add cheese, paprika, herb de Provence, pepper, and salt into the large mixing bowl. Place the chicken wings into the bowl and toss well to coat.
2. Preheat the Air Fryer to 350°F.
3. Place the chicken wings into the Air Fryer basket. Spray top of chicken wings with cooking spray.
4. Cook chicken wings for 15 minutes. Turn chicken wings halfway through. Serve and enjoy.

269. PERFECT CHICKEN THIGHS DINNER

PREPARATION: 10 MIN **COOKING:** 15 MIN **SERVINGS:** 4

INGREDIENTS

- 4 chicken thighs, bone-in & skinless
- 1/4 tsp. ground ginger
- 2 tsp. paprika
- 2 tsp. garlic powder
- salt and pepper

DIRECTIONS

1. Preheat the Air Fryer to 400°F.
2. In a bowl, mix ginger, paprika, garlic powder, pepper, and salt together and rub all over chicken thighs.
3. Spray chicken thighs with cooking spray.
4. Place chicken thighs into the Air Fryer basket and cook for 10 minutes.
5. Turn chicken thighs and cook for 5 minutes more. Serve and enjoy.

Nutrition: *Calories 286 Fat 11g Carbs 1.8g Protein 42.7g*

270. PERFECTLY SPICED CHICKEN TENDERS

PREPARATION: 10 MIN **COOKING:** 13 MIN **SERVINGS:** 4

INGREDIENTS

- 6 chicken tenders
- 1 tsp. onion powder
- 1 tsp. garlic powder
- 1 tsp. paprika
- 1 tsp. kosher salt

DIRECTIONS

1. Preheat the Air Fryer to 380°F.
2. In a bowl, mix onion powder, garlic powder, paprika, and salt together and rub all over chicken tenders.
3. Spray chicken tenders with cooking spray.
4. Place chicken tenders into the Air Fryer basket and cook for 13 minutes. Serve and enjoy.

Nutrition: *Calories 423 Fat 16.4g Carbs 1.5g Protein 63.7g*

MEAT

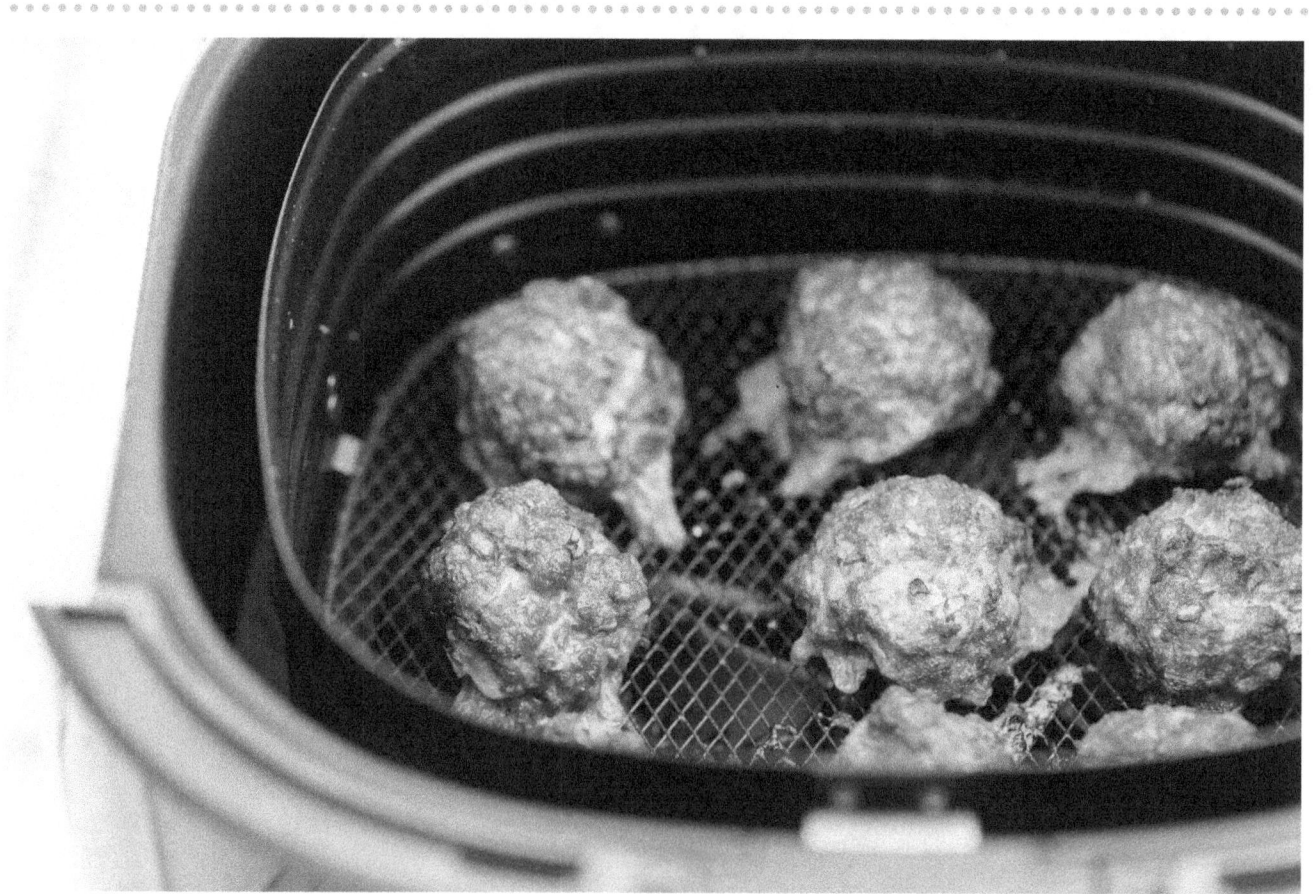

271. FLAVORFUL STEAK

PREPARATION: 10 MIN **COOKING:** 18 MIN **SERVINGS:** 2

INGREDIENTS

- 2 steaks, rinsed and pat dry
- ½ tsp. garlic powder
- 1 tsp. olive oil
- Pepper
- Salt

DIRECTIONS

1. Brush steaks with olive oil and season with garlic powder, pepper, and salt.
2. Preheat the Air Fryer oven to 400°F.
3. Place steaks on Air Fryer oven pan and air fry for 10-18 minutes. Turn halfway through. Serve and enjoy.

Nutrition: Calories 361 Fat 10.9g Carbs 0.5g Protein 61.6g

272. EASY ROSEMARY LAMB CHOPS

PREPARATION: 6 MIN **COOKING:** 10 MIN **SERVINGS:** 4

INGREDIENTS

- 4 lamb chops
- 2 tbsp. dried rosemary
- ¼ cup fresh lemon juice
- Pepper
- Salt

DIRECTIONS

1. In a small bowl, mix together lemon juice, rosemary, pepper, and salt.
2. Brush lemon juice rosemary mixture over lamb chops.
3. Place lamb chops on Air Fryer oven tray and air fry at 400°F for 3 minutes.
4. Turn lamb chops to the other side and cook for 3 minutes more. Serve and enjoy.

Nutrition: Calories 267 Fat 21.7g Carbs 1.4g Protein 16.9g

273. BBQ PORK RIBS

PREPARATION: 10 MIN **COOKING:** 12 MIN **SERVINGS:** 6

INGREDIENTS

- 1 slab baby back pork ribs, cut into pieces
- ½ cup BBQ sauce
- ½ tsp. paprika
- Salt

DIRECTIONS

1. Add pork ribs in a mixing bowl.
2. Add BBQ sauce, paprika, and salt over pork ribs and coat well and set aside for 30 minutes.
3. Preheat the Air Fryer oven to 350°F.
4. Arrange marinated pork ribs on Air Fryer oven pan and cook for 10-12 minutes. Turn halfway through. Serve and enjoy.

Nutrition: Calories 145 Fat 7g Carbs 10g Protein 9g

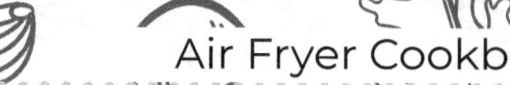
Air Fryer Cookbook

274. JUICY STEAK BITES

PREPARATION: 10 MIN **COOKING:** 9 MIN **SERVINGS:** 4

INGREDIENTS

- 1 lb. sirloin steak, sliced into bite-size pieces
- 1 tbsp. steak seasoning
- 1 tbsp. olive oil
- Pepper
- Salt

DIRECTIONS

1. Preheat the instant Air Fryer oven to 390°F.
2. Add steak pieces into the large mixing bowl. Add steak seasoning, oil, pepper, and salt over steak pieces and toss until well coated.
3. Transfer steak pieces on Air Fryer pan and air fry for 5 minutes.
4. Turn steak pieces to the other side and cook for 4 minutes more. Serve and enjoy.

Nutrition: Calories 241 Fat 10.6g Carbs 0g Protein 34.4g

275. GREEK LAMB CHOPS

PREPARATION: 10 MIN **COOKING:** 10 MIN **SERVINGS:** 4

INGREDIENTS

- 2 lbs. lamb chops
- 2 tsp. garlic, minced
- 1 ½ tsp. dried oregano
- ¼ cup fresh lemon juice
- salt and pepper

DIRECTIONS

1. Add lamb chops in a mixing bowl. Add remaining ingredients over the lamb chops and coat well.
2. Arrange lamb chops on the Air Fryer oven tray and cook at 400°F for 5 minutes.
3. Turn lamb chops and cook for 5 minutes more. Serve and enjoy.

Nutrition: Calories 538 Fat 29.4g Carbs 1.3g Protein 64g

276. EASY BEEF ROAST

PREPARATION: 10 MIN **COOKING:** 45 MIN **SERVINGS:** 6

INGREDIENTS

- 2 ½ lbs. beef roast
- 2 tbsp. Italian seasoning

DIRECTIONS

1. Arrange roast on the rotisserie spite.
2. Rub roast with Italian seasoning then insert into the Air Fryer oven.
3. Air fry at 350°F for 45 minutes or until the internal temperature of the roast reaches to 145°F. Slice and serve.

Nutrition: Calories 365 Fat 13.2g Carbs 0.5g Protein 57.4g

277. BEEF JERKY

PREPARATION: 10 MIN **COOKING:** 4 H **SERVINGS:** 4

INGREDIENTS

- 2 lbs. London broil, sliced thinly
- 1 tsp. onion powder
- 3 tbsp. brown sugar
- 3 tbsp. soy sauce
- 1 tsp. olive oil

Nutrition: Calories 133 Fat 4.7g Carbs 9.4g Protein 13.4g

DIRECTIONS

1. Add all ingredients except meat in the large zip-lock bag.
2. Mix until well combined. Add meat in the bag.
3. Seal bag and massage gently to cover the meat with marinade.
4. Let marinate the meat for 1 hour.
5. Arrange marinated meat slices on Air Fryer tray and dehydrate at 160°F for 4 hours.

278. SIMPLE BEEF PATTIES

PREPARATION: 10 MIN **COOKING:** 13 MIN **SERVINGS:** 4

INGREDIENTS

- 1 lb. ground beef
- ½ tsp. garlic powder
- ¼ tsp. onion powder
- Salt and Pepper

Nutrition: Calories 212 Fat 7.1g Carbs 0.4g Protein 34.5g

DIRECTIONS

1. Preheat the Air Fryer oven to 400°F.
2. Add ground meat, garlic powder, onion powder, pepper, and salt into the mixing bowl and mix until well combined.
3. Make even shape patties from meat mixture and arrange on Air Fryer pan.
4. Place pan in Air Fryer oven. Cook patties for 10 minutes. Turn patties after 5 minutes. Serve and enjoy.

279. PANKO-BREADED PORK CHOPS

PREPARATION: 5 MIN **COOKING:** 12 MIN **SERVINGS:** 6

INGREDIENTS

- 5 (3½- to 5 oz.) pork chops (bone-in or boneless)
- salt and pepper
- ¼ cup all-purpose flour
- 2 tbsp. panko bread crumbs
- Cooking oil

Nutrition: Calories 246 Fat 13g Carbs 11g Protein 26g

DIRECTIONS

1. Season the pork chops with salt and pepper to taste.
2. Sprinkle the flour on both sides of the pork chops, then coat both sides with panko bread crumbs.
3. Put the pork chops in the Air Fryer. Stacking them is okay.
4. Spray the pork chops with cooking oil. Cook for 6 minutes at 365°F.
5. Halfway through, flip the pork chops. Cook for an additional 6 minutes
6. Cool before serving.
7. Typically, bone-in pork chops are juicier than boneless. If you prefer really juicy pork chops, use bone-in.

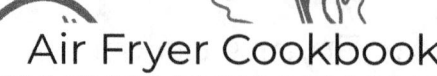

280. CRISPY ROAST GARLIC-SALT PORK

PREPARATION: 5 MIN   **COOKING:** 45 MIN   **SERVINGS:** 4

INGREDIENTS

- 1 tsp. Chinese five spice powder
- 1 tsp. white pepper
- 2 lb. pork belly
- 2 tsp.s garlic salt

DIRECTIONS

1. Preheat the Air Fryer to 390°F.
2. Mix all of the seasonings in a bowl to create the dry rub.
3. Score the skin of the pork belly with a knife and season the entire pork with the spice rub.
4. Place in the Air Fryer basket and cook for 40 to 45 minutes until the skin is crispy. Chop before serving.

Nutrition: *Calories 785 Fat 80.7g Carbs 7g Protein 14.2g*

281. BEEF ROLLS

PREPARATION: 10 MIN   **COOKING:** 14 MIN   **SERVINGS:** 4

INGREDIENTS

- 2 lb. beef steak, opened and flattened with a meat tenderizer
- Salt and black pepper to the taste
- 3 oz. red bell pepper, roasted and chopped
- 6 slices provolone cheese
- 3 tbsp. pesto

DIRECTIONS

1. Arrange flattened beef steak on a cutting board, spread pesto all over, add cheese in a single layer, add bell peppers, salt and pepper to the taste.
2. Roll your steak, secure with toothpicks, season again with salt and pepper, place roll in your Air Fryer's basket and cook at 400°F for 14 minutes, rotating roll halfway.
3. Leave aside to cool down, cut into 2-inch smaller rolls, arrange on a platter and serve them as an appetizer. Enjoy!

Nutrition: *Calories 230 Fat 17g Carbs 12g Protein 10g*

282. HOMEMADE CORNED BEEF WITH ONIONS

PREPARATION: 5 MIN   **COOKING:** 50 MIN   **SERVINGS:** 4

INGREDIENTS

- Salt and pepper to taste
- 1 cup water
- 1-lb. corned beef brisket, cut into chunks
- 1 tbsp. Dijon mustard
- 1 small onion, chopped

DIRECTIONS

1. Preheat the Air Fryer to 400°F.
2. Place all ingredients in a baking dish that will fit in the Air Fryer.
3. Cover with foil. Cook for 35 minutes.
4. Remove foil, mix well, turnover beef, and continue cooking for another 15 minutes.

Nutrition: *Calories 238 Carbs 3.1g Protein 17.2g Fat 17.1g*

283. CRISP RIBS

PREPARATION: 10 MIN **COOKING:** 50 MIN **SERVINGS:** 2

INGREDIENTS

- 1 rack of pork ribs
Rub:
- 1 1/2 cup broth
- 3 tbsp. Liquid Smoke
- 1 cup Barbecue Sauce

Nutrition: Calories 306 Fat 6.4g Carbs 46g Protein 14.7g

DIRECTIONS

1. Rub the rib rack with spice rub generously.
2. Pour the liquid into the Air Fryer. Set an Air Fryer Basket into the Pot and place the rib rack in the basket.
3. Put on the pressure-cooking lid (if available) and seal it.
4. Hit the "Pressure Button" and select 30 minutes of Cooking Time, then press "Start."
5. Once the Air Fryer, do a quick release and remove its lid.
6. Remove the ribs and rub them with barbecue sauce. Empty the pot and place the Air Fryer Basket in it.
7. Set the ribs in the basket, and Air fry them at 370°F for 20 minutes. Serve.

284. ROAST BEEF

PREPARATION: 10 MIN **COOKING:** 15 MIN **SERVINGS:** 4

INGREDIENTS

- 2 lb. beef roast top
- oil for spraying
- Rub
- Salt and pepper to taste
- 2 tsp. garlic powder
- 1 tsp. summer savory

Nutrition: Calories 427 Fat 14.2g Carbs 1.4g Protein 69.1g

DIRECTIONS

1. Whisk all the rub Ingredients: in a small bowl.
2. Liberally rub this mixture over the roast.
3. Place an Air Fryer Basket in the Air Fryer and layer it with cooking oil.
4. Set the seasoned roast in the Air Fryer Basket. Put on the Air Fryer lid and seal it.
5. Hit the "Air fry Button" and select 20 minutes of Cooking Time at 370°F, then press "Start."
6. Once the Air Fryer beeps, remove its lid. Turn the roast and continue Air Fryer for another 15 minutes. Serve warm.

285. BASIC PORK CHOPS

PREPARATION: 10 MIN **COOKING:** 15 MIN **SERVINGS:** 4

INGREDIENTS

- 4 pork chops, bone-in
- 1 tbsp. olive oil
- 1 tsp. kosher salt
- 1/2 tsp. black pepper

Nutrition: Calories 287 Fat 23.4g Carbs 0.2g Protein 18g

DIRECTIONS

1. Liberally season the pork chops with olive oil, salt, and black pepper.
2. Place the pork chops in the basket and spray them with cooking spray.
3. Set the Air Fryer Basket in the Air Fryer. Put on the Air Fryer lid and seal it.
4. Hit the "Air fry Button" and select 15 minutes of Cooking Time at 360°F, then press "Start."
5. Once the Air Fryer beeps, remove its lid, serve and enjoy.

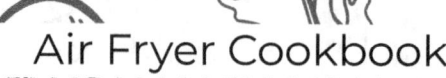

286. BREADED PORK CHOPS

PREPARATION: 10 MIN **COOKING:** 18 MIN **SERVINGS:** 4

INGREDIENTS

- 4 boneless, center-cut pork chops, 1-inch thick
- 1 tsp. Cajun seasoning
- 1 1/2 cups garlic-flavored croutons
- 2 eggs
- cooking spray

DIRECTIONS

1. Grind croutons in a food processor until it forms crumbs.
2. Season the pork chops with Cajun seasoning liberally.
3. Beat eggs in a shallow tray then dip the pork chops in the egg.
4. Coat the dipped chops in the crouton crumbs.
5. Place the breaded pork chops in the basket of the Air Fryer.
6. Set the Air Fryer Basket and spray the chops with cooking oil.
7. Put on the Air Fryer lid and seal it.
8. Hit the "Air fry Button" and select 18 minutes of Cooking Time at 370°F.
9. Once the Air Fryer beeps, remove its lid and serve.

Nutrition: Calories 301 Fat 12.4g Carbs 12.2g Protein 32.2g

287. BEEF AND BALSAMIC MARINADE

PREPARATION: 5 MIN **COOKING:** 40 MIN **SERVINGS:** 4

INGREDIENTS

- 4 medium beef steaks
- 3 garlic cloves; minced
- 1 cup balsamic vinegar
- 2 tbsp. olive oil
- Salt and black pepper to taste

DIRECTIONS

1. Take a bowl and mix steaks with the rest of the ingredients and toss.
2. Transfer the steaks to your Air Fryer's basket and cook at 390°F for 35 minutes, flipping them halfway
3. Divide among plates and serve with a side salad.

Nutrition: Calories 273 Fat 14g Carbs 6g Protein 19g

288. CRISPY BRATS

PREPARATION: 5 MIN **COOKING:** 15 MIN **SERVINGS:** 4

INGREDIENTS

- 4 x 3-oz. beef bratwursts

Nutrition: Calories 286 Fat 28g Protein 18g Carbs 0g

DIRECTIONS

1. Place brats into the Air Fryer basket.
2. Adjust the temperature to 375°F and set the timer for 15 minutes.

289. BASIL PORK CHOPS

PREPARATION: 5 MIN **COOKING:** 30 MIN **SERVINGS:** 4

INGREDIENTS

- 4 pork chops
- 2 tsp. basil; dried
- ½ tsp. chili powder
- 2 tbsp. olive oil
- A pinch of salt and black pepper

DIRECTIONS

1. In a pan that fits your Air Fryer, mix all the ingredients, toss.
2. Introduce in the fryer and cook at 400°F for 25 minutes. Divide everything between plates and serve

Nutrition: *Calories 274 Fat 13g Carbs 6g Protein 18g*

290. BEEF AND RADISHES

PREPARATION: 5 MIN **COOKING:** 15 MIN **SERVINGS:** 2

INGREDIENTS

- 1 lb. radishes, quartered
- 2 cups corned beef, cooked and shredded
- 2 spring onions; chopped
- 2 garlic cloves; minced
- A pinch of salt and black pepper

DIRECTIONS

1. In a pan that fits your Air Fryer, mix the beef with the rest of the ingredients, toss.
2. Put the pan in the fryer and cook at 390°F for 15 minutes
3. Divide everything into bowls and serve.

Nutrition: *Calories 267 Fat 13g Carbs 5g Protein 15g*

291. HERBED PORK CHOPS

PREPARATION: 5 MIN **COOKING:** 25 MIN **SERVINGS:** 4

INGREDIENTS

- 4 pork chops
- 2 tsp. basil; dried
- ½ tsp. chili powder
- 2 tbsp. olive oil
- A pinch of salt and black pepper

DIRECTIONS

1. In a pan that fits your Air Fryer, mix all the ingredients, toss.
2. Introduce in the fryer and cook at 400°F for 25 minutes. Divide everything between plates and serve

Nutrition: *Calories 274 Fat 13g Carbs 6g Protein 18g*

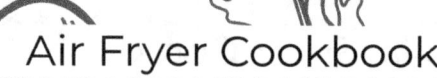 Air Fryer Cookbook

292. BEEF TENDERLOIN

PREPARATION: 5 MIN **COOKING:** 30 MIN **SERVINGS:** 6

INGREDIENTS

- 1 (2-lb. beef tenderloin, trimmed of visible fat
- 2 tbsp. salted butter; melted.
- 2 tsp. minced roasted garlic
- 3 tbsp. ground 4-peppercorn blend

DIRECTIONS

1. In a small bowl, mix the butter and roasted garlic. Brush it over the beef tenderloin.
2. Place the ground peppercorns onto a plate and roll the tenderloin through them, creating a crust. Place tenderloin into the Air Fryer basket
3. Adjust the temperature to 400°F and set the timer for 25 minutes. Flip the tenderloin halfway through cooking. Set aside for 10 minutes before slicing.

Nutrition: *Calories 289 Fat 18g Protein 37g Carbs 5g*

293. HONEY MUSTARD PORK TENDERLOIN

PREPARATION: 15 MIN **COOKING:** 25 MIN **SERVINGS:** 3

INGREDIENTS

- 1-lb. pork tenderloin
- 1 tbsp. garlic, minced
- 2 tbsp. soy sauce
- 2 tbsp. honey
- 1 tbsp. Dijon mustard
- 1 tbsp. grain mustard
- 1 tsp. Sriracha sauce

DIRECTIONS

1. In a large bowl, add all the ingredients except pork and mix well.
2. Add the pork tenderloin and coat with the mixture generously.
3. Refrigerate to marinate for 2-3 hours.
4. Remove the pork tenderloin from bowl, reserving the marinade.
5. Place the pork tenderloin onto the lightly greased cooking tray.
6. Arrange the drip pan in the bottom of the Air Fryer Oven cooking chamber.
7. Air fry for 25 minutes at 380°F.
8. Every few minutes, turn the pork and oat with the reserved marinade.
9. When cooking time is complete, remove the tray from Air Fryer and place the pork tenderloin onto a platter for about 10 minutes before slicing.
10. With a sharp knife, cut the pork tenderloin into desired sized slices and serve.

Nutrition: *Calories 277 Fat 5.7g Carbs 14.2g Protein 40.7g*

294. SEASONED PORK CHOPS

PREPARATION: 10 MIN   **COOKING:** 12 MIN   **SERVINGS:** 4

INGREDIENTS

- 4 (6 oz.) boneless pork chops
- 2 tbsp. pork rub
- 1 tbsp. olive oil

DIRECTIONS

1. Coat both sides of the pork chops with the oil and then, rub with the pork rub.
2. Place the pork chops onto the lightly greased cooking tray.
3. Arrange the drip pan in the bottom of the Air Fryer Oven cooking chamber.
4. Air fry for 12 minutes at 400°F.
5. After 4-5 minutes, turn the pork chops.
6. When cooking time is complete, remove the tray from Air Fryer and serve hot.

Nutrition: *Calories 285 Fat 9.5g Carbs 1.5g Protein 44.5g*

295. CRUSTED RACK OF LAMB

PREPARATION: 15 MIN   **COOKING:** 19 MIN   **SERVINGS:** 4

INGREDIENTS

- 1 rack of lamb, trimmed all fat and frenched
- Salt and ground black pepper, as required
- 1/3 cup pistachios, chopped finely
- 2 tbsp. panko breadcrumbs
- 2 tsp.s fresh thyme, chopped finely
- 1 tsp. fresh rosemary, chopped finely
- 1 tbsp. butter, melted
- 1 tbsp. Dijon mustard

DIRECTIONS

1. Insert the rotisserie rod through the rack on the meaty side of the ribs, right next to the bone.
2. Insert the rotisserie forks, one on each side of the rod to secure the rack.
3. Season the rack with salt and black pepper evenly.
4. Arrange the drip pan in the bottom of the Air Fryer Oven cooking chamber.
5. Set the timer for 12 minutes at 380°F.
6. When the display shows "Add Food" press the red lever down and load the left side of the rod into the Air Fryer.
7. Now, slide the rod's left side into the groove along the metal bar so it doesn't move. Then, close the door and touch "Rotate".
8. Meanwhile, in a small bowl, mix together the remaining ingredients except the mustard.
9. When cooking time is complete, remove the rack from Air Fryer and brush the meaty side with the mustard.
10. Then, coat the pistachio mixture on all sides of the rack and press firmly.
11. Now, place the rack of lamb onto the cooking tray, meat side up.
12. Air fry for 7 minutes at 380°F.
13. When cooking time is complete, remove the tray from Air Fryer and place the rack onto a cutting board for at least 10 minutes.
14. Cut the rack into individual chops and serve.

Nutrition: *Calories 824 Fat 39.3g Carbs 10.3g Protein 72g*

296. LAMB BURGERS

PREPARATION: 15 MIN **COOKING:** 8 MIN **SERVINGS:** 6

INGREDIENTS

- 2 lb. ground lamb
- 1 tbsp. onion powder
- Salt and ground black pepper, as required

Nutrition: Calories 285 Fat 11.1g Carbs 0.9g Protein 42.6g

DIRECTIONS

1. In a bowl, add all the ingredients and mix well.
2. Make 6 equal-sized patties from the mixture.
3. Arrange the patties onto a cooking tray.
4. Arrange the drip pan in the bottom of the Air Fryer Oven cooking chamber.
5. Air fry for 8 minutes at 360°F.
6. After 4 minutes, turn the burgers.
7. When cooking time is complete, remove the tray from Air Fryer and serve hot.

297. PORK TAQUITOS

PREPARATION: 10 MIN **COOKING:** 16 MIN **SERVINGS:** 8

INGREDIENTS

- 1 juiced lime
- 10 whole wheat tortillas
- 2 ½ C. shredded mozzarella cheese
- 30 oz. of cooked and shredded pork tenderloin

Nutrition: Calories 309 Fat 11g Protein 21g Sugar 2g

DIRECTIONS

1. Ensure your Air Fryer is preheated to 380°F.
2. Drizzle pork with lime juice and gently mix.
3. Heat up tortillas in the microwave with a dampened paper towel to soften.
4. Add about 3 oz. of pork and ¼ cup of shredded cheese to each tortilla. Tightly roll them up. Spray the Air Fryer basket with a bit of olive oil.
5. Set temperature to 380°F, and set time to 10 minutes. Air fry taquitos 7-10 minutes till tortillas turn a slight golden color, making sure to flip halfway through cooking process.

298. CAJUN BACON PORK LOIN FILLET

PREPARATION: 10 MIN **COOKING:** 20 MIN **SERVINGS:** 6

INGREDIENTS

- 1½ lb. pork loin fillet or pork tenderloin
- 3 tbsp. olive oil
- 2 tbsp. Cajun Spice Mix
- Salt
- 6 slices bacon
- Olive oil spray

Nutrition: Calories 355 Fat 22.88g Protein 34.83g Carbs 0.6g

DIRECTIONS

1. Cut the pork in half so that it will fit in the Air Fryer basket.
2. Place both pieces of meat in a resealable plastic bag. Add the oil, Cajun seasoning, and salt to taste, if using. Seal the bag and massage to coat all of the meat with the oil and seasonings. Marinate in the refrigerator for at least 1 hour or up to 24 hours.
3. Remove the pork from the bag and wrap 3 bacon slices around each piece. Spray the Air Fryer basket with olive oil spray. Place the meat in the Air Fryer. Set the Air Fryer to 350°F for 15 minutes. Increase the temperature to 400°F for 5 minutes. Use a meat thermometer to ensure the meat has reached an internal temperature of 145°F.
4. Let the meat rest for 10 minutes. Slice into 6 medallions and serve.

Air Fryer Cookbook

299. PORCHETTA-STYLE PORK CHOPS

PREPARATION: 10 MIN   **COOKING:** 15 MIN   **SERVINGS:** 2

INGREDIENTS

- 1 tbsp. extra-virgin olive oil
- Grated zest of 1 lemon
- 2 cloves garlic, minced
- 2 tsp.s chopped fresh rosemary
- 1 tsp. finely chopped fresh sage
- 1 tsp. fennel seeds, lightly crushed
- ¼ to ½ tsp. red pepper flakes
- 1 tsp. kosher salt
- 1 tsp. black pepper
- (8 oz.) center-cut bone-in pork chops, about 1 inch thick

DIRECTIONS

1. In a small bowl, combine the olive oil, zest, garlic, rosemary, sage, fennel seeds, red pepper, salt, and black pepper. Stir, crushing the herbs with the back of a spoon, until a paste forms. Spread the seasoning mix on both sides of the pork chops.
2. Place the chops in the Air Fryer basket. Set the Air Fryer to 375°F for 15 minutes. Use a meat thermometer to ensure the chops have reached an internal temperature of 145°F.

Nutrition: *Calories 200 Fat 9.69g Protein 23.45g Carbs 4.46g*

300. APRICOT GLAZED PORK TENDERLOINS

PREPARATION: 5 MIN   **COOKING:** 30 MIN   **SERVINGS:** 3

INGREDIENTS

- 1 tsp. salt
- 1/2 tsp. pepper
- 1 lb. pork tenderloin
- 2 tbsp. minced fresh rosemary or 1 tbsp. dried rosemary, crushed
- 2 tbsp. olive oil, divided
- 1 garlic cloves, minced
- Apricot Glaze Ingredients
- 1 cup apricot preserves
- 3 garlic cloves, minced
- 4 tbsp. lemon juice

DIRECTIONS

1. Mix well pepper, salt, garlic, oil, and rosemary. Brush all over pork. If needed cut pork crosswise in half to fit in Air Fryer. Lightly grease baking pan of Air Fryer with cooking spray. Add pork.
2. For 3 minutes per side, brown pork in a preheated 390°F Air Fryer. Meanwhile, mix well all glaze Ingredients in a small bowl. Baste pork every 5 minutes. Cook for 20 minutes at 330°F. Serve and enjoy.
3. or 6 minutes. Serve.

Nutrition: *Calories 454 Protein 43.76g Fat 16.71g Carbs 33.68g*

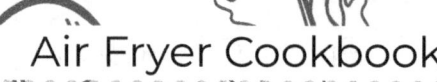

301. SWEET & SPICY COUNTRY-STYLE RIBS

PREPARATION: 10 MIN **COOKING:** 25 MIN **SERVINGS:** 4

INGREDIENTS

- 2 tbsp. brown sugar
- 2 tbsp. smoked paprika
- 1 tsp. garlic powder, 1 tsp. onion powder
- 1 tsp. dry mustard
- 1 tsp. ground cumin
- 1 tsp. kosher salt, 1 tsp. black pepper
- ¼ to ½ tsp. cayenne pepper
- 1½ lb. boneless country-style pork ribs
- 1 cup barbecue sauce

DIRECTIONS

1. In a small bowl, stir together the brown sugar, paprika, garlic powder, onion powder, dry mustard, cumin, salt, black pepper, and cayenne. Mix until well combined.
2. Pat the ribs dry with a paper towel. Generously sprinkle the rub evenly over both sides of the ribs and rub in with your fingers.
3. Place the ribs in the Air Fryer basket. Set the Air Fryer to 350°F for 15 minutes. Turn the ribs and brush with ½ cup of the barbecue sauce. Cook for an additional 10 minutes. Use a meat thermometer to ensure the pork has reached an internal temperature of 145°F. Serve with remaining barbecue sauce.

Nutrition: *Calories 416 Fat 12.19g Protein 38.39g Carbs 36.79g*

302. PORK TENDERS WITH BELL PEPPERS

PREPARATION: 5 MIN **COOKING:** 15 MIN **SERVINGS:** 4

INGREDIENTS

- 11 Oz Pork Tenderloin
- 1 Bell Pepper, in thin strips
- 1 Red Onion, sliced
- 2 Tsps. Provencal Herbs
- Black Pepper to taste
- 1 tbsp. Olive Oil
- 1/2 tbsp. Mustard

DIRECTIONS

1. Preheat the Air Fryer to 390°F.
2. In the oven dish, mix the bell pepper strips with the onion, herbs, and some salt and pepper to taste.
3. Add half a tbsp. of olive oil to the mixture
4. Cut the pork tenderloin into four pieces and rub with salt, pepper and mustard.
5. Thinly coat the pieces with remaining olive oil and place them upright in the oven dish on top of the pepper mixture
6. Place the bowl into the Air Fryer. Set the timer to 15 minutes and roast the meat and the vegetables
7. Turn the meat and mix the peppers halfway through. Serve with a fresh salad

Nutrition: *Calories 220 Fat 12.36g Protein 23.79g Carbs 2.45g*

303. WONTON MEATBALLS

PREPARATION: 15 MIN **COOKING:** 10 MIN **SERVINGS:** 4

INGREDIENTS

- 1-lb. ground pork
- 2 large eggs
- ¼ cup chopped green onions (white and green parts)
- ¼ cup chopped fresh cilantro or parsley
- 1 tbsp. minced fresh ginger
- 3 cloves garlic, minced
- 2 tsp.s soy sauce
- 1 tsp. oyster sauce
- ½ tsp. kosher salt
- 1 tsp. black pepper

DIRECTIONS

1. In the bowl of a stand mixer fitted with the paddle attachment, combine the pork, eggs, green onions, cilantro, ginger, garlic, soy sauce, oyster sauce, salt, and pepper. Mix on low speed until all of the ingredients are incorporated, 2 to 3 minutes.
2. Form the mixture into 12 meatballs and arrange in a single layer in the Air Fryer basket.
3. Set the Air Fryer to 350°F for 10 minutes. Use a meat thermometer to ensure the meatballs have reached an internal temperature of 145°F.
4. Transfer the meatballs to a bowl and serve.

Nutrition: *Calories 402 Fat 27.91g Carbs 3.1g Protein 32.69g*

304. BARBECUE FLAVORED PORK RIBS

PREPARATION: 5 MIN **COOKING:** 15 MIN **SERVINGS:** 6

INGREDIENTS

- ¼ cup honey, divided
- ¾ cup BBQ sauce
- 2 tbsp. tomato ketchup
- 1 tbsp. Worcestershire sauce
- 1 tbsp. soy sauce
- ½ tsp. garlic powder
- Freshly ground white pepper, to taste
- 1¾ lb. pork ribs

DIRECTIONS

1. In a large bowl, mix together 3 tbsp. of honey and remaining ingredients except pork ribs. Refrigerate to marinate for about 20 minutes. Preheat the Air Fryer to 355°F. Place the ribs in an Air Fryer basket.
2. Cook for about 13 minutes. Remove the ribs from the Air Fryer and coat with remaining honey. Serve hot.

Nutrition: *Calories 265 Fat 9.04g Protein 29.47g Carbs 15.87g*

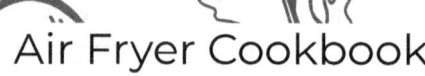

305. EASY AIR FRYER MARINATED PORK TENDERLOIN

PREPARATION: 1H 10M **COOKING:** 30 MIN **SERVINGS:** 4 TO 6

INGREDIENTS

- ¼ cup olive oil
- ¼ cup soy sauce
- ¼ cup freshly squeezed lemon juice
- 1 garlic clove, minced
- 1 tbsp. Dijon mustard
- 1 tsp. salt
- ½ tsp. freshly ground black pepper
- 2 lb. pork tenderloin

DIRECTIONS

1. In a large mixing bowl, make the marinade. Mix together the olive oil, soy sauce, lemon juice, minced garlic, Dijon mustard, salt, and pepper. Reserve ¼ cup of the marinade.
2. Place the tenderloin in a large bowl and pour the remaining marinade over the meat. Cover and marinate in the refrigerator for about 1 hour. Place the marinated pork tenderloin into the Air Fryer basket.
3. Set the temperature of your Air Fryer to 400°F. Set the timer and roast for 10 minutes. Using tongs, flip the pork and baste it with half of the reserved marinade. Reset the timer and roast for 10 minutes more.
4. Using tongs, flip the pork, then baste with the remaining marinade.
5. Reset the timer and roast for another 10 minutes, for a total cooking time of 30 minutes.

Nutrition: Calories 345 Fat 17.35g Carbs 3.66g Protein 41.56g

306. BALSAMIC GLAZED PORK CHOPS

PREPARATION: 5 MIN **COOKING:** 50 MIN **SERVINGS:** 4

INGREDIENTS

- ¾ cup balsamic vinegar
- 1 ½ tbsp. sugar
- 1 tbsp. butter
- 3 tbsp. olive oil
- 3 tbsp. salt
- 3 pork rib chops

DIRECTIONS

1. Place all ingredients in bowl and allow the meat to marinate in the fridge for at least 2 hours. Preheat the Air Fryer to 390°F. Place the grill pan accessory in the Air Fryer.
2. Grill the pork chops for 20 minutes making sure to flip the meat every 10 minutes for even grilling. Meanwhile, pour the balsamic vinegar on a saucepan and allow to simmer for at least 10 minutes until the sauce thickens. Brush the meat with the glaze before serving.

Nutrition: Calories 274 Fat 18g Carbs 7g Protein17g

307. PERFECT AIR FRIED PORK CHOPS

PREPARATION: 5 MIN   **COOKING:** 17 MIN   **SERVINGS:** 4

INGREDIENTS

- 3 cups bread crumbs
- ½ cup grated Parmesan cheese
- 2 tbsp. vegetable oil
- 2 tsp.s salt
- 2 tsp.s sweet paprika
- ½ tsp. onion powder
- ¼ tsp. garlic powder
- 6 (½-inch-thick) bone-in pork chops

DIRECTIONS

1. Spray the Air Fryer basket with olive oil. In a large resealable bag, combine the bread crumbs, Parmesan cheese, oil, salt, paprika, onion powder, and garlic powder. Seal the bag and shake it a few times in order for the spices to blend together. Place the pork chops, one by one, in the bag and shake to coat.
2. Place the pork chops in the greased Air Fryer basket in a single layer. Be careful not to overcrowd the basket. Spray the chops generously with olive oil to avoid powdery, uncooked breading.
3. Set the temperature of your Air Fryer to 360°F. Set the timer and roast for 10 minutes.
4. Using tongs, flip the chops. Spray them generously with olive oil. Reset the timer and roast for 7 minutes more.
5. Check that the pork has reached an internal temperature of 145°F. Add cooking time if needed.

Nutrition: Calories 513 Fat 23g Carbs 22g Protein 50g

308. RUSTIC PORK RIBS

PREPARATION: 5 MIN   **COOKING:** 15 MIN   **SERVINGS:** 4

INGREDIENTS

- 1 rack of pork ribs
- 3 tbsp. dry red wine
- 1 tbsp. soy sauce
- 1/2 tsp. dried thyme
- 1/2 tsp. onion powder
- 1/2 tsp. garlic powder
- 1/2 tsp. ground black pepper
- 1 tsp. smoked salt
- 1 tbsp. cornstarch
- 1/2 tsp. olive oil

DIRECTIONS

1. Begin by preheating your Air Fryer to 390°F. Place all ingredients in a mixing bowl and let them marinate for at least 1 hour.
2. Cook the marinated ribs approximately 25 minutes at 390°F. Serve hot.

Nutrition: Calories 119 Protein 12.26g Fat 5.61g Carbs 3.64g

309. AIR FRYER BABY BACK RIBS

PREPARATION: 5 MIN **COOKING:** 25 MIN **SERVINGS:** 4

INGREDIENTS

- 1 rack baby back ribs
- 1 tbsp. garlic powder
- 1 tsp. freshly ground black pepper
- 2 tbsp. salt
- 1 cup barbecue sauce (any type)

Nutrition: Calories 422 Fat 27g Carbs 25g Protein 18g

DIRECTIONS

1. Dry the ribs with a paper towel.
2. Season the ribs with the garlic powder, pepper, and salt. Place the seasoned ribs into the Air Fryer.
3. Set the temperature of your Air Fryer to 400°F. Set the timer and grill for 10 minutes.
4. Using tongs, flip the ribs. Reset the timer and grill for another 10 minutes.
5. Once the ribs are cooked, use a pastry brush to brush on the barbecue sauce, then set the timer and grill for a final 3 to 5 minutes.

310. PARMESAN CRUSTED PORK CHOPS

PREPARATION: 10 MIN **COOKING:** 15 MIN **SERVINGS:** 8

INGREDIENTS

- 3 tbsp. grated parmesan cheese
- 1 C. pork rind crumbs
- 2 beaten eggs
- ¼ tsp. chili powder
- ½ tsp. onion powder
- 1 tsp. smoked paprika
- ¼ tsp. pepper
- ½ tsp. salt
- 4-6 thick boneless pork chops

Nutrition: Calories 422 Fat 19g Carbs 16g Protein 38g

DIRECTIONS

1. Ensure your Air Fryer is preheated to 400°F.
2. With pepper and salt, season both sides of pork chops.
3. In a food processor, pulse pork rinds into crumbs. Mix crumbs with other seasonings.
4. Beat eggs and add to another bowl. Dip pork chops into eggs then into pork rind crumb mixture.
5. Spray down Air Fryer with olive oil and add pork chops to the basket. Set temperature to 400°F, and set time to 15 minutes.

311. CRISPY DUMPLINGS

PREPARATION: 10 MIN **COOKING:** 10 MIN **SERVINGS:** 8

INGREDIENTS

- .5 lb. Ground pork
- 1 tbsp. Olive oil
- .5 tsp. each Black pepper and salt
- Half of 1 pkg. Dumpling wrappers

Nutrition: Calories 110 Fat 8.34g Carbs 0.27g Protein 8.1g

DIRECTIONS

1. 1. Set the Air Fryer temperature setting at 390°F.
2. 2.Mix the fixings together. Prepare each dumpling using two tsp.s of the pork mixture.
3. 3.Seal the edges with a portion of water to make the triangle form.
4. 4. Lightly spray the Air Fryer basket using a cooking oil spray as needed. Add the dumplings to air-fry for eight minutes.
5. 5.Serve when they're ready.

312. PORK JOINT

PREPARATION: 10 MIN **COOKING:** 20 MIN **SERVINGS:** 10

INGREDIENTS

- 3 cups Cooked shredded pork tenderloin or chicken
- 2 cups Fat-free shredded mozzarella
- 10 small Flour tortillas
- Lime juice

DIRECTIONS

1. Set the Air Fryer at 380°F. Sprinkle the juice over the pork.
2. Microwave five of the tortillas at a time (putting a damp paper towel over them for 10 seconds). Add three oz. of pork and ¼ of a cup of cheese to each tortilla.
3. Tightly roll the tortillas. Line the tortillas onto a greased foil-lined pan.
4. Spray an even coat of cooking oil spray over the tortillas.
5. Air Fry for 7 to 10 minutes or until the tortillas are a golden color, flipping halfway through.

Nutrition: Calories 334 Fat 6.87g Protein 32.03g Carbs 33.92g

313. PORK SATAY

PREPARATION: 15 MIN **COOKING:** 9-14 MIN **SERVINGS:** 4

INGREDIENTS

- 1 (1-lb.) pork tenderloin, cut into 1½-inch cubes
- ¼ cup minced onion
- garlic cloves, minced
- 1 jalapeño pepper, minced
- tbsp. freshly squeezed lime juice
- tbsp. coconut milk
- tbsp. unsalted peanut butter
- tsp.s curry powder

DIRECTIONS

1. In a medium bowl, mix the pork, onion, garlic, jalapeño, lime juice, coconut milk, peanut butter, and curry powder until well combined. Let stand for 10 minutes at room temperature.
2. With a slotted spoon, remove the pork from the marinade. Reserve the marinade.
3. Thread the pork onto about 8 bamboo (see Tip, here) or metal skewers. Grill for 9 to 14 minutes, brushing once with the reserved marinade, until the pork reaches at least 145°F on a meat thermometer. Discard any remaining marinade. Serve immediately.

Nutrition: Calories 194 Fat 7g Carbs 7g Protein 25g

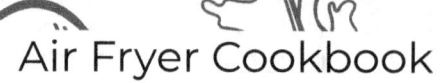

314. PORK BURGERS WITH RED CABBAGE SALAD

PREPARATION: 20 MIN   **COOKING:** 7-9 MIN   **SERVINGS:** 4

INGREDIENTS

- ½ cup Greek yogurt
- 2 tbsp. low-sodium mustard, divided
- 1 tbsp. lemon juice
- ¼ cup sliced red cabbage
- ¼ cup grated carrots
- 1-lb. lean ground pork
- ½ tsp. paprika
- 1 cup mixed baby lettuce greens
- small tomatoes, sliced
- small low-sodium whole-wheat sandwich buns, cut in half

DIRECTIONS

1. In a small bowl, combine the yogurt, 1 tbsp. mustard, lemon juice, cabbage, and carrots; mix and refrigerate.
2. In a medium bowl, combine the pork, remaining 1 tbsp. mustard, and paprika. Form into 8 small patties.
3. Put the sliders into the Air Fryer basket. Grill for 7 to 9 minutes at 370°F, or until the sliders register 165°F as tested with a meat thermometer.
4. Assemble the burgers by placing some of the lettuce greens on a bun bottom. Top with a tomato slice, the ¬burgers, and the cabbage mixture. Add the bun top and serve immediately.

Nutrition: Calories 472 Fat 15g Carbs 15g Protein 35g

315. CRISPY MUSTARD PORK TENDERLOIN

PREPARATION: 10 MIN   **COOKING:** 12-16 MIN   **SERVINGS:** 4

INGREDIENTS

- tbsp. low-sodium grainy mustard
- tsp.s olive oil
- ¼ tsp. dry mustard powder
- 1 (1-lb.) pork tenderloin, silver skin and excess fat trimmed and discarded (see Tip, here)
- slices low-sodium whole-wheat bread, crumbled
- ¼ cup ground walnuts
- tbsp. cornstarch

DIRECTIONS

1. In a small bowl, stir together the mustard, olive oil, and mustard powder. Spread this mixture over the pork.
2. On a plate, mix the bread crumbs, walnuts, and cornstarch. Dip the mustard-coated pork into the crumb ¬mixture to coat.
3. Air fry the pork for 12 to 16 minutes at 370°F, or until it registers at least 145°F on a meat thermometer. Slice to serve.

Nutrition: Calories 239 Fat 9g Carbs 15g Protein 26g

316. APPLE PORK TENDERLOIN

PREPARATION: 10 MIN **COOKING:** 14-19 MIN **SERVINGS:** 4

INGREDIENTS

- 1 (1-lb.) pork tenderloin, cut into 4 pieces
- 1 tbsp. apple butter
- 2 tsp.s olive oil
- 2 Granny Smith apples or Jonagold apples, sliced
- 3 celery stalks, sliced
- 1 onion, sliced
- ½ tsp. dried marjoram
- ⅓ cup apple juice

DIRECTIONS

1. Rub each piece of pork with the apple butter and olive oil.
2. In a medium metal bowl, mix the pork, apples, celery, onion, marjoram, and apple juice.
3. Place the bowl into the Air Fryer and roast for 14 to 19 minutes at 365°F, or until the pork reaches at least 145°F on a meat thermometer and the apples and vegetables are tender. Stir once during cooking. Serve immediately.

Nutrition: Calories 213 Fat 5g Carbs 20g Protein 24g

317. ESPRESSO-GRILLED PORK TENDERLOIN

PREPARATION: 15 MIN **COOKING:** 9-11 MIN **SERVINGS:** 4

INGREDIENTS

- 1 tbsp. packed brown sugar
- 2 tsp.s espresso powder
- 1 tsp. ground paprika
- ½ tsp. dried marjoram
- 1 tbsp. honey
- 1 tbsp. freshly squeezed lemon juice
- 2 tsp.s olive oil
- 1 (1-lb.) pork tenderloin

DIRECTIONS

1. In a small bowl, mix the brown sugar, espresso powder, paprika, and marjoram.
2. Stir in the honey, lemon juice, and olive oil until well mixed.
3. Spread the honey mixture over the pork and let stand for 10 minutes at room temperature.
4. Roast the tenderloin in the Air Fryer basket for 9 to 11 minutes at 365°F, or until the pork registers at least 145°F on a meat thermometer. Slice the meat to serve.

Nutrition: Calories 177 Fat 5g Carbs 10g Protein 23g

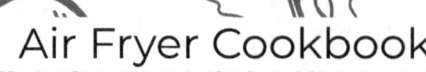

318. PORK AND POTATOES

PREPARATION: 5 MIN **COOKING:** 25 MIN **SERVINGS:** 4

INGREDIENTS

- 2 cups creamer potatoes, rinsed and dried
- 2 tsp.s olive oil
- 1 (1-lb.) pork tenderloin, cut into 1-inch cubes
- 1 onion, chopped
- 1 red bell pepper, chopped
- 2 garlic cloves, minced
- ½ tsp. dried oregano
- 2 tbsp. low-sodium chicken broth

Nutrition: Calories 235 Fat 5g Carbs 22g Protein 26g

DIRECTIONS

1. In a medium bowl, toss the potatoes and olive oil to coat.
2. Transfer the potatoes to the Air Fryer basket. Roast for 15 minutes at 380°F.
3. In a medium metal bowl, mix the potatoes, pork, onion, red bell pepper, garlic, and oregano.
4. Drizzle with the chicken broth. Put the bowl in the Air Fryer basket. Roast for about 10 minutes more, shaking the basket once during cooking, until the pork reaches at least 145°F on a meat thermometer and the potatoes are tender. Serve immediately.

319. PORK AND FRUIT KEBABS

PREPARATION: 15 MIN **COOKING:** 9-12 MIN **SERVINGS:** 4

INGREDIENTS

- ⅓ cup apricot jam
- 2 tbsp. freshly squeezed lemon juice
- 2 tsp.s olive oil
- ½ tsp. dried tarragon
- 1 (1-lb.) pork tenderloin, cut into 1-inch cubes
- 4 plums, pitted and quartered
- 4 small apricots, pitted and halved

Nutrition: Calories 256 Fat 5g Carbs 30g Protein 24g

DIRECTIONS

1. In a large bowl, mix the jam, lemon juice, olive oil, and tarragon.
2. Add the pork and stir to coat. Let stand for 10 minutes at room temperature.
3. Alternating the items, thread the pork, plums, and ¬apricots onto 4 metal skewers that fit into the Air Fryer. Brush with any remaining jam mixture. Discard any remaining marinade.
4. Grill the kebabs in the Air Fryer for 9 to 12 minutes 365°F, or until the pork reaches 145°F on a meat thermometer and the fruit is tender. Serve immediately.

320. STEAK AND VEGETABLE KEBABS

PREPARATION: 15 MIN **COOKING:** 5 TO 7 MIN **SERVINGS:** 4

INGREDIENTS

- 2 tbsp. balsamic vinegar
- 2 tsp.s olive oil
- ½ tsp. dried marjoram
- ⅛ tsp. freshly ground black pepper
- ¾ lb. round steak, cut into 1-inch pieces
- 1 red bell pepper, sliced
- 16 button mushrooms
- 1 cup cherry tomatoes

Nutrition: Calories 194 Fat 6g Carbs 7g Protein 31g

DIRECTIONS

1. In a medium bowl, stir together the balsamic vinegar, olive oil, marjoram, and black pepper.
2. Add the steak and stir to coat. Let stand for 10 minutes at room temperature.
3. Alternating items, thread the beef, red bell pepper, mushrooms, and tomatoes onto 8 bamboo (see Tip, here) or metal skewers that fit in the Air Fryer.
4. Grill in the Air Fryer for 5 to 7 minutes at 370°F, or until the beef is browned and reaches at least 145°F on a meat thermo¬meter. Serve immediately.

321. SPICY GRILLED STEAK

PREPARATION: 7 MIN   **COOKING:** 6-9 MIN   **SERVINGS:** 4

INGREDIENTS

- 2 tbsp. low-sodium salsa
- 1 tbsp. minced chipotle pepper
- 1 tbsp. apple cider vinegar
- 1 tsp. ground cumin
- ⅛ tsp. freshly ground black pepper
- ⅛ tsp. red pepper flakes
- ¾ lb. sirloin tip steak, cut into 4 pieces and gently pounded to about ⅓ inch thick

DIRECTIONS

1. In a small bowl, thoroughly mix the salsa, chipotle pepper, cider vinegar, cumin, black pepper, and red pepper flakes. Rub this mixture into both sides of each steak piece. Let stand for 15 minutes at room temperature.
2. Grill the steaks in the Air Fryer at 365°F, two at a time, for 6 to 9 minutes, or until they reach at least 145°F on a meat thermometer.
3. Remove the steaks to a clean plate and cover with aluminum foil to keep warm. Repeat with the remaining steaks.
4. Slice the steaks thinly against the grain and serve.

Nutrition: Calories 160 Fat 6g Carbs 1g Protein 24g

322. GREEK VEGETABLE SKILLET

PREPARATION: 10 MIN   **COOKING** 9-19 MIN   **SERVINGS:** 4

INGREDIENTS

- ½ lb. 96 percent lean ground beef
- 2 medium tomatoes, chopped
- 1 onion, chopped
- 2 garlic cloves, minced
- 2 cups fresh baby spinach
- 2 tbsp. freshly squeezed lemon juice
- ⅓ cup low-sodium beef broth
- 2 tbsp. crumbled low-sodium feta cheese

DIRECTIONS

1. In a 6-by-2-inch metal pan, crumble the beef. Cook in the Air Fryer for 3 to 7 minutes at 370°F, stirring once during cooking, until browned. Drain off any fat or liquid.
2. Add the tomatoes, onion, and garlic to the pan. Air-fry for 4 to 8 minutes more, or until the onion is tender.
3. Add the spinach, lemon juice, and beef broth. Air-fry for 2 to 4 minutes more, or until the spinach is wilted.
4. Sprinkle with the feta cheese and serve immediately

Nutrition: Calories 97 Fat 1g Carbs 5g Protein 15g

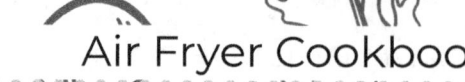
Air Fryer Cookbook

323. LIGHT HERBED MEATBALLS

PREPARATION: 10 MIN **COOKING:** 12-17 MIN **SERVINGS:** 24

INGREDIENTS

- 1 medium onion, minced
- 2 garlic cloves, minced
- 1 tsp. olive oil
- 1 slice low-sodium whole-wheat bread, crumbled
- 3 tbsp. 1 percent milk
- 1 tsp. dried marjoram
- 1 tsp. dried basil
- 1-lb. 96 percent lean ground beef

DIRECTIONS

1. In a 6-by-2-inch pan, combine the onion, garlic, and olive oil. Air-fry for 2 to 4 minutes at 370°F, or until the vegetables are crisp-tender.
2. Transfer the vegetables to a medium bowl, and add the bread crumbs, milk, marjoram, and basil. Mix well.
3. Add the ground beef. With your hands, work the mixture gently but thoroughly until combined. Form the meat mixture into about 24 (1-inch) meatballs.
4. Bake the meatballs, in batches, in the Air Fryer basket for 12 to 17 minutes, or until they reach 160°F on a meat thermometer. Serve immediately.

Nutrition: Calories 190 Fat 6g Carbs 8g Protein 25g

324. BROWN RICE AND BEEF-STUFFED BELL PEPPERS

PREPARATION: 10 MIN **COOKING:** 11-16 MIN **SERVINGS:** 4

INGREDIENTS

- 4 medium bell peppers, any colors, rinsed, tops removed
- 1 medium onion, chopped
- ½ cup grated carrot
- 2 tsp.s olive oil
- 2 medium beefsteak tomatoes, chopped
- 1 cup cooked brown rice
- 1 cup chopped cooked low-sodium roast beef
- 1 tsp. dried marjoram

DIRECTIONS

1. Remove the stems from the bell pepper tops and chop the tops.
2. In a 6-by-2-inch pan, combine the chopped bell pepper tops, onion, carrot, and olive oil. Cook for 2 to 4 minutes, or until the vegetables are crisp-tender.
3. Transfer the vegetables to a medium bowl. Add the ¬tomatoes, brown rice, roast beef, and marjoram. Stir to mix.
4. Stuff the vegetable mixture into the bell peppers. Place the bell peppers in the Air Fryer basket. Bake for 11 to 16 minutes at 355°F, or until the peppers are tender and the filling is hot. Serve immediately.

Nutrition: Calories 206 Fat 6g Carbs 20g Protein 18g

Air Fryer Cookbook

325. BEEF AND BROCCOLI

PREPARATION: 10 MIN   **COOKING:** 14-18 MIN   **SERVINGS:** 4

INGREDIENTS

- 2 tbsp. cornstarch
- ½ cup low-sodium beef broth
- 1 tsp. low-sodium soy sauce
- 12 oz. sirloin strip steak, cut into 1-inch cubes
- 2½ cups broccoli florets
- 1 onion, chopped
- 1 cup sliced cremini mushrooms
- 1 tbsp. grated fresh ginger
- Brown rice, cooked (optional)

DIRECTIONS

1. In a medium bowl, stir together the cornstarch, beef broth, and soy sauce.
2. Add the beef and toss to coat. Let stand for 5 minutes at room temperature.
3. With a slotted spoon, transfer the beef from the broth mixture into a medium metal bowl. Reserve the broth.
4. Add the broccoli, onion, mushrooms, and ginger to the beef. Place the bowl into the Air Fryer and cook for 12 to 15 minutes at 370°F, or until the beef reaches at least 145°F on a meat thermometer and the vegetables are tender.
5. Add the reserved broth and cook for 2 to 3 minutes more, or until the sauce boils.
6. Serve immediately over hot cooked brown rice, if desired.

Nutrition: Calories 240 Fat 6g Carbs 11g Protein 19g

326. BEEF AND FRUIT STIR-FRY

PREPARATION: 5 MIN   **COOKING:** 25 MIN   **SERVINGS:** 2

INGREDIENTS

- 12 oz. sirloin tip steak, thinly sliced
- 1 tbsp. freshly squeezed lime juice
- 1 cup canned mandarin orange segments, drained, juice reserved
- 1 cup canned pineapple chunks, drained, juice reserved
- 1 tsp. low-sodium soy sauce
- 1 tbsp. cornstarch
- 1 tsp. olive oil
- 2 scallions, white and green parts, sliced
- Brown rice, cooked (optional)

DIRECTIONS

1. In a medium bowl, mix the steak with the lime juice. Set aside.
2. In a small bowl, thoroughly mix 3 tbsp. of reserved mandarin orange juice, 3 tbsp. of reserved pineapple juice, the soy sauce, and cornstarch.
3. Drain the beef and transfer it to a medium metal bowl, reserving the juice. Stir the reserved juice into the mandarin-pineapple juice mixture. Set aside.
4. Add the olive oil and scallions to the steak. Place the metal bowl in the Air Fryer and cook for 3 to 4 minutes at 365°F, or until the steak is almost cooked, shaking the basket once during cooking.
5. Stir in the mandarin oranges, pineapple, and juice ¬mixture. Cook for 3 to 7 minutes more, or until the sauce is bubbling and the beef is tender and reaches at least 145°F on a meat thermometer.
6. Stir and serve over hot cooked brown rice, if desired.

Nutrition: Calories 212 Fat 4g Carbs 28g Protein 19g

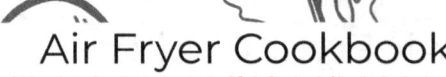

Air Fryer Cookbook

327. GARLIC PUTTER PORK CHOPS

PREPARATION: 10 MIN **COOKING:** 10 MIN **SERVINGS:** 4

INGREDIENTS

- tsp. parsley
- tsp. grated garlic cloves
- 1 tbsp. coconut oil
- 1 tbsp. coconut butter
- pork chops

Nutrition: Calories 526 Fat 23g Carbs 10g Protein 41g

DIRECTIONS

1. Ensure your Air Fryer is preheated to 350°F.
2. Mix butter, coconut oil, and all seasoning together. Then rub seasoning mixture over all sides of pork chops. Place in foil, seal, and chill for 1 hour.
3. Remove pork chops from foil and place into Air Fryer.
4. Set temperature to 350°F, and set time to 7 minutes. Cook 7 minutes on one side and 8 minutes on the other.
5. Drizzle with olive oil and serve alongside a green salad.

328. CAJUN PORK STEAKS

PREPARATION: 5 MIN **COOKING:** 20 MIN **SERVINGS:** 6

INGREDIENTS

- 4-6 pork steaks
- BBQ sauce:
- Cajun seasoning
- 1 tbsp. vinegar
- 1 tsp. low-sodium soy sauce
- ½ C. brown sugar

Nutrition: Calories 209 Fat 11g Carbs 7g Protein 28g

DIRECTIONS

1. Ensure your Air Fryer is preheated to 290°F.
2. Sprinkle pork steaks with Cajun seasoning.
3. Combine remaining ingredients and brush onto steaks. Add coated steaks to Air Fryer.
4. Set temperature to 290°F, and set time to 20 minutes. Cook 15-20 minutes till just browned.

329. CAJUN SWEET-SOUR GRILLED PORK

PREPARATION: 5 MIN **COOKING:** 12 MIN **SERVINGS:** 3

INGREDIENTS

- ¼ cup brown sugar
- 1/4 cup cider vinegar
- 1-lb pork loin, sliced into 1-inch cubes
- 2 tbsp. Cajun seasoning
- 3 tbsp. brown sugar

Nutrition: Calories 428 Fat 16.7g Carbs 5g Protein 39g

DIRECTIONS

1. In a shallow dish, mix well pork loin, 3 tbsp. brown sugar, and Cajun seasoning. Toss well to coat. Marinate in the ref for 3 hours.
2. In a medium bowl mix well, brown sugar and vinegar for basting.
3. Thread pork pieces in skewers. Baste with sauce and place on skewer rack in Air Fryer.
4. For 12 minutes, cook on 360°F. Halfway through Cooking Time, turnover skewers and baste with sauce. If needed, cook in batches.
5. Serve and enjoy.

330. PORK LOIN WITH POTATOES

PREPARATION: 5 MIN **COOKING:** 40 MIN **SERVINGS:** 6

INGREDIENTS

- 2 lb. pork loin
- large red potatoes, chopped
- ½ tsp. garlic powder
- ½ tsp. red pepper flakes, crushed
- Salt and black pepper, to taste

Nutrition: Calories 260 Fat 8g Carbs 27g Protein 21g

DIRECTIONS

1. In a large bowl, put all of the ingredients together except glaze and toss to coat well. Preheat the Air Fryer to 325°F. Place the loin in the Air Fryer basket.
2. Arrange the potatoes around pork loin.
3. Cook for about 25 minutes.

331. ROASTED CHAR SIEW (PORK BUTT)

PREPARATION: 10 MIN **COOKING:** 25 MIN **SERVINGS:** 4

INGREDIENTS

- 1 strip of pork shoulder butt with a good amount of fat marbling

Marinade:
- 1 tsp. sesame oil
- tbsp. raw honey
- 1 tsp. light soy sauce
- 1 tbsp. rose wine

Nutrition: Calories 289 Fat 13g Carbs 6g Protein 33g

DIRECTIONS

1. Mix all of the marinade ingredients together and put it to a Ziploc bag. Place pork in bag, making sure all sections of pork strip are engulfed in the marinade. Chill 3-24 hours.
2. Take out the strip 30 minutes before planning to cook and preheat your Air Fryer to 350°F.
3. Place foil on small pan and brush with olive oil. Place marinated pork strip onto prepared pan.
4. Set temperature to 350°F, and set time to 20 minutes. Roast 20 minutes.
5. Glaze with marinade every 5-10 minutes.
6. Remove strip and leave to cool a few minutes before slicing.

332. ASIAN PORK CHOPS

PREPARATION: 2H 10M **COOKING:** 15 MIN **SERVINGS:** 2

INGREDIENTS

- 1/2 cup hoisin sauce
- tbsp. cider vinegar
- 1 tbsp. Asian sweet chili sauce
- (1/2-inch-thick) boneless pork chops
- salt and pepper

Nutrition: Calories 338 Fat 21g Carbs 28g Protein 19g

DIRECTIONS

1. Stir together hoisin, chili sauce, and vinegar in a large mixing bowl. Separate a quarter cup of this mixture, then add pork chops to the bowl and let it sit in the fridge for 2 hours. Take out the pork chops and place them on a plate. Sprinkle each side of the pork chop evenly with salt and pepper.
2. Cook at 360°F or 14 minutes, flipping half way through. Brush with reserved marinade and serve.

333. MARINATED PORK CHOPS

PREPARATION: 10 MIN **COOKING:** 30 MIN **SERVINGS:** 2

INGREDIENTS

- pork chops, boneless
- 1 tsp. garlic powder
- ½ cup flour
- 1 cup buttermilk
- Salt and pepper

DIRECTIONS

1. Add pork chops and buttermilk in a zip-lock bag. Seal the bag and set aside in the refrigerator overnight.
2. In another zip-lock bag add flour, garlic powder, pepper, and salt.
3. Remove marinated pork chops from buttermilk and add in flour mixture and shake until well coated.
4. Preheat the Air Fryer oven to 380°F.
5. Spray Air Fryer tray with cooking spray.
6. Arrange pork chops on a tray and Air Fryer for 28-30 minutes. Turn pork chops after 18 minutes.
7. Serve and enjoy.

Nutrition: Calories 424 Fat 21.3g Carbs 30.8g Protein 25.5g

334. STEAK WITH CHEESE BUTTER

PREPARATION: 10 MIN **COOKING:** 8-10 MIN **SERVINGS:** 2

INGREDIENTS

- 2 rib-eye steaks
- tsp. garlic powder
- 1/2 tbsp. blue cheese butter
- 1 tsp. pepper
- tsp. kosher salt

Nutrition: Calories 830 Fat 60g Carbs 3g Protein 70g

DIRECTIONS

1. Preheat the Air Fryer to 400°F.
2. Mix together garlic powder, pepper, and salt and rub over the steaks.
3. Spray Air Fryer basket with cooking spray.
4. Put the steak in the Air Fryer basket and cook for 4-5 minutes on each side.
5. Top with blue butter cheese.
6. Serve and enjoy.

335. MADEIRA BEEF

PREPARATION: 5 MIN **COOKING:** 20 MIN **SERVINGS:** 4

INGREDIENTS

- 1 cup Madeira
- 1 and ½ lb. beef meat, cubed
- Salt and black pepper to the taste
- 1 yellow onion, thinly sliced
- 1 chili pepper, sliced

Nutrition: Calories 295 Fat 16 Carbs 20 Protein 15

DIRECTIONS

1. Put the reversible rack in the Air Fryer, add the baking pan inside and mix all the ingredients in it.
2. Cook on Baking mode at 380°F for 25 minutes, divide the mix into bowls and serve.

336. CREAMY PORK AND ZUCCHINIS

PREPARATION: 5 MIN   **COOKING:** 25 MIN   **SERVINGS:** 4

INGREDIENTS

- 1 and ½ lb. pork stew meat, cubed
- 1 cup tomato sauce
- 1 tbsp. olive oil
- 2 zucchinis, sliced
- Salt and black pepper to the taste

DIRECTIONS

1. Put the reversible rack in the Air Fryer, add the baking pan inside and mix all the ingredients in it.
2. Cook on Baking mode at 380°F, divide the mix into bowls and serve.

Nutrition: Calories 284 Fat 12 Carbs 17 Protein 12

337. BULLET-PROOF BEEF ROAST

PREPARATION: 2 H   **COOKING:** 2H 5M   **SERVINGS:** 2

INGREDIENTS

- 1 cup of organic beef
- tbsp. olive oil
- 1 lb. beef round roast
- Salt and pepper, to taste

DIRECTIONS

1. Place all of the ingredients in a resealable bag and let it marinate in the fridge for about two hours.
2. Fix the temperature to 400°F and preheat the Air Fryer for 5 minutes.
3. Place the ingredients in the Ziploc bag in a baking tray that will fit the Air Fryer.
4. Let it cook for 2 hours at a temperature of 400°F.
5. Serve while it is warm.

Nutrition: Calories 280 Fat 15g Carbs 13g Protein 26g

338. LAMB BURGERS

PREPARATION: 15 MIN   **COOKING:** 8 MIN   **SERVINGS:** 6

INGREDIENTS

- 2 lb. ground lamb
- 1 tbsp. onion powder
- Salt and ground black pepper, as required

DIRECTIONS

1. In a bowl, add all the ingredients and mix well.
2. Make 6 equal-sized patties from the mixture. Arrange the patties onto a cooking tray.
3. Arrange the drip pan in the bottom of the Air Fryer.
4. Air fry for 8 minutes at 360°F and turn the burgers after 4 minutes
5. When cooking time is complete, remove the tray from Air Fryer and serve hot.

Nutrition: Calories 285 Carbs 0.9g Fat 11.1g Protein 42.6g

FISH AND SEAFOOD

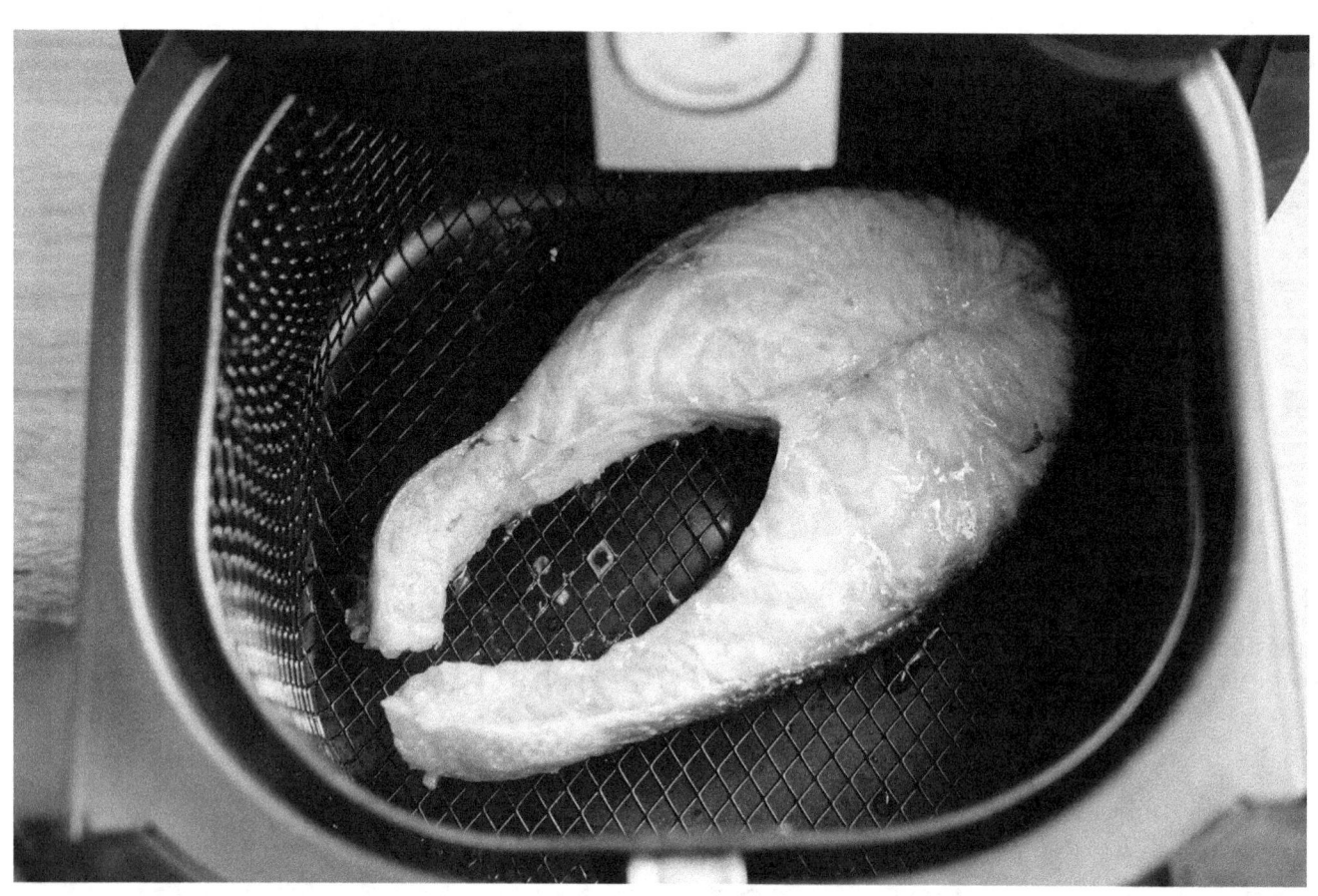

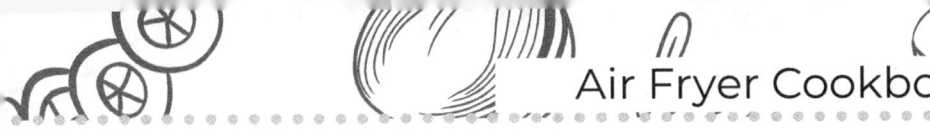

339. LEMON BUTTER SCALLOPS

PREPARATION: 1H 5M   **COOKING:** 10 MIN   **SERVINGS:** 4

INGREDIENTS

- 1 lemon
- 1 lb. scallops
- ½ cup butter
- ¼ cup parsley, chopped

DIRECTIONS

1. Juice the lemon into a Ziploc bag.
2. Wash your scallops, dry them, and season to taste. Put them in the bag with the lemon juice. Refrigerate for an hour.
3. Remove the bag from the refrigerator and leave for about twenty minutes until it returns to room temperature. Transfer the scallops into a foil pan that is small enough to be placed inside the fryer.
4. Pre-heat the fryer at 400°F and put the rack inside.
5. Place the foil pan on the rack, and cook for five minutes.
6. In the meantime, melt the butter in a saucepan over a medium heat. Zest the lemon over the saucepan, then add in the chopped parsley. Mix well.
7. Take care when removing the pan from the fryer. Transfer the contents to a plate and drizzle with the lemon-butter mixture. Serve hot.

Nutrition: Calories 412 Fat 17g Carbs 18g Protein 26g

340. CHEESY LEMON HALIBUT

PREPARATION: 5 MIN   **COOKING:** 10 MIN   **SERVINGS:** 4

INGREDIENTS

- 1 lb. halibut fillet
- ½ cup butter
- 2 ½ tbsp. mayonnaise
- 2 ½ tbsp. lemon juice
- ¾ cup parmesan cheese, grated

DIRECTIONS

1. Pre-heat your fryer at 375°F.
2. Spritz the halibut fillets with cooking spray and season as desired.
3. Put the halibut in the fryer and cook for twelve minutes.
4. In the meantime, combine the butter, mayonnaise, and lemon juice in a bowl with a hand mixer. Ensure a creamy texture is achieved.
5. Stir in the grated parmesan.
6. When the halibut is ready, open the drawer and spread the butter over the fish with a butter knife. Let it cook for a couple more minutes, then serve hot.

Nutrition: Calories 354 Fat 21g Carbs 23g Protein 19g

341. SPICY MACKEREL

PREPARATION: 5 MIN **COOKING:** 10 MIN **SERVINGS:** 4

INGREDIENTS

- 2 mackerel fillets
- 2 tbsp. red chili flakes
- 2 tsp. garlic, minced
- 1 tsp. lemon juice

Nutrition: Calories 393 Fat 12g Carbs 13g Protein 35g

DIRECTIONS

1. Season the mackerel fillets with the red pepper flakes, minced garlic, and a drizzle of lemon juice. Allow to sit for five minutes.
2. Preheat your fryer at 350°F.
3. Cook the mackerel for five minutes, before opening the drawer, flipping the fillets, and allowing to cook on the other side for another five minutes.
4. Plate the fillets, making sure to spoon any remaining juice over them before serving.

342. THYME SCALLOPS

PREPARATION: 5 MIN **COOKING:** 10 MIN **SERVINGS:** 4

INGREDIENTS

- 1 lb. scallops
- Salt and pepper
- ½ tbsp. butter
- ½ cup thyme, chopped

Nutrition: Calories 454 Fat 18g Carbs 27g Protein 34g

DIRECTIONS

1. Wash the scallops and dry them completely. Season with pepper and salt, then set aside while you prepare the pan.
2. Grease a foil pan in several spots with the butter and cover the bottom with the thyme. Place the scallops on top.
3. Pre-heat the fryer at 400°F and set the rack inside.
4. Place the foil pan on the rack and allow to cook for seven minutes.
5. Take care when removing the pan from the fryer and transfer the scallops to a serving dish. Spoon any remaining butter in the pan over the fish and enjoy.

343. CHINESE STYLE COD

PREPARATION: 5 MIN **COOKING:** 10 MIN **SERVINGS:** 2

INGREDIENTS

- 2 medium cod fillets; boneless
- 1 tbsp. light soy sauce
- 1/2 tsp. ginger; grated
- 1 tsp. peanuts; crushed
- 2 tsp. garlic powder

Nutrition: Calories 254 Fat 10g Carbs 14g Protein 23g

DIRECTIONS

1. Put fish fillets in a heat proof dish that fits your Air Fryer, add garlic powder, soy sauce and ginger; toss well, put in your Air Fryer and cook at 350°F, for 10 minutes.
2. Divide fish on plates, sprinkle peanuts on top and serve.

344. MUSTARD SALMON RECIPE

| PREPARATION: 5 MIN | COOKING: 10 MIN | SERVINGS: 4 |

INGREDIENTS

- 1 big salmon fillet; boneless
- 2 tbsp. mustard
- 1 tbsp. coconut oil
- 1 tbsp. maple extract
- Salt and black pepper to the taste

DIRECTIONS

1. In a bowl; mix maple extract with mustard, whisk well, season salmon with salt and pepper and brush salmon with this mix.
2. Spray some cooking spray over fish; place in your Air Fryer and cook at 370°F, for 10 minutes; flipping halfway. Serve with a tasty side salad.

Nutrition: Calories 300 Fat 7g Carbs 16g Protein 20g

345. SALMON AND ORANGE MARMALADE RECIPE

| PREPARATION: 5 MIN | COOKING: 20 MIN | SERVINGS: 4 |

INGREDIENTS

- 1 lb. wild salmon; skinless, boneless and cubed
- 1/4 cup orange juice
- 1/3 cup orange marmalade
- 1/4 cup balsamic vinegar
- A pinch of salt and black pepper

DIRECTIONS

1. Heat up a pot with the vinegar over medium heat; add marmalade and orange juice; stir, bring to a simmer, cook for 1 minute and take off heat.
2. Thread salmon cubes on skewers, season with salt and black pepper, brush them with half of the orange marmalade mix, arrange in your Air Fryer's basket and cook at 360°F, for 3 minutes on each side. Brush skewers with the rest of the vinegar mix; divide among plates and serve right away with a side salad.

Nutrition: Calories 240 Fat 9g Carbs 14g Protein 10g

346. TILAPIA & CHIVES SAUCE

| PREPARATION: 5 MIN | COOKING: 10 MIN | SERVINGS: 4 |

INGREDIENTS

- 4 medium tilapia fillets
- 2 tsp. honey
- Juice from 1 lemon
- 2 tbsp. chives; chopped
- Salt and black pepper to the taste

DIRECTIONS

1. Flavor fish with salt and pepper, spray with cooking spray, place in preheated Air Fryer 350°F and cook for 8 minutes; flipping halfway.
2. Meanwhile; in a bowl, mix honey, salt, pepper, chives and lemon juice and whisk really well. Divide Air Fryer fish on plates, drizzle yogurt sauce all over and serve right away.

Nutrition: Calories 261g Fat 8g Carbs 24g Protein 21g

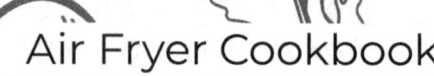

Air Fryer Cookbook

347. BUTTERY SHRIMP SKEWERS

PREPARATION: 5 MIN   **COOKING:** 10 MIN   **SERVINGS:** 4

INGREDIENTS

- 8 shrimps; peeled and deveined
- 8 green bell pepper slices
- 1 tbsp. butter; melted
- 4 garlic cloves; minced
- Salt and black pepper to the taste

DIRECTIONS

1. In a bowl; mix shrimp with garlic, butter, salt, pepper and bell pepper slices; toss to coat and leave aside for 10 minutes.
2. Arrange 2 shrimp and 2 bell pepper slices on a skewer and repeat with the rest of the shrimp and bell pepper pieces.
3. Place them all in your Air Fryer's basket and cook at 360°F for 6 minutes. Divide among plates and serve right away.

Nutrition: Calories 140 Fat 1g Carbs 15g Protein 7g

348. MARINATED SALMON RECIPE

PREPARATION: 1H 5M   **COOKING:** 30 MIN   **SERVINGS:** 4

INGREDIENTS

- 1 whole salmon
- 1 tbsp. tarragon; chopped
- 1 tbsp. garlic; minced
- Juice from 2 lemons
- A pinch of salt and black pepper

DIRECTIONS

1. In a large fish, mix fish with salt, pepper and lemon juice; toss well and keep in the fridge for 1 hour.
2. Stuff salmon with garlic and place in your Air Fryer's basket and cook at 320°F for 25 minutes. Divide among plates and serve with a tasty coleslaw on the side.

Nutrition: Calories 300 Fat 8g Carbs 19g Protein 27g

349. TASTY GRILLED RED MULLET

PREPARATION: 5 MIN   **COOKING:** 10 MIN   **SERVINGS:** 8

INGREDIENTS

- 8 whole red mullets, gutted and scales removed
- Salt and pepper to taste
- Juice from 1 lemon
- 1 tbsp. olive oil

DIRECTIONS

1. Preheat the Air Fryer at 390°F.
2. Place the grill pan attachment in the Air Fryer.
3. Season the red mullet with salt, pepper, and lemon juice.
4. Brush with olive oil.
5. Grill for 15 minutes.

Nutrition: Calories 152 Fat 6.2g Carbs 0.9g Protein 23.1g

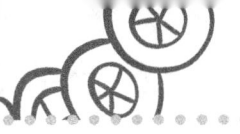 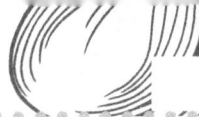 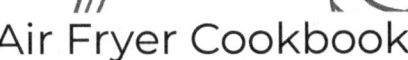

Air Fryer Cookbook

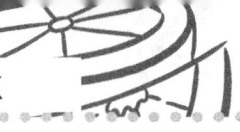 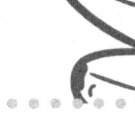

350. GARLICKY-GRILLED TURBOT

PREPARATION: 5 MIN   **COOKING:** 20 MIN   **SERVINGS:** 2

INGREDIENTS

- 2 whole turbot, scaled and head removed
- Salt and pepper to taste
- 1 clove of garlic, minced
- ½ cup chopped celery leaves
- 2 tbsp. olive oil

DIRECTIONS

1. Preheat the Air Fryer at 390°F.
2. Place the grill pan attachment in the Air Fryer.
3. Flavor the turbot with salt, pepper, garlic, and celery leaves.
4. Brush with oil.
5. Cook in the grill pan for 20 minutes until the fish becomes flaky.

Nutrition: Calories 269 Fat 25.6g Carbs 3.3g Protein 66.2g

351. CHAR-GRILLED SPICY HALIBUT

PREPARATION: 5 MIN   **COOKING:** 20 MIN   **SERVINGS:** 4

INGREDIENTS

- 3 lb. halibut fillet, skin removed
- Salt and pepper to taste
- 4 tbsp. olive oil
- 2 cloves of garlic, minced
- 1 tbsp. chili powder

DIRECTIONS

1. Place all ingredients in a Ziploc bag.
2. Keep it in the fridge for at least 2 hours.
3. Preheat the Air Fryer at 390°F.
4. Place the grill pan attachment in the Air Fryer.
5. Grill the fish for 20 minutes while flipping every 5 minutes.

Nutrition: Calories 385 Fat 40.6g Carbs 1.7g Protein 33g

352. SWORDFISH WITH CHARRED LEEKS

PREPARATION: 5 MIN   **COOKING:** 20 MIN   **SERVINGS:** 4

INGREDIENTS

- 4 swordfish steaks
- Salt and pepper to taste
- 3 tbsp. lime juice
- 2 tbsp. olive oil
- 4 medium leeks, cut into an inch long

DIRECTIONS

1. Preheat the Air Fryer at 390°F. Place the grill pan attachment in the Air Fryer.
2. Season the swordfish with salt, pepper and lime juice.
3. Brush the fish with olive oil. Place fish fillets on grill pan and top with leeks.
4. Grill for 20 minutes.

Nutrition: Calories 611 Fat 40g Carbs 14.6g Protein 48g

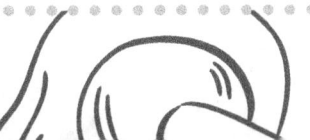 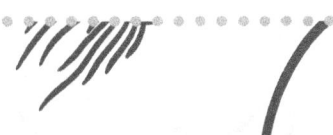

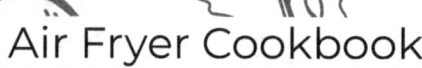
Air Fryer Cookbook

353. BREADED COCONUT SHRIMP

PREPARATION: 5 MIN **COOKING:** 15 MIN **SERVINGS:** 4

INGREDIENTS

- Shrimp (1 lb.)
- Panko breadcrumbs (1 cup)
- Shredded coconut (1 cup)
- Eggs (2)
- All-purpose flour (.33 cup)

Nutrition: Calories 285 Fat 12.8g Carbs 3.7g Protein 38.1g

DIRECTIONS

1. Fix the temperature of the Air Fryer at 360°F.
2. Peel and devein the shrimp.
3. Whisk the seasonings with the flour as desired. In another dish, whisk the eggs, and in the third container, combine the breadcrumbs and coconut.
4. Dip the cleaned shrimp into the flour, egg wash, and finish it off with the coconut mixture.
5. Lightly spray the basket of the fryer and set the timer for 10-15 minutes.
6. Air-fry until it's a golden brown before serving.

354. BREADED COD STICKS

PREPARATION: 5 MIN **COOKING:** 20 MIN **SERVINGS:** 4

INGREDIENTS

- Large eggs (2)
- Milk (3 tbsp.)
- Breadcrumbs (2 cups)
- Almond flour (1 cup)
- Cod (1 lb.)

Nutrition: Calories 254 Fat 14.2g Carbs 5.7g Protein 39.1g

DIRECTIONS

1. Heat the Air Fryer at 350°F.
2. Prepare three bowls; one with the milk and eggs, one with the breadcrumbs (salt and pepper if desired), and another with almond flour.
3. Dip the sticks in the flour, egg mixture, and breadcrumbs.
4. Place in the basket and set the timer for 12 minutes. Toss the basket halfway through the cooking process.
5. Serve with your favorite sauce.

355. CAJUN SALMON

PREPARATION: 5 MIN **COOKING:** 20 MIN **SERVINGS:** 4

INGREDIENTS

- Salmon fillet (1 - 7 oz.) 0.75-inches thick
- Cajun seasoning
- Juice (¼ of a lemon)
- Optional: Sprinkle of sugar

Nutrition: Calories 285 Fat 17.8g Carbs 6.8g Protein 42.1g

DIRECTIONS

1. Set the Air Fryer at 356°F to preheat for five minutes.
2. Rinse and dry the salmon with a paper towel. Cover the fish with the Cajun coating mix.
3. Place the fillet in the Air Fryer for seven minutes with the skin side up.
4. Serve with a sprinkle of lemon and dusting of sugar if desired.

356. CAJUN SHRIMP

PREPARATION: 5 MIN **COOKING:** 5 MIN **SERVINGS:** 6

INGREDIENTS

- Tiger shrimp (16-20/1.25 lb.)
- Olive oil (1 tbsp.)
- Old Bay seasoning (.5 tsp.)
- Smoked paprika (.25 tsp.)
- Cayenne pepper (.25 tsp.)

DIRECTIONS

1. Set the Air Fryer at 390°F.
2. Cover the shrimp using the oil and spices.
3. Toss them into the Air Fryer basket and set the timer for five minutes.
4. Serve with your favorite side dish.

Nutrition: Calories 356 Fat 18g Carbs 5g Protein 34g

357. CODFISH NUGGETS

PREPARATION: 5 MIN **COOKING:** 20 MIN **SERVINGS:** 4

INGREDIENTS

- Cod fillet (1 lb.)
- Eggs (3)
- Olive oil (4 tbsp.)
- Almond flour (1 cup)
- Gluten-free breadcrumbs (1 cup)

DIRECTIONS

1. Warm the Air Fryer at 390°F.
2. Slice the cod into nuggets.
3. Prepare three bowls. Whisk the eggs in one. Combine the salt, oil, and breadcrumbs in another. Sift the almond flour into the third one.
4. Cover each of the nuggets with the flour, dip in the eggs, and the breadcrumbs.
5. Arrange the nuggets in the basket and set the timer for 20 minutes.
6. Serve the fish with your favorite dips or sides.

Nutrition: Calories 334 Fat 10g Carbs 8g Protein 32g

358. CREAMY SALMON

PREPARATION: 5 MIN **COOKING:** 20 MIN **SERVINGS:** 4

INGREDIENTS

- Chopped dill (1 tbsp.)
- Olive oil (1 tbsp.)
- Sour cream (3 tbsp.)
- Plain yogurt (1.76 oz.)
- Salmon (6 pieces)/.75 lb.)

DIRECTIONS

1. Heat the Air Fryer and wait for it to reach 285°F.
2. Shake the salt over the salmon and add them to the fryer basket with the olive oil to air-fry for 10 minutes.
3. Whisk the yogurt, salt, and dill.
4. Serve the salmon with the sauce with your favorite sides.

Nutrition: Calories 340 Carbs 5g Fat 16g Protein 32g

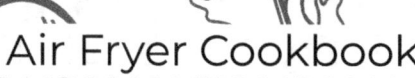

359. CRUMBLED FISH

PREPARATION: 5 MIN   **COOKING:** 15 MIN   **SERVINGS:** 4

INGREDIENTS

- Breadcrumbs (.5 cup)
- Vegetable oil (4 tbsp.)
- Egg (1)
- Fish fillets (4)
- Lemon (1)

Nutrition: Calories 320 Carbs 8g Fat 10g Protein 28g

DIRECTIONS

1. Heat the Air Fryer to reach 356°F.
2. Whisk the oil and breadcrumbs until crumbly.
3. Dip the fish into the egg, then the crumb mixture.
4. Arrange the fish in the cooker and air-fry for 12 minutes.
5. Garnish using the lemon.

360. EASY CRAB STICKS

PREPARATION: 5 MIN   **COOKING:** 10 MIN   **SERVINGS:** 4

INGREDIENTS

- Crab sticks (1 package)
- Cooking oil spray (as needed)

Nutrition: Calories 285 Fat 12.8g Carbs 3.7g Protein 38.1g

DIRECTIONS

1. Take each of the sticks out of the package and unroll it until the stick is flat. Tear the sheets into thirds.
2. Arrange them on the Air Fryer basket and lightly spritz using cooking spray. Set the timer for 10 minutes at 360°F.
3. Note: If you shred the crab meat, you can cut the time in half, but they will also easily fall through the holes in the basket.

361. FRIED CATFISH

PREPARATION: 5 MIN   **COOKING:** 15 MIN   **SERVINGS:** 4

INGREDIENTS

- Olive oil (1 tbsp.)
- Seasoned fish fry (.25 cup)
- Catfish fillets (4)

Nutrition: Calories 376 Fat 9g Carbs 10g Protein 28g

DIRECTIONS

1. Heat the Air Fryer to reach 400°F before fry time.
2. Rinse the catfish and pat dry using a paper towel.
3. Dump the seasoning into a sizeable zipper-type bag. Add the fish and shake to cover each fillet. Spray with a spritz of cooking oil spray and add to the basket.
4. Set the timer for 10 minutes. Flip and reset the timer for ten additional minutes. Turn the fish once more and cook for 2-3 minutes.
5. Once it reaches the desired crispiness, transfer to a plate, and serve.

362. Grilled Sardines

PREPARATION: 5 MIN **COOKING:** 20 MIN **SERVINGS:** 4

INGREDIENTS
- 5 sardines
- Herbs of Provence

DIRECTIONS
1. Preheat the Air Fryer to 320°F.
2. Spray the basket and place your sardines in the basket of your fryer.
3. Set the timer for 14 minutes. After 7 minutes, remember to turn the sardines so that they are roasted on both sides.

Nutrition: Calories 189 Fat 10g Carbs 0g Protein 22g

363. ZUCCHINI WITH TUNA

PREPARATION: 10 MIN **COOKING:** 30 MIN **SERVINGS:** 4

INGREDIENTS
- 4 medium zucchinis
- 4 oz. of tuna in oil (canned) drained
- 1 oz. grated cheese
- 1 tsp. pine nuts
- Salt, pepper to taste

DIRECTIONS
1. Cut the zucchini in half laterally and empty it with a small spoon (set aside the pulp that will be used for the filling); place them in the basket.
2. In a food processor, put the zucchini pulp, drained tuna, pine nuts and grated cheese. Mix everything until you get a homogeneous and dense mixture.
3. Fill the zucchini. Set the Air Fryer to 360°F.
4. Air fry for 20 min. depending on the size of the zucchini. Let cool before serving

Nutrition: Calories 389 Carbs 10g Fat 29g Protein 23g

364. CARAMELIZED SALMON FILLET

PREPARATION: 5 MIN **COOKING:** 25 MIN **SERVINGS:** 4

INGREDIENTS
- 2 salmon fillets
- 2 oz. cane sugar
- 4 tbsp. soy sauce
- 1.7 oz. sesame seeds
- Unlimited Ginger

DIRECTIONS
1. Preheat the Air Fryer at 360°F for 5 minutes.
2. Put the sugar and soy sauce in the basket. Cook everything for 5 minutes.
3. In the meantime, wash the fish well, pass it through sesame to cover it completely and place it inside the tank and add the fresh ginger.
4. Cook for 12 minutes. Turn the fish over and finish cooking for another 8 minutes.

Nutrition: Calories 569 Fat 14.9g Carbs 40g Protein 66.9g

Air Fryer Cookbook

365. DEEP FRIED PRAWNS

PREPARATION: 15 MIN **COOKING:** 10 MIN **SERVINGS:** 6

INGREDIENTS

- 12 prawns
- 2 eggs
- Flour to taste
- Breadcrumbs
- 1 tsp. oil

DIRECTIONS

1. Remove the head of the prawns and shell carefully.
2. Pass the prawns first in the flour, then in the beaten egg and then in the breadcrumbs.
3. Preheat the Air Fryer for 1 minute at 300°F.
4. Add the prawns and cook for 4 minutes. If the prawns are large, it will be necessary to cook 6 at a time.
5. Turn the prawns and cook for another 4 minutes.
6. They should be served with a yogurt or mayonnaise sauce.

Nutrition: Calories 2385 Fat 23g Carbs 52.3g Protein 21.4g

366. MUSSELS WITH PEPPER

PREPARATION: 5 MIN **COOKING:** 12 MIN **SERVINGS:** 5

INGREDIENTS

- 25 oz. mussels
- 1 clove garlic
- 1 tsp. oil
- Pepper to taste
- Parsley Taste

DIRECTIONS

1. Clean and scrape the mold cover and remove the byssus (the "beard" that comes out of the mold).
2. Pour the oil, clean the mussels and the crushed garlic in the Air Fryer basket. Set the temperature to 390°F and simmer for 12 minutes. Towards the end of cooking, add black pepper and chopped parsley.
3. Finally, distribute the mussel juice well at the bottom of the basket, stirring the basket.

Nutrition: Calories 150 Carbs 2g Fat 8g Protein 15g

367. MONKFISH WITH OLIVES AND CAPERS

PREPARATION: 25 MIN **COOKING:** 40 MIN **SERVINGS:** 4

INGREDIENTS

- 1 monkfish
- 10 cherry tomatoes
- 1.75 oz. cailletier olives
- 5 capers

DIRECTIONS

1. Spread aluminum foil inside the Air Fryer basket and place the monkfish clean and skinless.
2. Add chopped tomatoes, olives, capers, oil, and salt.
3. Set the temperature to 320°F.
4. Cook the monkfish for about 40 minutes.

Nutrition: Calories 404 Fat 29g Carbs 36g Protein 24g

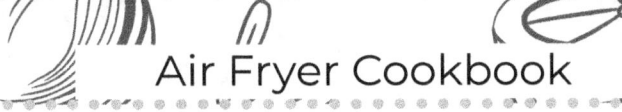

Air Fryer Cookbook

368. SHRIMP, ZUCCHINI AND CHERRY TOMATO SAUCE

PREPARATION: 5 MIN **COOKING:** 25 MIN **SERVINGS:** 4

INGREDIENTS

- 2 zucchinis
- 10 oz. shrimp
- 7 cherry tomatoes
- Salt and pepper to taste
- 1 clove garlic

DIRECTIONS

1. Pour the oil in the Air Fryer, add the garlic clove and diced zucchini.
2. Cook for 15 minutes at 300°F. Add the shrimps and the pieces of tomato, salt, and spices.
3. Cook for another 5 to 10 minutes or until the shrimp water evaporates.

Nutrition: Calories 214.3 Fat 8.6g Carbs 7.8g Protein 27.0g

369. SALMON WITH PISTACHIO BARK

PREPARATION: 10 MIN **COOKING:** 30 MIN **SERVINGS:** 4

INGREDIENTS

- 20 oz. salmon fillet
- 1.75 oz. pistachios
- Salt to taste

DIRECTIONS

1. Put the parchment paper on the bottom of the Air Fryer basket and place the salmon fillet in it (it can be cooked whole or already divided into four portions).
2. Cut the pistachios in thick pieces; grease the top of the fish, salt (little because the pistachios are already salted) and cover everything with the pistachios.
3. Set the Air Fryer to 360°F and simmer for 25 minutes.

Nutrition: Calories 371.7 Fat 21.8g Carbs 9.4g Protein 34.7g

370. SALTED MARINATED SALMON

PREPARATION: 10 MIN **COOKING:** 30 MIN **SERVINGS:** 4

INGREDIENTS

- 17 oz. salmon fillet
- 2 lb. coarse salt

DIRECTIONS

1. Place the baking paper on the Air Fryer basket and the salmon on top (skin side up) covered with coarse salt.
2. Set the Air Fryer to 300°F.
3. Cook everything for 25 to 30 minutes. At the end of cooking, remove the salt from the fish and serve with a drizzle of oil.

Nutrition: Calories 290 Fat 13g Carbs 3g Protein 40g

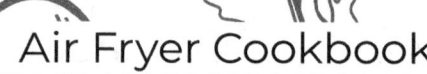
Air Fryer Cookbook

371. SAUTÉED TROUT WITH ALMONDS

PREPARATION: 35 MIN **COOKING:** 20 MIN **SERVINGS:** 4

INGREDIENTS

- 25 oz. salmon trout
- 15 black peppercorns
- Dill leaves to taste
- 1 oz. almonds
- Salt to taste

DIRECTIONS

1. Cut the trout into cubes and marinate it for half an hour with the rest of the ingredients (except salt).
2. Cook in Air Fryer for 17 minutes at 320°F. Pour a drizzle of oil and serve.

Nutrition: Calories 238.5 Fat 20.1g Carbs 11.5g Protein 4.0g

372. RABAS

PREPARATION: 5 MIN **COOKING:** 12 MIN **SERVINGS:** 4

INGREDIENTS

- 16 rabas
- 1 egg
- Breadcrumbs
- Salt, pepper, sweet paprika

DIRECTIONS

1. Put the rabas in the Air Fryer to boil for 2 minutes.
2. Remove and dry well. Beat the egg and season to taste. You can put salt, pepper and sweet paprika. Place in the egg.
3. Bread with breadcrumbs. Place in sticks.
4. Air fry for 10 minutes at 360°F

Nutrition: Calories 356 Fat 18g Carbs 5 g Protein 34g

373. HONEY GLAZED SALMO

PREPARATION: 10 MIN **COOKING:** 8 MIN **SERVINGS:** 2

INGREDIENTS

- 2 (6 oz.) salmon fillets
- Salt, as required
- 2 tbsp. honey

DIRECTIONS

1. Sprinkle the salmon fillets with salt and then, coat with honey.
2. Preheat at 355°F.
3. Arrange the salmon fillets in greased Air Fryer basket and insert in the Air Fryer. Cook for 8 minutes. Serve hot.

Nutrition: Calories 289 Fat 10.5g Carbs 17.3g Protein 33.1g

374. SWEET & SOUR GLAZED SALMON

PREPARATION: 12 MIN **COOKING:** 20 MIN **SERVINGS:** 2

INGREDIENTS

- 1/3 cup soy sauce
- 1/3 cup honey
- 3 tsp.s rice wine vinegar
- 1 tsp. water
- 4 (3½-oz.) salmon fillets

DIRECTIONS

1. Mix the soy sauce, honey, vinegar, and water together in a bowl.
2. In another small bowl, reserve about half of the mixture.
3. Add salmon fillets in the remaining mixture and coat well.
4. Cover the bowl and refrigerate to marinate for about 2 hours.
5. Preheat at 355°F.
6. Arrange the salmon fillets in greased Air Fryer basket and insert in the Air Fryer. Cook for 12 minutes
7. Flip the salmon fillets once halfway through and coat with the reserved marinade after every 3 minutes.
8. Serve hot.

Nutrition: Calories 462 Fat 12.3g Carbs 49.8g Protein 41.3g

375. RANCH TILAPIA

PREPARATION: 15 MIN **COOKING:** 13 MIN **SERVINGS:** 4

INGREDIENTS

- ¾ cup cornflakes, crushed
- 1 (1-oz.) packet dry ranch-style dressing mix
- 2½ tbsp. vegetable oil
- 2 eggs
- 4 (6-oz.) tilapia fillets

DIRECTIONS

1. In a shallow bowl, beat the eggs.
2. In another bowl, add the cornflakes, ranch dressing, and oil and mix until a crumbly mixture form.
3. Dip the fish fillets into egg and then, coat with the bread crumbs mixture.
4. Preheat at 356°F.
5. Arrange the tilapia fillets in greased Air Fryer basket and insert in the Air Fryer. Cook for 13 minutes. Serve hot.

Nutrition: Calories 267 Fat 12.2g Carbs 5.1g Protein 34.9g

376. BREADED FLOUNDER

PREPARATION: 15 MIN **COOKING:** 12 MIN **SERVINGS:** 3

INGREDIENTS

- 1 egg
- 1 cup dry breadcrumbs
- ¼ cup vegetable oil
- 3 (6-oz.) flounder fillets
- 1 lemon, sliced

DIRECTIONS

1. In a shallow bowl, beat the egg
2. In another bowl, add the breadcrumbs and oil and mix until a crumbly mixture is formed.
3. Dip flounder fillets into the beaten egg and then coat with the breadcrumb mixture.
4. Preheat at 355°F.
5. Arrange the flounder fillets in greased Air Fryer basket and insert in the Air Fryer. Cook for 12 minutes
6. Plate with lemon slices and serve hot.

Nutrition: Calories 524 Fat 24.2g Carbs 26.5g Protein 47.8g

377. SIMPLE HADDOCK

PREPARATION: 5 MIN **COOKING:** 40 MIN **SERVINGS:** 6

INGREDIENTS

- 2 (6-oz.) haddock fillets
- 1 tbsp. olive oil
- Salt and ground black pepper, as required

DIRECTIONS

1. Coat the fish fillets with oil and then, sprinkle with salt and black pepper.
2. Preheat at 355°F.
3. Arrange the haddock fillets in greased Air Fryer basket and insert in the Air Fryer. Cook for 8 minutes. Serve hot.

Nutrition: Calories 251 Fat 8.6g Saturated Fat 1.3g Carbs 0g Protein 41.2g

378. BREADED HAKE

PREPARATION: 15 MIN **COOKING:** 12 MIN **SERVINGS:** 4

INGREDIENTS

- 1 egg
- 4 oz. breadcrumbs
- 2 tbsp. vegetable oil
- 4 (6-oz.) hake fillets
- 1 lemon, cut into wedges

DIRECTIONS

1. In a shallow bowl, whisk the egg.
2. In another bowl, add the breadcrumbs, and oil and mix until a crumbly mixture forms.
3. Dip fish fillets into the egg and then, coat with the bread crumbs mixture.
4. Preheat at 350°F.
5. Arrange the hake fillets in greased Air Fryer basket and insert in the Air Fryer. Cook for 12 minutes. Serve hot.

Nutrition: Calories 297 Fat 10.6g Carbs 22g Protein 29.2g

379. SESAME SEEDS COATED TUNA

PREPARATION: 15 MIN **COOKING:** 6 MIN **SERVINGS:** 2

INGREDIENTS

- 1 egg white
- ¼ cup white sesame seeds
- 1 tbsp. black sesame seeds
- Salt and ground black pepper, as required
- 2 (6-oz.) tuna steaks

DIRECTIONS

1. In a bowl, beat the egg white.
2. In another bowl, mix together the sesame seeds, salt, and black pepper.
3. Dip the tuna steaks into the egg white and then coat with the sesame seeds mixture.
4. Preheat at 355°F. Arrange the tuna steak fillets in greased Air Fryer basket and insert in the Air Fryer. Cook for 8 minutes
5. Flip the tuna steaks once halfway through. Serve hot.

Nutrition: Calories 450 Fat 21.9g Carbs 5.4g Protein 56.7g

Air Fryer Cookbook

380. CHEESE AND HAM PATTIES

PREPARATION: 10 MIN **COOKING:** 10 MIN **SERVINGS:** 4

INGREDIENTS

- 1 puff pastry sheet
- 4 handfuls mozzarella cheese, grated
- 4 tsp.s mustard
- 8 ham slices, chopped

DIRECTIONS

1. Spread out puff pastry on a clean surface and cut it in 12 squares.
2. Divide cheese, ham, and mustard on half of them, top with the other halves, and seal the edges.
3. Place all the patties in your Air Fryer's basket and cook at 370°F for 10 minutes.
4. Divide the patties between plates and serve.

Nutrition: Calories 212 Fat 12g Carbs 14g Protein 8g

381. AIR-FRIED SEAFOOD

PREPARATION: 10 MIN **COOKING:** 10 MIN **SERVINGS:** 4

INGREDIENTS

- 1 lb. fresh scallops, mussels, fish fillets, prawns, shrimp
- 2 eggs, lightly beaten
- Salt and black pepper
- 1 cup breadcrumbs mixed with the zest of 1 lemon
- Cooking spray

DIRECTIONS

1. Clean the seafood as needed.
2. Dip each piece into the egg and season with salt and pepper.
3. Coat in the crumbs and spray with oil.
4. Arrange into the Air Fryer and cook for 6 minutes at 400°F turning once halfway through. Serve and Enjoy!

Nutrition: Calories 133 Protein 17.4g Fat 3.1g Carbs 8.2g

382. FISH WITH CHIPS

PREPARATION: 5 MIN **COOKING:** 20 MIN **SERVINGS:** 2

INGREDIENTS

- 1 cod fillet (6 oz.)
- 3 cups salt
- 3 cups vinegar-flavored kettle cooked chips
- ¼ cup buttermilk
- salt and pepper to taste

DIRECTIONS

1. Mix to combine the buttermilk, pepper, and salt in a bowl. Put the cod and leave to soak for 5 minutes
2. Put the chips in a food processor and process until crushed. Transfer to a shallow bowl. Coat the fillet with the crushed chips.
3. Put the coated fillet in the air frying basket. Cook for 12 minutes at 400°F. Serve and Enjoy!

Nutrition: Calories 646 Fat 33g Protein 41g Carbs 48g

383. CRUMBLY FISHCAKES

PREPARATION: 5 MIN   **COOKING:** 10 MIN   **SERVINGS:** 4

INGREDIENTS

- 8 oz. salmon, cooked
- 1 ½ oz. potatoes, mashed
- A handful of parsley, chopped
- Zest of 1 lemon
- 1 ¾ oz. plain flour

DIRECTIONS

1. Carefully flakes the salmon. In a bowl, mix flaked salmon, zest, capers, dill, and mashed potatoes.
2. From small cakes using the mixture and dust the cakes with flour; refrigerate for 60 minutes.
3. Preheat your Air Fryer to 350°F. and cook the cakes for 7 minutes. Serve chilled.

Nutrition: Calories 210 Protein 10g Fat 7g Carbs 25g

384. BACON WRAPPED SHRIMP

PREPARATION: 10 MIN   **COOKING:** 20 MIN   **SERVINGS:** 4

INGREDIENTS

- 16 thin slices of bacon
- 16 pieces of tiger shrimp (peeled and deveined)

DIRECTIONS

1. With a slice of bacon, wrap each shrimp. Put all the finished pieces in tray and chill for 20 minutes.
2. Arrange the bacon-wrapped shrimp in the air frying basket. Cook for 7 minutes at 390°F. Transfer to a plate lined with paper towels to drain before serving.

Nutrition: Calories 436 Protein 32g Fat 41.01g Carbs 0.8g

385. CRAB LEGS

PREPARATION: 10 MIN   **COOKING:** 10 MIN   **SERVINGS:** 4

INGREDIENTS

- 3 lb. crab legs
- ¼ cup salted butter, melted and divided
- ½ lemon, juiced
- ¼ tsp. garlic powder

DIRECTIONS

1. In a bowl, toss the crab legs and two tbsp. of the melted butter together. Place the crab legs in the basket of the fryer.
2. Cook at 400°F for fifteen minutes, giving the basket a good shake halfway through.
3. Combine the remaining butter with the lemon juice and garlic powder.
4. Crack open the cooked crab legs and remove the meat. Serve with the butter dip on the side, and enjoy!

Nutrition: Calories 27 Fat 19g Carbs 18g Protein 12g

Air Fryer Cookbook

386. FISH STICKS

PREPARATION: 5 MIN   **COOKING:** 10 MIN   **SERVINGS:** 4

INGREDIENTS

- 1 lb. whitefish
- 2 tbsp. Dijon mustard
- ¼ cup mayonnaise
- 1 ½ cup pork rinds, finely ground
- ¾ tsp. Cajun seasoning

DIRECTIONS

1. Place the fish on a tissue to dry it off, then cut it up into slices about two inches thick.
2. In one bowl, combine the mustard and mayonnaise, and in another, the Cajun seasoning and pork rinds.
3. Coat the fish firstly in the mayo-mustard mixture, then in the Cajun-pork rind mixture. Give each slice a shake to remove any surplus. Then place the fish sticks in the basket of the air flyer.
4. Cook at 400°F for five minutes. Turn the fish sticks over and cook for another five minutes on the other side.
5. Serve warm with a dipping sauce of your choosing and enjoy.

Nutrition: Calories 212 Fat 12g Carbs 14g Protein 8g

387. CRUSTY PESTO SALMON

PREPARATION: 5 MIN   **COOKING:** 10 MIN   **SERVINGS:** 2

INGREDIENTS

- ¼ cup almonds, roughly chopped
- ¼ cup pesto
- 2 x 4-oz. salmon fillets
- 2 tbsp. unsalted butter, melted

DIRECTIONS

1. Mix the almonds and pesto together.
2. Place the salmon fillets in a round baking dish, roughly six inches in diameter.
3. Brush the fillets with butter, followed by the pesto mixture, ensuring to coat both the top and bottom. Put the baking dish inside the fryer.
4. Cook for twelve minutes at 390°F.
5. The salmon is ready when it flakes easily when prodded with a fork. Serve warm.

Nutrition: Calories 354 Fat 21g Carbs 23g Protein 19g

388. SALMON PATTIES

PREPARATION: 5 MIN   **COOKING:** 10 MIN   **SERVINGS:** 4

INGREDIENTS

- 1 tsp. chili powder
- tbsp. full-fat mayonnaise
- ¼ cup ground pork rinds
- x 5-oz. pouches of cooked pink salmon
- 1 egg

DIRECTIONS

1. Stir everything together to prepare the patty mixture. If the mixture is dry or falling apart, add in more pork rinds as necessary.
2. Take equal-sized amounts of the mixture to form four patties, before placing the patties in the basket of your Air Fryer.
3. Cook at 400°F for eight minutes.
4. Halfway through cooking, flip the patties over. Once they are crispy, serve with the toppings of your choice and enjoy.

Nutrition: Calories 325 Fat 21g Carbs 18g Protein 29g

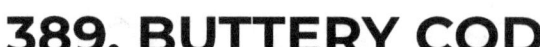

389. BUTTERY COD

PREPARATION: 5 MIN   **COOKING:** 10 MIN   **SERVINGS:** 4

INGREDIENTS

- 2 x 4-oz. cod fillets
- 2 tbsp. salted butter, melted
- 1 tsp. Old Bay seasoning
- ½ medium lemon, sliced

Nutrition: Calories 354 Fat 21g Carbs 23g Protein 19g

DIRECTIONS

1. Place the cod fillets in a dish.
2. Brush with melted butter, season with Old Bay, and top with some lemon slices.
3. Wrap the fish in aluminum foil and put into your fryer.
4. Cook for eight minutes at 350°F.
5. The cod is ready when it flakes easily. Serve hot.

390. SESAME TUNA STEAK

PREPARATION: 5 MIN   **COOKING:** 10 MIN   **SERVINGS:** 4

INGREDIENTS

- 1 tbsp. coconut oil, melted
- 2 x 6-oz. tuna steaks
- ½ tsp. garlic powder
- 2 tsp. black sesame seeds
- 2 tsp. white sesame seeds

Nutrition: Calories 343 Fat 11g Carbs 27g Protein 25g

DIRECTIONS

1. Apply the coconut oil to the tuna steaks with a brunch, then season with garlic powder.
2. Combine the black and white sesame seeds. Embed them in the tuna steaks, covering the fish all over. Place the tuna into your Air Fryer.
3. Cook for eight minutes at 400°F, turning the fish halfway through.
4. The tuna steaks are ready when they have reached a temperature of 145°F. Serve straight away.

391. LEMON GARLIC SHRIMP

PREPARATION: 5 MIN   **COOKING:** 10 MIN   **SERVINGS:** 4

INGREDIENTS

- 1 medium lemon
- ½ lb. medium shrimp, shelled and deveined
- ½ tsp. Old Bay seasoning
- 2 tbsp. unsalted butter, melted
- ½ tsp. minced garlic

Nutrition: Calories 374 Fat 14g Carbs 18g Protein 21g

DIRECTIONS

1. Grate the lemon rind into a bowl. Cut the lemon in half then juice it over the same bowl. Toss in the shrimp, Old Bay, and butter, mixing everything to make sure the shrimp is completely covered.
2. Transfer to a round baking dish roughly six inches wide, then place this dish in your Air Fryer.
3. Cook at 400°F for six minutes. The shrimp is ready when it becomes a bright pink color.
4. Serve hot, drizzling any leftover sauce over the shrimp.

392. FOIL PACKET SALMON

PREPARATION: 5 MIN   **COOKING:** 10 MIN   **SERVINGS:** 4

INGREDIENTS

- 2 x 4-oz. skinless salmon fillets
- 2 tbsp. unsalted butter, melted
- ½ tsp. garlic powder
- 1 medium lemon
- ½ tsp. dried dill

Nutrition: Calories 365 Fat 16g Carbs 18g Protein 23g

DIRECTIONS

1. Take a sheet of foil and cut into two squares measuring roughly 5" x 5". Lay each of the salmon fillets at the center of each piece. Brush both fillets with a tbsp. of bullet and season with a quarter-tsp. of garlic powder.
2. Halve the lemon and grate the skin of one half over the fish. Cut four half-slices of lemon, using two to top each fillet. Season each fillet with a quarter-tsp. of dill.
3. Fold the tops and sides of the aluminum foil over the fish to create a kind of packet. Place each one in the fryer.
4. Cook for twelve minutes at 400°F.
5. The salmon is ready when it flakes easily. Serve hot.

393. FOIL PACKET LOBSTER TAIL

PREPARATION: 5 MIN   **COOKING:** 10 MIN   **SERVINGS:** 4

INGREDIENTS

- 2 x 6-oz. lobster tail halves
- 2 tbsp. salted butter, melted
- ½ medium lemon, juiced
- ½ tsp. Old Bay seasoning
- 1 tsp. dried parsley

Nutrition: Calories 369 Fat 19g Carbs 25g Protein 28g

DIRECTIONS

1. Lay each lobster on a sheet of aluminum foil. Pour a light drizzle of melted butter and lemon juice over each one, and season with Old Bay.
2. Fold down the sides and ends of the foil to seal the lobster. Place each one in the fryer.
3. Cook at 375°F for twelve minutes.
4. Just before serving, top the lobster with dried parsley.

394. AVOCADO SHRIMP

PREPARATION: 5 MIN   **COOKING:** 20 MIN   **SERVINGS:** 4

INGREDIENTS

- ½ cup onion, chopped
- 2 lb. shrimp
- 1 tbsp. seasoned salt
- 1 avocado
- ½ cup pecans, chopped

Nutrition: Calories 384 Fat 24g Carbs 13g Protein 39g

DIRECTIONS

1. Pre-heat the fryer at 400°F.
2. Put the chopped onion in the basket of the fryer and spritz with some cooking spray. Leave to cook for five minutes.
3. Add the shrimp and set the timer for a further five minutes. Sprinkle with some seasoned salt, then allow to cook for an additional five minutes.
4. During these last five minutes, halve your avocado and remove the pit. Cube each half, then scoop out the flesh.
5. Take care when removing the shrimp from the fryer. Place it on a dish and top with the avocado and the chopped pecans.

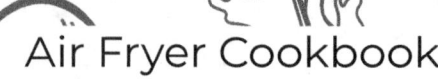

395. CITRUSY BRANZINI ON THE GRILL

PREPARATION: 5 MIN   **COOKING:** 15 MIN   **SERVINGS:** 4

INGREDIENTS

- 4 branzini fillets
- Salt and pepper to taste
- 2 lemons, juice freshly squeezed
- 2 oranges, juice freshly squeezed

DIRECTIONS

1. Place all ingredients in a Ziploc bag. Keep it in the fridge for 2 hours.
2. Preheat the Air Fryer at 390°F. Place the grill pan attachment in the Air Fryer.
3. Place the fish on the grill pan and cook for 15 minutes until the fish is flaky.

Nutrition: Calories 318 Fat 15.6g Carbs 20.8g Protein 23.5g

396. CAJUN-SEASONED LEMON SALMON

PREPARATION: 5 MIN   **COOKING:** 10 MIN   **SERVINGS:** 4

INGREDIENTS

- 1 salmon fillet
- 1 tsp. Cajun seasoning
- lemon wedges, for serving
- 1 tsp. liquid stevia
- ½ lemon, juiced

DIRECTIONS

1. Preheat your Air Fryer to 350°F. Combine lemon juice and liquid stevia and coat salmon with this mixture. Sprinkle Cajun seasoning all over salmon. Place salmon on parchment paper in Air Fryer and cook for 7-minutes. Serve with lemon wedges.

Nutrition: Calories 287 Fat 9.3g Carbs 8.4g Protein 15.3g

397. GRILLED SALMON FILLETS

PREPARATION: 5 MIN   **COOKING:** 10 MIN   **SERVINGS:** 4

INGREDIENTS

- salmon fillets
- tbsp. olive oil
- 1/3 cup of light soy sauce
- 1/3 cup of water
- Salt and black pepper to taste

DIRECTIONS

1. Season salmon fillets with salt and pepper. Mix what's left of the ingredients in a bowl. Allow the salmon fillets to marinate in mixture for 2-hours. Preheat your Air Fryer to 355°F for 5-minutes. Drain salmon fillets and air fry for 8-minutes.

Nutrition: Calories 302 Fat 8.6g Carbs 7.3g Protein 15.3g

398. CHEESY BREADED SALMON

PREPARATION: 5 MIN **COOKING:** 20 MIN **SERVINGS:** 4

INGREDIENTS

- cups breadcrumbs
- salmon fillets
- eggs, beaten
- 1 cup Swiss cheese, shredded

DIRECTIONS

1. Preheat your Air Fryer to 390°F. Dip each salmon filet into eggs. Top with Swiss cheese. Dip into breadcrumbs, coating entire fish. Put into an oven-safe dish and cook for 20-minutes.

Nutrition: Calories 296 Fat 9.2g Carbs 8.7g Protein 15.2g

399. COCONUT CRUSTED SHRIMP

PREPARATION: 15 MIN **COOKING:** 40 MIN **SERVINGS:** 4

INGREDIENTS

- oz. coconut milk
- ½ cup sweetened coconut, shredded
- ½ cup panko breadcrumbs
- 1-lb. large shrimp, peeled and deveined
- Salt and black pepper, to taste

DIRECTIONS

1. Preheat the Air Fryer to 350°F and grease an Air Fryer basket.
2. Place the coconut milk in a shallow bowl.
3. Mix coconut, breadcrumbs, salt, and black pepper in another bowl.
4. Dip each shrimp into coconut milk and finally, dredge in the coconut mixture.
5. Arrange half of the shrimps into the Air Fryer basket and cook for about 20 minutes.
6. Dish out the shrimps onto serving plates and repeat with the remaining mixture to serve.

Nutrition: Calories 408 Fats: 23.7g Carbs 11.7g Proteins: 31g,

400. RICE FLOUR COATED SHRIMP

PREPARATION: 20 MIN **COOKING:** 20 MIN **SERVINGS:** 3

INGREDIENTS

- tbsp. rice flour
- 1-lb. shrimp, peeled and deveined
- tbsp. olive oil
- 1 tsp. powdered sugar
- Salt and black pepper, as required

DIRECTIONS

1. Preheat the Air Fryer to 325°F and grease an Air Fryer basket.
2. Mix rice flour, olive oil, sugar, salt, and black pepper in a bowl.
3. Stir in the shrimp and transfer half of the shrimp to the Air Fryer basket.
4. Cook for about 10 minutes, flipping once in between.
5. Dish out the mixture onto serving plates and repeat with the remaining mixture.

Nutrition: Calories 299 Fat 12g Carbs 11.1g Protein 35g

401. BUTTERED SCALLOPS

PREPARATION: 15 MIN   **COOKING:** 4 MIN   **SERVINGS:** 2

INGREDIENTS

- ¾ lb. sea scallops, cleaned and patted very dry
- 1 tbsp. butter, melted
- ½ tbsp. fresh thyme, minced
- Salt and black pepper, as required

Nutrition: Calories 202 Fat 7.1g Carbs 4.4g Protein 28.7g

DIRECTIONS

1. Preheat the Air Fryer to 390°F and grease an Air Fryer basket.
2. Mix scallops, butter, thyme, salt, and black pepper in a bowl.
3. Arrange scallops in the Air Fryer basket and cook for about 4 minutes.
4. Dish out the scallops in a platter and serve hot.

402. BUTTER TROUT

PREPARATION: 5 MIN   **COOKING:** 20 MIN   **SERVINGS:** 4

INGREDIENTS

- trout fillets; boneless
- Juice of 1 lime
- 1 tbsp. parsley; chopped.
- tbsp. butter; melted
- Salt and black pepper to taste.

Nutrition: Calories 221 Fat 11g Carbs 6g Protein 9g

DIRECTIONS

1. Mix the fish fillets with the melted butter, salt and pepper, rub gently, put the fish in your Air Fryer's basket and cook at 390°F for 6 minutes on each side.
2. Divide between plates and serve with lime juice drizzled on top and with parsley sprinkled at the end.

403. PESTO ALMOND SALMON

PREPARATION: 5 MIN   **COOKING:** 15 MIN   **SERVINGS:** 4

INGREDIENTS

- 2 1 ½-inch-thick salmon fillets: about 4 oz. each
- ¼ cup sliced almonds, roughly chopped
- ¼ cup pesto
- tbsp. unsalted butter; melted.

Nutrition: Calories 433 Fat 34.0g Protein 23.3g Carbs 6.1g

DIRECTIONS

1. In a small bowl, mix pesto and almonds. Set aside. Place fillets into a 6-inch round baking dish
2. Brush each fillet with butter and place half of the pesto mixture on the top of each fillet. Place dish into the Air Fryer basket. Set the temperature to 390°F and set the timer for 12 minutes
3. Salmon will easily flake when fully cooked and reach an internal temperature of at least 145°F. Serve warm.

404. GARLIC LEMON SHRIMP

PREPARATION: 5 MIN **COOKING:** 10 MIN **SERVINGS:** 4

INGREDIENTS

- 8 oz. medium shelled and deveined shrimp
- 1 medium lemon.
- 2 tbsp. unsalted butter; melted.
- ½ tsp. minced garlic
- ½ tsp. Old Bay seasoning

DIRECTIONS

1. Zest lemon and then cut in half. Place shrimp in a large bowl and squeeze juice from ½ lemon on top of them.
2. Add lemon zest to bowl along with remaining ingredients. Toss shrimp until fully coated
3. Pour bowl contents into 6-inch round baking dish. Place into the Air Fryer basket.
4. Adjust the temperature to 400°F and set the timer for 6 minutes. Shrimp will be bright pink when fully cooked. Serve warm with pan sauce.

Nutrition: Calories 190 Fat 11.8g Protein 16.4g Carbs 2.9g

405. AIR-FRIED CRAB STICKS

PREPARATION: 5 MIN **COOKING:** 10 MIN **SERVINGS:** 4

INGREDIENTS

- Crab sticks: 1 package
- Cooking oil spray: as needed

DIRECTIONS

1. Take each of the sticks out of the package and unroll until flat. Tear the sheets into thirds.
2. Arrange them on a plate and lightly spritz using cooking spray. Set the timer for 10 minutes at 360°F.
3. Note: If you shred the crab meat; you can cut the time in half, but they will also easily fall through the holes in the basket.

Nutrition: Calories 220 Fat 13g Carbs 11g Protein 23g

406. E-Z CATFISH

PREPARATION: 5 MIN **COOKING:** 25 MIN **SERVINGS:** 3

INGREDIENTS

- Olive oil: 1 tbsp.
- Seasoned fish fry: .25 cup
- Catfish fillets: 4

DIRECTIONS

1. Prepare the fryer to 400°F.
2. First, wash the fish, and dry with a paper towel.
3. Dump the seasoning into a large zip-type baggie. Add the fish and shake to cover each fillet. Spray with a spritz of cooking oil spray. Add to the basket.
4. Set the timer for ten minutes. Flip, and reset the timer for ten more minutes. Flip once more and cook for two to three minutes.
5. Once it reaches the desired crispiness, transfer to a plate to serve.

Nutrition: Calories 290 Carbs 14g Fat 16g Protein 30g

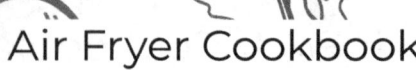
Air Fryer Cookbook

407. FISH NUGGETS

PREPARATION: 5 MIN   **COOKING:** 20 MIN   **SERVINGS:** 4

INGREDIENTS

- Cod fillet: 1 lb.
- Eggs: 3
- Olive oil: 4 tbsp.
- Almond flour: 1 cup
- Gluten-free breadcrumbs: 1 cup

Nutrition: Calories 220 Carbs 10g Fat 12g Protein 23g

DIRECTIONS

1. Fix the temperature of the Air Fryer at 390°F.
2. Cut the cod into nuggets.
3. Prepare three dishes. Beat the eggs in one. Combine the oil and breadcrumbs in another. The last one will be almond flour.
4. Cover each of the nuggets using the flour, a dip in the eggs, and the breadcrumbs.
5. Arrange the prepared nuggets in the basket and set the timer for 20 minutes. Serve.

408. GRILLED SHRIMP

PREPARATION: 5 MIN   **COOKING:** 10 MIN   **SERVINGS:** 4

INGREDIENTS

- Medium shrimp/prawns: 8
- Melted butter: 1 tbsp.
- Rosemary: 1 sprig
- Pepper and salt: as desired
- Minced garlic cloves: 3

DIRECTIONS

1. Combine all of the fixings in a mixing bowl. Toss well and arrange in the fryer basket.
2. Set the timer for 7 minutes: 356°F and serve.

Nutrition: Calories 180 Fat 10g Carbs 2g Protein 15g

409. HONEY & SRIRACHA TOSSED CALAMARI

PREPARATION: 10 MIN   **COOKING:** 20 MIN   **SERVINGS:** 2

INGREDIENTS

- Calamari tubes - tentacles if you prefer: .5 lb.
- Club soda: 1 cup
- Flour: 1 cup
- Salt - red pepper & black pepper: 2 dashes each
- Honey: .5 cup+ 1-2 tbsp. Sriracha

DIRECTIONS

1. Fully rinse the calamari and blot it dry using a bunch of paper towels. Slice into rings: .25-inch wide). Toss the rings into a bowl. Pour in the club soda and stir until all are submerged. Wait for about 10 minutes.
2. Sift the salt, flour, red & black pepper. Set aside for now.
3. Dredge the calamari into the flour mixture and set on a platter until ready to fry.
4. Spritz the basket of the Air Fryer with a small amount of cooking oil spray. Arrange the calamari in the basket, careful not to crowd it too much.
5. Set the temperature at 375°F and the timer for 11 minutes.
6. Shake the basket twice during the cooking process, loosening any rings that may stick.
7. Remove from the basket, toss with the sauce, and return to the fryer for two more minutes.
8. Serve with additional sauce as desired.
9. Make the sauce by combining honey, and sriracha, in a small bowl, mix until fully combined.

Nutrition: Calories 210 Fat 12g Carbs 5g Protein 19g

410. SALMON CROQUETTES

PREPARATION: 5 MIN   **COOKING:** 10 MIN   **SERVINGS:** 4

INGREDIENTS

- Red salmon: 1 lb. can
- Breadcrumbs: 1 cup
- Vegetable oil: .33 cup
- Chopped parsley: half of 1 bunch
- Eggs: 2

DIRECTIONS

1. Set the Air Fryer at 392°F.
2. Drain and mash the salmon. Whisk and add the eggs and parsley.
3. In another dish, mix the breadcrumbs and oil.
4. Prepare 16 croquettes using the breadcrumb mixture.
5. Arrange in the preheated fryer basket for 7 minutes.
6. Serve.

Nutrition: Calories 240 Fat 16g Carbs 7g Protein 30g

411. SPICY COD

PREPARATION: 5 MIN   **COOKING:** 10 MIN   **SERVINGS:** 4

INGREDIENTS

- 4 cod fillets; boneless
- 2 tbsp. assorted chili peppers
- 1 lemon; sliced
- Juice of 1 lemon
- Salt and black pepper to taste

DIRECTIONS

1. In your Air Fryer, mix the cod with the chili pepper, lemon juice, salt and pepper
2. Arrange the lemon slices on top and cook at 360°F for 10 minutes. Divide the fillets between plates and serve.

Nutrition: Calories 250 Fat 13g Carbs 13g Protein 29g

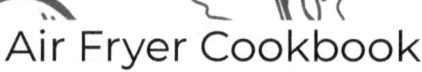

412. AIR FRIED LOBSTER TAILS

PREPARATION: 5 MIN **COOKING:** 10 MIN **SERVINGS:** 2

INGREDIENTS

- 2 tbsp. unsalted butter, melted
- 1 tbsp. minced garlic
- 1 tsp. salt
- 1 tbsp. minced fresh chives
- 2 (4- to 6 oz.) frozen lobster tails

DIRECTIONS

1. In a bowl, put the butter, garlic, salt, and chives then mix.
2. Butterfly the lobster tail: Starting at the meaty end of the tail, use kitchen shears to cut down the center of the top shell. Stop when you reach the fanned, wide part of the tail. Carefully spread apart the meat and the shell along the cut line, but keep the meat attached where it connects to the wide part of the tail. Use your hand to gently disconnect the meat from the bottom of the shell. Lift the meat up and out of the shell (keeping it attached at the wide end). Close the shell under the meat, so the meat rests on top of the shell.
3. Place the lobster in the Air Fryer basket and generously brush the butter mixture over the meat.
4. Set the temperature of your Air Fryer to 380°F. Set the timer and steam for 4 minutes.
5. Open the Air Fryer and rotate the lobster tails. Brush them with more of the butter mixture. Reset the timer and steam for 4 minutes more. The lobster is done when the meat is opaque.

Nutrition: Calories 255 Fat 13g Carbs 2g Protein 32g

413. AIR FRYER SALMON

PREPARATION: 5 MIN **COOKING:** 10 MIN **SERVINGS:** 2

INGREDIENTS

- ½ tsp. salt
- ½ tsp. garlic powder
- ½ tsp. smoked paprika
- Salmon

DIRECTIONS

1. Mix spices together and sprinkle onto salmon. Place seasoned salmon into the Air Fryer.
2. Close crisping lid. Set temperature to 400°F, and set time to 10 minutes.

Nutrition: Calories 185 Fat 11g Carbs 12g Protein 21g

414. SIMPLE SCALLOPS

PREPARATION: 5 MIN **COOKING:** 5 MIN **SERVINGS:** 4

INGREDIENTS

- 12 medium sea scallops
- 1 tsp. fine sea salt
- ground black pepper as desired
- Fresh thyme leaves, for garnish (optional)

Nutrition: Calories 170 Fat 11g Carbs 8g Protein 17g

DIRECTIONS

1. Grease the Air Fryer basket with avocado oil. Preheat the Air Fryer to 390°F. Rinse the scallops and pat completely dry. Spray avocado oil on the scallops and season them with the salt and pepper.
2. Place them in the Air Fryer basket, spacing them apart (if you're using a smaller Air Fryer, work in batches if necessary). Flip the scallops after cooking for 2 minutes, and cook for another 2 minutes, or until cooked through and no longer translucent. Garnish with ground black pepper and thyme leaves, if desired. Best served fresh.

415. 3-INGREDIENT AIR FRYER CATFISH

PREPARATION: 5 MIN **COOKING:** 15 MIN **SERVINGS:** 4

INGREDIENTS

- 1 tbsp. chopped parsley
- 1 tbsp. olive oil
- ¼ C. seasoned fish fry
- 4 catfish fillets

Nutrition: Calories 208 Fat 5g Carbs 5g Protein 17g

DIRECTIONS

1. Ensure your Air Fryer is preheated to 400°F.
2. Rinse off catfish fillets and pat dry. Add fish fry seasoning to Ziploc baggie, then catfish. Shake bag and ensure fish gets well coated. Spray each fillet with olive oil. Add fillets to Air Fryer basket.
3. Set temperature to 400°F, and set time to 10 minutes. Cook 10 minutes. Then flip and cook another 2-3 minutes.

416. PECAN-CRUSTED CATFISH

PREPARATION: 5 MIN **COOKING:** 12 MIN **SERVINGS:** 4

INGREDIENTS

- ½ cup pecan meal
- 1 tsp. fine sea salt
- ¼ tsp. ground black pepper
- 4 (4 oz.) catfish fillets
- For garnish (optional) Fresh oregano

Nutrition: Calories 162 Fat 11g Carbs 1g Protein 17g

DIRECTIONS

1. Grease the Air Fryer basket with avocado oil. Preheat the Air Fryer to 375°F. In a large bowl, mix the pecan meal, salt, and pepper. One at a time, dredge the catfish fillets in the mixture, coating them well. Use your hands to press the pecan meal into the fillets. Spray the fish with avocado oil and place them in the Air Fryer basket.
2. Cook the coated catfish for 12 minutes, or until it flakes easily and is no longer translucent in the center, flipping halfway through. Garnish with oregano sprigs and pecan halves, if desired.

Air Fryer Cookbook

417. FLYING FISH

PREPARATION: 5 MIN **COOKING:** 12 MIN **SERVINGS:** 4

INGREDIENTS

- Tbsp. Oil
- 3–4 oz Breadcrumbs
- 1 Whisked Whole Egg in a Saucer/Soup Plate
- 4 Fresh Fish Fillets
- Fresh Lemon (For serving)

DIRECTIONS

1. Warm up the Air Fryer to 350°F. Mix the crumbs and oil until it looks nice and loose. Dip the fish in the egg and coat lightly, then move on to the crumbs. Make sure the fillet is covered evenly.
2. Cook in the Air Fryer basket for roughly 12 minutes – depending on the size of the fillets you are using. Serve with fresh lemon & chips to complete the duo.

Nutrition: Calories 180 Fat 12g Carbs 9g Protein 19g

418. AIR FRYER FISH TACOS

PREPARATION: 5 MIN **COOKING:** 15 MIN **SERVINGS:** 4

INGREDIENTS

- 1 lb. cod
- 1 tbsp. cumin
- ½ tbsp. chili powder
- 1 ½ C. coconut flour
- 10 oz. Mexican beer
- 2 eggs

DIRECTIONS

1. Whisk beer and eggs together. Whisk flour, pepper, salt, cumin, and chili powder together. Slice cod into large pieces and coat in egg mixture then flour mixture.
2. Spray bottom of your Air Fryer basket with olive oil and add coated codpieces. Cook 15 minutes at 375°F.
3. Serve on lettuce leaves topped with homemade salsa.

Nutrition: Calories 178 Fat 10g Carbs 61g Protein 19g

41. BACON WRAPPED SCALLOPS

PREPARATION: 5 MIN **COOKING:** 5 MIN **SERVINGS:** 4

INGREDIENTS

- 1 tsp. paprika
- 1 tsp. lemon pepper
- 5 slices of center-cut bacon
- 20 raw sea scallops

DIRECTIONS

1. Rinse and drain scallops, placing on paper towels to soak up excess moisture. Cut slices of bacon into 4 pieces. With a piece of bacon, wrap each scallop, then using toothpicks to secure. Sprinkle wrapped scallops with paprika and lemon pepper.
2. Spray Air Fryer basket with olive oil and add scallops.
3. Cook 5-6 minutes at 400°F, making sure to flip halfway through.

Nutrition: Calories 389 Fat 17g Carbs 63g Protein 21g;

420. QUICK FRIED CATFISH

PREPARATION: 5 MIN   **COOKING:** 15 MIN   **SERVINGS:** 4

INGREDIENTS

- 3/4 cups Original Bisquick™ mix
- 1/2 cup yellow cornmeal
- 1 tbsp. seafood seasoning
- 4 catfish fillets (4-6 oz. each)
- 1/2 cup ranch dressing

DIRECTIONS

1. In a bowl mix the Bisquick mix, cornmeal, and seafood seasoning together. Pat the filets dry, then brush them with ranch dressing. Press the filets into the Bisquick mix on both sides until the filet is evenly coated.
2. Cook in your Air Fryer at 360°F for 15 minutes, flip the filets halfway through. Serve.

Nutrition: Calories 372 Fat 16g Carbs 14g Protein 28g

421. AIR-FRIED HERBED SHRIMP

PREPARATION: 2 MIN   **COOKING:** 5 MIN   **SERVINGS:** 4

INGREDIENTS

- One ¼ lb. shrimp, peeled and deveined
- ½ tsp. paprika
- One tbsp. olive oil
- ¼ cayenne pepper
- ½ tsp. Old Bay seasoning

DIRECTIONS

1. Preheat Air Fryer to 400°F. Mix all the ingredients in a bowl. Place the seasoned shrimp into the Air Fryer basket and cook for 5-minutes.

Nutrition: Calories 300 Fat 9.3g Carbs 8.2g Protein 14.6g

422. WILD CAUGHT SALMON

PREPARATION: 5 MIN   **COOKING:** 12 MIN   **SERVINGS:** 2

INGREDIENTS

- 2 salmon fillets, wild-caught, each about 1 ½ inch thick
- 1 tsp. ground black pepper
- 2 tsp. paprika
- 1 tsp. salt
- 2 tsp. olive oil

DIRECTIONS

1. Switch on the air fryer, insert fryer basket, grease it with olive oil, then shut with its lid, set the fryer at 390°F and preheat for 5 minutes. Meanwhile, rub each salmon fillet with oil and then season with black pepper, paprika, and salt.
2. Open the fryer, add seasoned salmon in it, close with its lid and cook for 7 minutes until nicely golden and cooked, flipping the fillets halfway through the frying. when air fryer beeps, open its lid, transfer salmon onto a serving plate and serve.

Nutrition: Calories 288 Carbs 1.4g Fat 18.9g Protein 28.3g

BONUS KETO AIR FRYER RECIPES

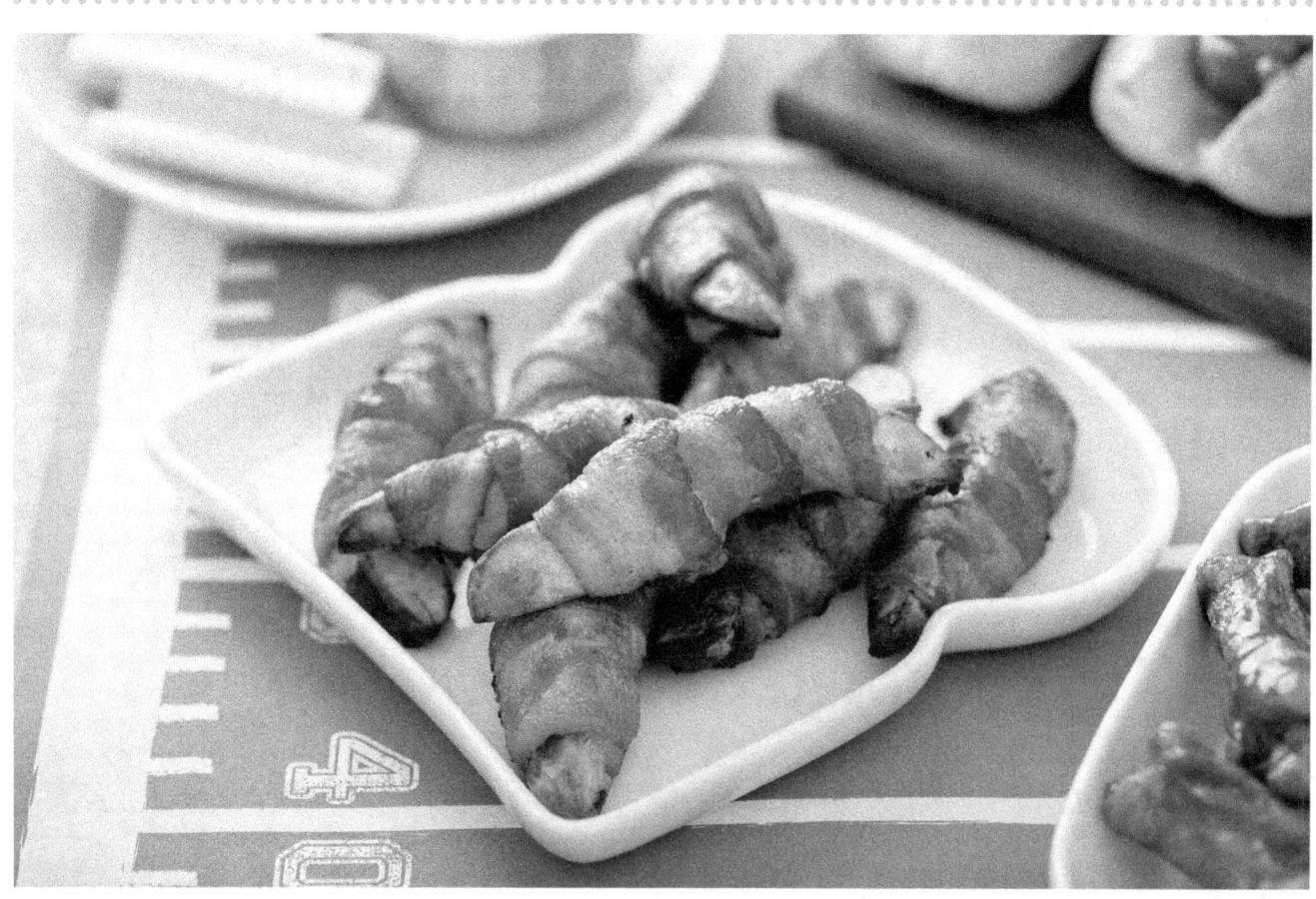

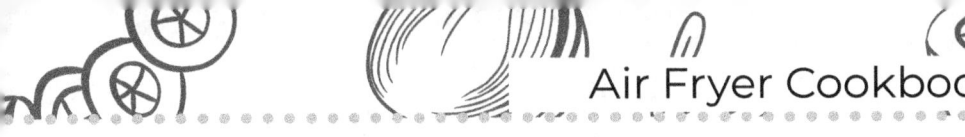

Air Fryer Cookbook

423. CRISPY KETO PORK BITES

PREPARATION: 5 MIN **COOKING:** 25 MIN **SERVINGS:** 2

INGREDIENTS

- 1 medium onion
- ½ lb. pork belly
- tbsp. coconut cream
- 1 tbsp. butter
- Salt & pepper, to taste

DIRECTIONS

1. Slice the pork belly into even and thin strips
2. The onion has to be diced.
3. Transfer all the ingredients into a mixing bowl and allow it to marinate in the fridge for the next two hours.
4. Fix the temperature to 350°F and preheat the Air Fryer for 5 minutes.
5. Keep the pork strips inside the Air Fryer and let it cook for 25 minutes at a temperature of 350°F.
6. Enjoy!

Nutrition: Calories 448 Fat 42g Carbs 2g Protein 20g

424. KETO AIR BREAD

PREPARATION: 10 MIN **COOKING:** 25 MIN **SERVINGS:** 19

INGREDIENTS

- 1 cup almond flour
- ¼ sea salt
- 1 tsp. baking powder
- ¼ cup butter
- 3 eggs

DIRECTIONS

1. Crack the eggs into a bowl then using a hand blender mix them up. Melt the butter at room temperature. Take the melted butter and add it to the egg mixture. Add the salt, baking powder and almond flour to egg mixture and knead the dough.
2. Cover the prepared dough with a towel for 10-minutes to rest. Meanwhile, preheat your Air Fryer to 360°F.
3. Place the prepared dough in the Air Fryer tin and cook the bread for 10-minutes. Then reduce the heat to 350°F and cook the bread for additional 15-minutes you can use a toothpick to check to make sure the bread is cooked.
4. Transfer the bread to a wooden board to allow it to chill. Once the bread has chilled, then slice and serve it.

Nutrition: Calories 40 Fat 3.9g Carbs 0.5g Protein 1.2g

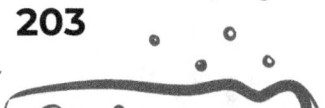

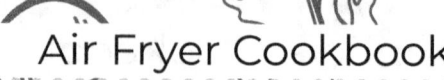

425. HERBED BREAKFAST EGGS

PREPARATION: 10 MIN **COOKING:** 17 MIN **SERVINGS:** 2

INGREDIENTS

- 4 eggs
- 1 tsp. oregano
- 1 tsp. parsley, dried
- ½ tsp. sea salt
- 1 tbsp. chives, chopped
- 1 tbsp. cream
- 1 tsp. paprika

DIRECTIONS

1. Place the eggs in the Air Fryer basket and cook them for 17-minutes at 320°F. Meanwhile, combine the parsley, oregano, cream, and salt in shallow bowl.
2. Chop the chives and add them to cream mixture. When the eggs are cooked, place them in cold water and allow them to chill. After this, peel the eggs and cut them into halves.
3. Remove the egg yolks and add yolks to cream mixture and mash to blend well with a fork. Then fill the egg whites with the cream-egg yolk mixture. Serve immediately.

Nutrition: Calories 136 Fat 9.3g Carbs 2.1g Protein 11.4g

426. EGGS IN ZUCCHINI NESTS

PREPARATION: 10 MIN **COOKING:** 7 MIN **SERVINGS:** 2

INGREDIENTS

- 4 tsp.s butter
- ½ tsp. paprika
- ½ tsp. black pepper
- ¼ tsp. sea salt
- 4 oz. cheddar cheese, shredded
- 4 eggs
- 8 oz. zucchini, grated

DIRECTIONS

1. Grate the zucchini and place the butter in ramekins. Add the grated zucchini in ramekins in the shape of nests. Sprinkle the zucchini nests with salt, pepper, and paprika. Beat the eggs and pour over zucchini nests.
2. Top egg mixture with shredded cheddar cheese. Preheat the Air Fryer basket at 360°F and cook the dish for 7-minutes. When the zucchini nests are cooked, chill them for 3 minutes and serve them in the ramekins.

Nutrition: Calories 221 Fat 17.7g Carbs 2.9g Protein 13.4g

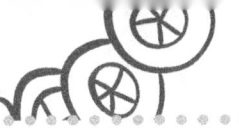 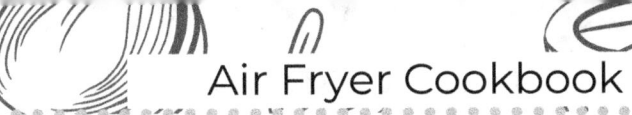

Air Fryer Cookbook

427. BREAKFAST LIVER PATE

PREPARATION: 5 MIN **COOKING:** 10 MIN **SERVINGS:** 7

INGREDIENTS

- 1 lb. chicken liver
- 1 tsp. salt
- ½ tsp. cilantro, dried
- 1 yellow onion, diced
- 1 tsp. ground black pepper
- 1 cup water
- 4 tbsp. butter

DIRECTIONS

1. Chop the chicken liver roughly and place it in the Air Fryer basket tray. Add water to Air Fryer basket tray and add diced onion. Preheat your Air Fryer to 360°F and cook chicken liver for 10-minutes. Dry out the chicken liver when it is finished cooking.
2. Transfer the chicken liver to blender, add butter, ground black pepper and dried cilantro and blend. Once you get a pate texture, transfer to liver pate bowl and serve immediately or keep in the fridge for later.

Nutrition: Calories 173 Fat 10.8g Carbs 2.2g Protein 16.1g

428. BREAD-FREE BREAKFAST SANDWICH

PREPARATION: 10 MIN **COOKING:** 10 MIN **SERVINGS:** 2

INGREDIENTS

- 6 oz. ground chicken
- 2 slices of cheddar cheese
- 2 lettuce leaves
- 1 tbsp. dill, dried
- ½ tsp. sea salt
- 1 egg
- 1 tsp. cayenne pepper
- 1 tsp. tomato puree

DIRECTIONS

1. Combine the ground chicken with the pepper and sea salt. Add the dried dill and stir. Beat the egg into the ground chicken mixture. Make 2 medium-sized burgers from the ground chicken mixture.
2. Preheat your Air Fryer to 380°F. Spray the Air Fryer basket tray with olive oil and place the ground chicken burgers inside of it. Cook the chicken burgers for 10-minutes Flip over burgers and cook for an additional 6-minutes. When the burgers are cooked, transfer them to the lettuce leaves.
3. Sprinkle the top of them with tomato puree and with a slice of cheddar cheese. Serve immediately!

Nutrition: Calories 324 Fat 19.2g Carbs 2.3g Protein 34.8g

429. EGG BUTTER

PREPARATION: 5 MIN   **COOKING:** 17 MIN   **SERVINGS:** 2

INGREDIENTS

- 4 eggs
- 4 tbsp. butter
- 1 tsp. salt

Nutrition: Calories 164 Fat 8.5g Carbs 2.67g Protein 3g

DIRECTIONS

1. Cover the Air Fryer basket with foil and place the eggs there. Transfer the Air Fryer basket into the Air Fryer and cook the eggs for 17 minutes at 320°F.
2. When the time is over, remove the eggs from the Air Fryer basket and put them in cold water to chill them. After this, peel the eggs and chop them up finely. Combine the chopped eggs with butter and add salt.
3. Mix it until you get the spread texture. Serve the egg butter with the keto almond bread.

430. AWESOME LEMON BELL PEPPERS

PREPARATION: 10 MIN   **COOKING:** 5 MIN   **SERVINGS:** 4

INGREDIENTS

- 4 bell peppers
- 1 tsp. olive oil
- 1 tbsp. lemon juice
- 1/4 tsp. garlic, minced
- 1 tsp. parsley, chopped
- 1 pinch sea salt
- Pinch of pepper

Nutrition: Calories 59 Fat 4g Carbs 6g Protein 2g

DIRECTIONS

1. Preheat your Air Fryer to 390°F
2. Add bell pepper in the Air Fryer. Drizzle with it with the olive oil and air fry for 5 minutes
3. Take a serving plate and transfer it. Take a small bowl and add garlic, parsley, lemon juice, salt, and pepper
4. Mix them well and Drizzle with the mixture over the peppers. Serve and enjoy!

431. CREAMY POTATOES

PREPARATION: 10 MIN   **COOKING:** 20 MIN   **SERVINGS:** 2

INGREDIENTS

- ¾ lb. potatoes, peeled and cubed
- 1 tbsp. olive oil
- Salt and black pepper, to taste
- ½ tbsp. hot paprika
- ½ cup Greek yogurt

Nutrition: Calories 170 Fat 3g Carb: 2g Protein 5g

DIRECTIONS

1. Place potatoes in a bowl, pour water to cover, and leave aside for 10 minutes. Drain, pat dry, then transfer to another bowl.
2. Add salt, pepper, paprika, and half of the oil to the potatoes and mix.
3. Put potatoes in the Air Fryer basket and cook at 360°F for 20 minutes.
4. In a bowl, mix yogurt with salt, pepper, and the rest of the oil and whisk.
5. Divide potatoes onto plates, drizzle with yogurt dressing, mix, and serve.

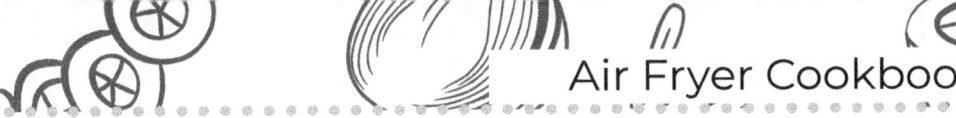

432. GREEN BEANS AND CHERRY TOMATOES

PREPARATION: 10 MIN   **COOKING:** 15 MIN   **SERVINGS:** 2

INGREDIENTS

- 8 oz. cherry tomatoes
- 8 oz. green beans
- 1 tbsp. olive oil
- Salt and black pepper, to taste

DIRECTIONS

1. In a bowl, mix cherry tomatoes with green beans, olive oil, salt, and pepper. Mix.
2. Cook in the Air Fryer at 400°F for 15 minutes. Shake once. Serve.

Nutrition: Calories 162 Fat 6g Carb: 8g Protein 9g

433. CRISPY BRUSSELS SPROUTS AND POTATOES

PREPARATION: 10 MIN   **COOKING:** 8 MIN   **SERVINGS:** 2

INGREDIENTS

- ¾ lb. brussels sprouts, washed and trimmed
- ½ cup new potatoes, chopped
- 2 tsp.s bread crumbs
- Salt and black pepper, to taste
- 2 tsp.s butter

DIRECTIONS

1. In a bowl, add Brussels sprouts, potatoes, bread crumbs, salt, pepper, and butter. Mix well.
2. Place in the Air Fryer and cook at 400°F for 8 minutes. Serve.

Nutrition: Calories 152 Fat 3g Carb: 7g Protein 4g

434. HERBED TOMATOES

PREPARATION: 10 MIN   **COOKING:** 15 MIN   **SERVINGS:** 2

INGREDIENTS

- 2 big tomatoes, halved and insides scooped out
- Salt and black pepper, to taste
- ½ tbsp. olive oil
- 1 clove garlic, minced
- ¼ tsp. thyme, chopped

DIRECTIONS

1. In the Air Fryer, mix tomatoes with thyme, garlic, oil, salt, and pepper.
2. Mix and cook at 390°F for 15 minutes. Serve.

Nutrition: Calories 112 Fat 1g Carb: 4g Protein 4g

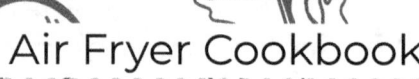
Air Fryer Cookbook

435. AIR FRIED LEEKS

PREPARATION: 10 MIN **COOKING:** 7 MIN **SERVINGS:** 2

INGREDIENTS

- 2 leeks, washed, ends cut, and halved
- Salt and black pepper, to taste
- ½ tbsp. butter, melted
- ½ tbsp. lemon juice

Nutrition: Calories 100 Fat 4g Carb: 6g Protein 2g

DIRECTIONS

1. Rub leeks with melted butter and season with salt and pepper.
2. Lay it inside the Air Fryer and cook at 350F for 7 minutes.
3. Arrange on a platter. Drizzle with lemon juice and serve.

436. CRISPY BROCCOLI

PREPARATION: 10 MIN **COOKING:** 10 MIN **SERVINGS:** 4

INGREDIENTS

- 1 large head fresh broccoli
- 2 tsp.s olive oil
- tbsp. lemon juice

Nutrition: Calories 63 Fat 2g Carbs 10g Protein 4g

DIRECTIONS

1. Rinse the broccoli and pat dry. Cut off the florets and separate them. You can also use the broccoli stems too; cut them into 1" chunks and peel them.
2. Toss the broccoli, olive oil, and lemon juice in a large bowl until coated.
3. Roast the broccoli in the Air Fryer at 365°F, in batches, for 10 to 14 minutes or until the broccoli is crisp-tender and slightly brown around the edges. Repeat with the remaining broccoli. Serve immediately.

437. GARLIC-ROASTED BELL PEPPERS

PREPARATION: 5 MIN **COOKING:** 20 MIN **SERVINGS:** 4

INGREDIENTS

- 4 bell peppers, any colors, stemmed, seeded, membranes removed, and cut into fourths
- 1 tsp. olive oil
- 4 garlic cloves, minced
- ½ tsp. dried thyme

DIRECTIONS

1. Put the peppers in the basket of the Air Fryer and drizzle with olive oil. Toss gently. Roast for 15 minutes at 365°F.
2. Sprinkle with the garlic and thyme. Roast for 3 to 5 minutes more, or until tender. Serve immediately.

Nutrition: Calories 36 Fat 1g Carbs 5g Protein 1g

438. ASPARAGUS WITH GARLIC

PREPARATION: 5 MIN **COOKING:** 10 MIN **SERVINGS:** 4

INGREDIENTS

- 1-lb. asparagus, rinsed, ends snapped off where they naturally break
- 2 tsp.s olive oil
- 3 garlic cloves, minced
- 2 tbsp. balsamic vinegar
- ½ tsp. dried thyme

Nutrition: Calories 41 Fat 1g Carbs 6g Protein 3g

DIRECTIONS

1. In a huge bowl, mix the asparagus with olive oil. ¬Transfer to the Air Fryer basket.
2. Sprinkle with garlic. Roast for 4 to 5 minutes at 375°F for crisp-tender or for 8 to 11 minutes for asparagus that is crisp on the outside and tender on the inside.
3. Drizzle with the balsamic vinegar and sprinkle with the thyme leaves. Serve immediately.

439. INSTANT LAMB STEAK WITH APPLES AND PEARS

PREPARATION: 10 MIN **COOKING:** 1 H **SERVINGS:** 3

INGREDIENTS

- 2 lamb steaks
- 3 Arkansas Black apples, sliced
- 2 pears, sliced
- 3 tbsp. melted butter
- 4 kale leaves
- 2 tbsp. apple cider
- ½ tsp. ground black pepper
- 1 medium white onion, cut into 8 wedges
- ½ tsp. ground allspice
- 1 tsp. black pepper

Nutrition: Calories 379 Fat 79g Carbs 279g Protein 68g

DIRECTIONS

1. In a skillet, melt the butter and Put the Air Fryer to sauté mode and spoon the melted butter.
2. Add in the lamb steaks and sauté for around 20 minutes.
3. Transfer the lamb to a plate.
4. Add in the onion, apples and pears in the Air Fryer and allow them to sauté for 10 minutes until the apples are somewhat browned and caramelized.
5. Add in the lamb and pour the apple cider on top. Combine all the ingredients (except kale) and close the lid to cook for 20-30 minutes on a HIGH pressure.
6. Portion the lamb into two plates. Serve the lamb with the apples and fresh kale.

440. ADOBO CHICKEN

PREPARATION: 5 MIN **COOKING:** 30 MIN **SERVINGS:** 6

INGREDIENTS

- 2 lbs. Chicken, Boneless
- 1 Tbsp. Turmeric
- 1 Tbsp. Garlic
- 4 Tomatoes, Chopped
- 7 Oz. Green Chilies
- ½ Cup Water

Nutrition: Calories 342 Fat 19g Carbs 2g Protein 32g

DIRECTIONS

1. Put your chicken into your Air Fryer and then seasoning it. Add in your chilies and tomatoes.
2. Empty your water in, and then cook for twenty-five minutes before using a quick release. Serve on its own or over rice.

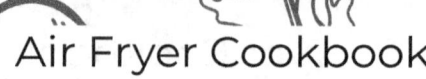

Air Fryer Cookbook

441. TOMATO & FETA SHRIMP

PREPARATION: 5 MIN   **COOKING:** 25 MIN   **SERVINGS:** 6

INGREDIENTS

- 1 ½ Cups Onion, Chopped
- ½ Tsp. Red Pepper Flakes
- 1 Tbsp. Garlic
- 3 Tbsp. Butter, Unsalted
- Oz. Tomatoes, Canned, Diced & Undrained
- 1 Tsp. Oregano
- 1 Tsp. Sea Salt, Fine
- 1 Cup Feta Cheese, Crumbled
- ½ Cup Black Olives, Sliced
- ¼ Cup Parsley, Chopped
- 1 lb. Shrimp, Frozen & Peeled

DIRECTIONS

1. Press sauté, and then add in your butter. Once the butter begins to bubble and get foamy, add in your red pepper flakes and garlic, cooking for a minute. They should become fragrant.
2. Mix in your oregano, tomatoes, salt, and onion. Stir well, and then add your frozen shrimp.
3. Secure your lid, and then cook on low pressure for a minute. Use a quick release, and then add in your tomato broth.
4. Let this mixture to cool for a while, and then scatter olives, feta cheese and parsley over. You can serve this warm on its own or over mashed cauliflower.

Nutrition: Calories 120 Fat 3g Carbs 7g Protein 15g

442. ROASTED CHICKEN

PREPARATION: 10 MIN   **COOKING:** 45 MIN   **SERVINGS:** 4

INGREDIENTS

- 2 Tbsp. Rosemary, Fresh
- 1 Tbsp. Sea Salt, Fine
- ½ Tbsp. Black Pepper
- 1 Bay leaf
- 1 Tbsp. Thyme
- 1 tbsp. Olive Oil
- 1 Chicken, Whole
- 1 Tbsp. Lemon Juice, Fresh

DIRECTIONS

1. Press sauté, and then drizzle your olive oil. Cook your chicken, flipping once before placing it to the side.
2. Add in your stand, and then add in your lemon juice, rosemary, chicken stock, and thyme. Season with salt and pepper.
3. Press poultry, and close the lid. Cook for 25 to 30 minutes.
4. Allow to cool before serving. Remember to remove your bay leaf.

Nutrition: Calories 250 Fat 31g Carbs 1g Protein 30g

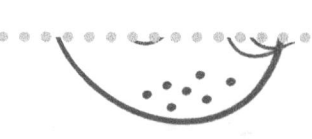

443. SALSA CHICKEN

PREPARATION: 5 MIN **COOKING:** 15 MIN **SERVINGS:** 6

INGREDIENTS

- ½ Tsp. Chili
- 1 Tbsp. Paprika
- ½ Tbsp. Cumin
- 17 Oz. Salsa Verde
- 2 lbs. chicken Breasts, Boneless & Skinless
- 1 Tbsp. Black Pepper
- 1 Tbsp. sea Salt
- ½ Onion, Diced
- 1 Jalapeno, Diced
- ¼ Cup Cilantro, Fresh & Chopped
- 1 Lime, Fresh

DIRECTIONS

1. Put half of your salsa into the Air Fryer, and then season with salt and pepper. Add in your cilantro, jalapeno, and onion. Add in your chicken, and mix well.
2. Add in another quarter of salsa, and then place your other ¼ cup to the side. Close the lid, and cook on high heat for 10 minutes. Use a quick release, and then shred your chicken.
3. Put it back in your pot, and then add in your lime juice and salsa.

Nutrition: Calories 96 Fat 9g Carbs 3g Protein 11g

444. ITALIAN SHREDDED CHICKEN

PREPARATION: 5 MIN **COOKING:** 15 MIN **SERVINGS:** 8

INGREDIENTS

- 1 Tbsp. Italian Seasoning
- 4 lbs. Chicken Breasts
- ½ Tsp. Sea Salt, Fine
- ½ Tsp. Ground Black Pepper
- 1 Cup Chicken Broth

DIRECTIONS

1. Lay your chicken in the Air Fryer, and then add in your seasoning. Spice it well, and then pour your broth over your chicken.
2. Cook on high pressure for 10 minutes, and then shred into strips before serving with broth

Nutrition: Calories 170 Fat 7g Carbs 1g Protein 27g

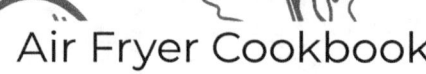 Air Fryer Cookbook

445. ZOODLE SOUP

PREPARATION: 5 MIN **COOKING:** 25 MIN **SERVINGS:** 6

INGREDIENTS

- 1 Tbsp. Olive oil
- 1 Onion, Diced
- 1 lb. Chicken Breasts, Boneless, Skinless & Sliced
- 2 Cloves Garlic, Minced
- 3 Carrots, Sliced
- 1 Bay leaf
- 6 Cups Chicken Broth
- 3 Stalks Celery, Sliced
- 1 Jalapeno Pepper, Diced
- 2 Tbsp. Apple Cider Vinegar
- 4 Zucchinis, Spiralized
- Sea Salt & Black Pepper to Taste

DIRECTIONS

1. Choose sauté, and then add in your garlic and onion. Cook until you can smell the aroma, and then add in your celery, carrots, jalapeno and chicken breasts. Stir for a minute before seasoning with salt and pepper.
2. Mix in your bay leaf, chicken broth, and apple cider vinegar. Close the lid, and cook on high pressure for 20 minutes before using a quick release.
3. Choose sauté again, and then add in your zucchini, cooking for another three minutes. Serve warm.

Nutrition: Calories 164 Fat 5g Carbs 10g Protein 19g

446. CABBAGE SOUP

PREPARATION: 10 MIN **COOKING:** 35 MIN **SERVINGS:** 6

INGREDIENTS

- 1 Onion, Chopped
- 1 Tbsp. Avocado Oil
- 1 lb. Ground Beef
- ½ Tsp. Garlic Powder
- 1 Can Tomatoes, diced
- Sea Salt & Black Pepper to Taste
- 6 Cups Bone Broth
- 1 lb. Cabbage, Shredded
- 2 Bay Leaves

DIRECTIONS

1. Choose sauté, and then add in your oil. Once it heats up, sauté your beef and onions. Flavor with garlic, salt and pepper. Cook for 2 minutes, and then add in your bone broth, , cabbage, bay leaves and diced tomatoes.
2. Cook on high pressure for thirty minutes.
3. Use a quick release, and serve warm.

Nutrition: Calories 428 Fat 24.8 Carbs 9.2g Protein 26.3g

447. MOJO CHICKEN

PREPARATION: 5 MIN   **COOKING:** 45 MIN   **SERVINGS:** 4

INGREDIENTS

- 1 Tbsp. Lemon Juice, Fresh
- 1 Tbsp. Olive oil
- 1 Whole chicken
- 2 Tbsp. Rosemary, Fresh & Chopped
- 1 Tbsp., Fresh & Chopped
- Sea Salt & Black Pepper to Taste

Nutrition: Calories 250 Fat 31g Carbs 1g Protein 30g

DIRECTIONS

1. Choose sauté, and then add in your olive oil. Mix in your chicken, and sauté on both sides. Set aside, and then add in your trivet.
2. Mix in your lemon juice, chicken stock, rosemary and thyme. Flavor with salt and pepper, and then press your poultry button.
3. Cook for 25-30 mins., and then remove the bay leaf before serving.

448. SPICED ALMONDS

PREPARATION: 5 MIN   **COOKING:** 12 MIN   **SERVINGS:** 4

INGREDIENTS

- ½ tsp. ground cinnamon
- ½ tsp. smoked paprika
- 1 cup almonds
- 1 egg white
- Sea salt to taste

Nutrition: Calories 90 Fat 2g Carbs 3g Protein 5g

DIRECTIONS

1. Preheat Air Fryer to 310°F. Grease the Air Fryer basket with cooking spray. In a bowl, beat the egg white with cinnamon and paprika and stir in almonds.
2. Spread the almonds on the bottom of the frying basket and Air Fry for 12 minutes, shaking once or twice. Remove and sprinkle with sea salt to serve.

449. CRISPY CAULIFLOWER BITES

PREPARATION: 5 MIN   **COOKING:** 15 MIN   **SERVINGS:** 4

INGREDIENTS

- 1 tbsp. Italian seasoning
- 1 cup flour
- 1 cup milk
- 1 egg, beaten
- 1 head cauliflower, cut into florets

Nutrition: Calories 70 Fat 1g Carbs 2g Protein 3g

DIRECTIONS

1. Preheat Air Fryer to 390°F. Grease the Air Fryer basket with cooking spray. In a bowl, mix the flour, milk, egg, and Italian seasoning. Coat the cauliflower in the mixture and drain the excess liquid.
2. Place the florets in the frying basket, spray them with cooking spray, and Air Fry for 7 minutes. Shake and continue cooking for another 5 minutes. Allow to cool before serving.

450. ROASTED COCONUT CARROTS

PREPARATION: 5 MIN   **COOKING:** 10 MIN   **SERVINGS:** 4

INGREDIENTS

- 1 tbsp. coconut oil, melted
- 1 lb. horse carrots, sliced
- Salt and black pepper to taste
- ½ tsp. chili powder

DIRECTIONS

1. Preheat Air Fryer to 400°F.
2. In a bowl, mix the carrots with coconut oil, chili powder, salt, and pepper. Place in the Air Fryer and Air Fry for 7 minutes. Shake the basket and cook for another 5 minutes until golden brown. Serve.

Nutrition: Calories 80 Fat 1g Carbs 3g Protein 4g

451. BAKED POTATOES WITH BACON

PREPARATION: 5 MIN   **COOKING:** 30 MIN   **SERVINGS:** 4

INGREDIENTS

- 4 potatoes, scrubbed, halved, cut lengthwise
- 1 tbsp. olive oil
- Salt and black pepper to taste
- 4 oz bacon, chopped

DIRECTIONS

1. Preheat Air Fryer to 390°F. Brush the potatoes with olive oil and season with salt and pepper. Arrange them in the greased frying basket, cut-side down.
2. Bake for 15 minutes, flip them, top with bacon and bake for 12-15 minutes or until potatoes are golden and bacon is crispy. Serve warm.

Nutrition: Calories 150 Fat 7g Carbs 9g Protein 12g

452. WALNUT & CHEESE FILLED MUSHROOMS

PREPARATION: 5 MIN   **COOKING:** 10 MIN   **SERVINGS:** 4

INGREDIENTS

- 4 large portobello mushroom caps
- ⅓ cup walnuts, minced
- 1 tbsp. canola oil
- ½ cup mozzarella cheese, shredded
- 2 tbsp. fresh parsley, chopped

DIRECTIONS

1. Preheat Air Fryer to 350°F. Grease the Air Fryer basket with cooking spray.
2. Rub the mushrooms with canola oil and fill them with mozzarella cheese. Top with minced walnuts and arrange on the bottom of the greased Air Fryer basket. Bake for 10 minutes or until golden on top. Remove, let cool for a few minutes and sprinkle with freshly chopped parsley to serve.

Nutrition: Calories 110 Fat 5g Carbs 6g Protein 8g

Air Fryer Cookbook

453. AIR-FRIED CHICKEN THIGHS

PREPARATION: 5 MIN **COOKING:** 15 MIN **SERVINGS:** 4

INGREDIENTS

- 1 ½ lb. chicken thighs
- 2 eggs, lightly beaten
- 1 cup seasoned breadcrumbs
- ½ tsp. oregano
- Salt and black pepper, to taste

DIRECTIONS

1. Preheat Air Fryer to 390°F. Season the chicken with oregano, salt, and pepper. In a bowl, add the beaten eggs. In a separate bowl, add the breadcrumbs. Dip chicken thighs in the egg wash, then roll them in the breadcrumbs and press firmly so the breadcrumbs stick well.
2. Spray the chicken with cooking spray and arrange on the frying basket in a single layer, skin-side up. Air Fry for 12 minutes, turn the chicken thighs over and continue cooking for 6-8 more minutes. Serve.

Nutrition: Calories 190 Fat 8g Carbs 11g Protein 16g

---

454. SIMPLE BUTTERED POTATOES

PREPARATION: 5 MIN **COOKING:** 30 MIN **SERVINGS:** 4

INGREDIENTS

- 1 lb. potatoes, cut into wedges
- 2 garlic cloves, grated
- 1 tsp. fennel seeds
- 2 tbsp. butter, melted
- Salt and black pepper to taste

DIRECTIONS

1. In a bowl, mix the potatoes, butter, garlic, fennel seeds, salt, and black pepper, until they are well-coated. Set up the potatoes in the Air Fryer basket.
2. Bake on 360°F for 25 minutes, shaking once during cooking until crispy on the outside and tender on the inside. Serve warm.

Nutrition: Calories 100 Fat 4g Carbs 8g Protein 7g

---

455. HOMEMADE PEANUT CORN NUTS

PREPARATION: 5 MIN **COOKING:** 20 MIN **SERVINGS:** 4

INGREDIENTS

- 6 oz dried hominy, soaked overnight
- 3 tbsp. peanut oil
- 2 tbsp. old bay seasoning
- Salt to taste

DIRECTIONS

1. Preheat Air Fryer to 390°F.
2. Pat dry hominy and season with salt and old bay seasoning. Drizzle with oil and toss to coat. Spread in the Air Fryer basket and Air Fry for 10-12 minutes. Remove to shake up and return to cook for 10 more minutes until crispy. Transfer to a towel-lined plate to soak up the excess fat. Let cool and serve.

Nutrition: Calories 100 Fat 3g Carbs 3g Protein 5g

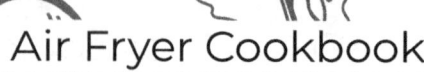

456. DUCK FAT ROASTED RED POTATOES

PREPARATION: 5 MIN   **COOKING:** 25 MIN   **SERVINGS:** 4

INGREDIENTS

- 4 red potatoes, cut into wedges
- 1 tbsp. garlic powder
- Salt and black pepper to taste
- 2 tbsp. thyme, chopped
- 3 tbsp. duck fat, melted

DIRECTIONS

1. Preheat Air Fryer to 380°F. In a bowl, mix duck fat, garlic powder, salt, and pepper. Add the potatoes and shake to coat.
2. Place in the basket and bake for 12 minutes, remove the basket, shake and continue cooking for another 8-10 minutes until golden brown. Serve warm topped with thyme.

Nutrition: Calories 110 Fat 5g Carbs 8g Protein 7g

457. CHICKEN WINGS WITH ALFREDO SAUCE

PREPARATION: 5 MIN   **COOKING:** 20 MIN   **SERVINGS:** 4

INGREDIENTS

- 1 ½ lb. chicken wings, pat-dried
- Salt to taste
- ½ cup Alfredo sauce

DIRECTIONS

1. Preheat Air Fryer to 370°F.
2. Season the wings with salt. Arrange them in the greased Air Fryer basket, without touching and Air Fry for 12 minutes until no longer pink in the center. Work in batches if needed. Flip them, increase the heat to 390°F and cook for 5 more minutes. Plate the wings and drizzle with Alfredo sauce to serve.

Nutrition: Calories 150 Fat 5g Carbs 7g Protein 14g

458. CRISPY KALE CHIPS

PREPARATION: 5 MIN   **COOKING:** 10 MIN   **SERVINGS:** 4

INGREDIENTS

- 4 cups kale leaves, stems removed, chopped
- 2 tbsp. olive oil
- 1 tsp. garlic powder
- Salt and black pepper to taste
- ¼ tsp. onion powder

DIRECTIONS

1. In a bowl, mix kale and olive oil. Add in garlic and onion powders, salt, and black pepper; toss to coat.
2. Arrange the kale in the frying basket and Air Fry for 8 minutes at 350°F, shaking once. Serve cool.

Nutrition: Calories 80 Fat 1g Carbs 3g Protein 3g

459. CRISPY SQUASH

PREPARATION: 5 MIN **COOKING:** 20 MIN **SERVINGS:** 4

INGREDIENTS

- 2 cups butternut squash, cubed
- 2 tbsp. olive oil
- Salt and black pepper to taste
- ¼ tsp. dried thyme
- 1 tbsp. fresh parsley, finely chopped

Nutrition: Calories 100 Fat 2g Carbs 5g Fat 2g Protein 3g

DIRECTIONS

1. In a bowl, add squash, olive oil, salt, pepper, and thyme, and toss to coat.
2. Place the squash in the Air Fryer and Air Fry for 14 minutes at 360°F, shaking once or twice. Serve sprinkled with fresh parsley.

460. KETOGENIC MAC & CHEESE

PREPARATION: 5 MIN **COOKING:** 20 MIN **SERVINGS:** 4

INGREDIENTS

- tbsp. avocado oil
- Sea salt & black pepper to taste
- 1 cauliflower, medium
- ¼ cup heavy cream
- ¼ cup almond milk, unsweetened
- 1 cup cheddar cheese, shredded

Nutrition: Calories 135.5 Fat 10.2g Carbs 1.4 g Protein 27g

DIRECTIONS

1. Start by preheating your Air Fryer to 400°F, and then make sure to grease your Air Fryer basket.
2. Chop your cauliflower into florets, and then Drizzle with oil over them. Toss until they're well coated, and then season with salt and pepper to taste.
3. Heat your cheddar, heavy cream, milk and avocado oil in a pot, pouring the mixture over your cauliflower.
4. Cook for fourteen minutes, and then serve warm.

461. SALMON PIE

PREPARATION: 5 MIN   **COOKING:** 45 MIN   **SERVINGS:** 8

INGREDIENTS

- 1 tsp. paprika
- ½ cup cream
- ½ tsp.s baking soda
- 1 ½ cups almond flour
- 1 onion, diced
- 1 tbsp. apple cider vinegar
- 1 lb. Salmon
- 1 tbsp. chives
- 1 tsp. dill
- 1 tsp. oregano
- 1 tsp. butter
- 1 tsp. parsley
- 1 egg

Nutrition: Calories 134 Fat 8.1g Carbs 2.2 g Protein 13.2 g

DIRECTIONS

1. Start by beating your eggs in a bowl, making sure they're whisked well. Add in your cream, whisking for another two minutes
2. Add in your apple cider vinegar and baking soda, stirring well.
3. Add in your almond flour, combining until it makes a non-stick, smooth dough.
4. Chop your salmon into pieces, and then sprinkle your seasoning over it.
5. Mix well, and then cut your dough into two parts.
6. Place parchment paper over your Air Fryer basket tray, placing the first part of your dough in the tray to form a crust. Add in your salmon filling.
7. Roll out the second part, covering your salmon filling. Secure the edges, and then heat your Air Fryer to 360°F.
8. Cook for 15 minutes, and then reduce the heat to 355°F, cooking for another 15 minutes
9. Slice and serve warm.

462. GARLIC CHICKEN STIR

PREPARATION: 5 MIN   **COOKING:** 20 MIN   **SERVINGS:** 4

INGREDIENTS

- ½ Cup coconut milk
- ½ cup chicken stock
- tbsp. curry paste
- 1 tbsp. lemongrass
- 1 tbsp. apple cider vinegar
- tsp.s garlic, minced
- 1 onion
- 1 lb. Chicken breast, skinless & boneless
- 1 tsp. olive oil

DIRECTIONS

1. Start by cubing your chicken, and then peel your onion before dicing it.
2. Combine your onion and chicken together in your Air Fryer basket, and then preheat it to 365°F. Cook for five minutes
3. Add in your garlic, apple cider vinegar, coconut milk, lemongrass, curry paste and chicken stock. Mix well, and cook for ten minutes more.
4. Stir well before serving.

Nutrition: Calories 275 Fat 15.7g Carbs 5.9 g Protein 25.6 g

Air Fryer Cookbook

463. CHICKEN STEW

PREPARATION: 5 MIN   **COOKING:** 25 MIN   **SERVINGS:** 4

INGREDIENTS

- 1 tsp. cilantro
- oz. chicken breast, boneless & skinless
- 1 onion
- ½ cup spinach
- cups chicken stock
- oz. cabbage
- oz. cauliflower
- 1 tsp. salt
- 1 green bell pepper
- 1/3 cup heavy cream
- 1 tsp. paprika
- 1 tsp. butter
- 1 tsp. cayenne pepper

DIRECTIONS

1. Start by cubing your chicken breast, and then sprinkling your cilantro, cayenne, salt and paprika over it.
2. Heat your Air Fryer to 365°F, and then melt your butter in your Air Fryer basket.
3. Add your chicken cubes in, cooking it for 4 minutes
4. Chop your spinach, and then dice your onion.
5. Shred your cabbage and cut your cauliflower into florets. Chop your green pepper next, and then add them into your Air Fryer.
6. Pour your chicken stock and heavy cream in, and then reduce your Air Fryer to 360°F. Cook for 8 minutes, and stir before serving.

Nutrition: Calories 102 Fat 4.5 g Carbs 4.1 g Protein 9.8 g

464. GOULASH

PREPARATION: 5 MIN   **COOKING:** 12 MIN   **SERVINGS:** 6

INGREDIENTS

- 1 white onion
- green peppers, chopped
- 1 tsp. olive oil
- 14 oz. ground chicken
- tomatoes
- ½ cup chicken stock
- 1 tsp. sea salt, fine
- cloves garlic, sliced
- 1 tsp. black pepper
- 1 tsp. mustard

DIRECTIONS

1. Peel your onion before chopping it roughly.
2. Spray your Air Fryer down with olive oil before preheating it to 365 °F.
3. Add in your chopped green pepper, cooking for five minutes
4. Add your ground chicken and cubed tomato next. Mix well, and cook for 6 minutes
5. Add in the chicken stock, salt, pepper, mustard and garlic. Mix well, and cook for 6 minutes more. Serve warm.

Nutrition: Calories 161 Fat 6.1 g Carbs 4.3 g Protein 20.3 g

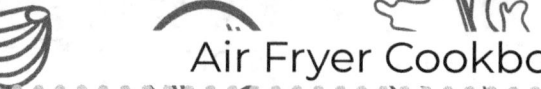
Air Fryer Cookbook

465. BEEF & BROCCOLI

PREPARATION: 5 MIN   **COOKING:** 20 MIN   **SERVINGS:** 4

INGREDIENTS

- 1 tsp. paprika
- 1 onion
- 1/3 cup water
- oz. broccoli
- oz. beef brisket
- 1 tsp. canola oil
- 1 tsp. butter
- ½ tsp. chili flakes
- 1 tbsp. flax seeds

DIRECTIONS

1. Start by chopping your beef brisket, and then sprinkle it with chili flakes and paprika. Mix your meat well, and then preheat your Air Fryer to 360°F.
2. Spray your Air Fryer down with canola oil, placing your beef in the basket tray. Cook for 7 minutes, and make sure to stir once while cooking.
3. Chop your broccoli into florets, and then add them into your Air Fryer basket next.
4. Add in your butter and flax seeds before mixing in your water. Slice your onion, adding it into it, and stir well.
5. Cook at 265°F for 6 minutes. Serve warm.

Nutrition: Calories 187 Fat 7.3g Carbs 3.8g Protein 23.4g

466. GROUND BEEF MASH

PREPARATION: 5 MIN   **COOKING:** 25 MIN   **SERVINGS:** 2

INGREDIENTS

- 1 lb. Ground beef
- 1 onion
- 1 tsp. garlic, sliced
- ¼ cup cream
- 1 tsp. white pepper
- 1 tsp. olive oil
- 1 tsp. dill
- tsp.s chicken stock
- green peppers
- 1 tsp. cayenne pepper

DIRECTIONS

1. Start by peeling your onion before grating it. Combine it with your sliced garlic, and then sprinkle your ground beef down with it. Add in your white pepper, and then add your cayenne and dill.
2. Coat your Air Fryer basket down with olive oil, heating it up to 365°F.
3. Place the spiced beef in the basket, cooking for 3 minutes before stirring. Add in the rest of your grated onion mixture and chicken stock, and then cook for 2 minutes more.
4. Chop your green peppers into small pieces, and then add them in.
5. Add in your cream, and stir well.
6. Allow it to cook for 10 minutes more.
7. Mash your mixture to make sure it's scrambled before serving warm.

Nutrition: Calories 25 Fat 9.3g Carbs 4.9g Protein 35.5g

467. CHICKEN CASSEROLE

PREPARATION: 5 MIN **COOKING:** 30 MIN **SERVINGS:** 4

INGREDIENTS

- 1 tbsp. butter
- oz. round chicken
- ½ onion
- oz. bacon
- Sea salt & black pepper to taste
- 1 tsp. turmeric
- 1 tsp. paprika
- oz. cheddar cheese, shredded
- 1 egg
- ½ cup cream
- 1 tbsp. almond flour

DIRECTIONS

1. Spread your butter into your Air Fryer tray, and then add in your ground chicken. Season it with salt and pepper, and then add in your turmeric and paprika. Stir well, and then add in your cheddar cheese.
2. Beat your egg into your ground chicken, and mix well. Whisk your cream and almond flour together.
3. Peel and dice your onion, and then add it into your Air Fryer too.
4. Layer your cheese and bacon, and then heat your Air Fryer to 380°F. Cook for 18 minutes, and then allow it to cool slightly before serving.

Nutrition: Calories 396 Fat 28.6g Carbs 2.8g Protein 30.4g

468. CHICKEN HASH

PREPARATION: 5 MIN **COOKING:** 20 MIN **SERVINGS:** 3

INGREDIENTS

- 1 Tbsp. Water
- 1 Green Pepper
- ½ Onion
- Oz. Cauliflower
- Chicken Fillet, 7 Oz.
- 1 Tbsp. cream
- Tbsp. Butter
- Black Pepper to taste

DIRECTIONS

1. Start by roughly chopping your cauliflower before placing it in a blender. Blend until you get a cauliflower rice.
2. Chop your chicken into small pieces, and then get out your chicken fillets. Sprinkle with black pepper.
3. Heat your Air Fryer to 380°F, and then put your chicken in the Air Fryer basket. Add in your water and cream, cooking for 6 minutes
4. Reduce the heat to 360°F, and then dice your green pepper and onion.
5. Add this to your cauliflower rice, and then add in your butter. Mix well, and then add it to your chicken. Cook for 8 minutes
6. Serve warm.

Nutrition: Calories 261 Fat 16.8g Carbs 4.4g Protein 21g

VEGETABLES AND VEGETARIAN

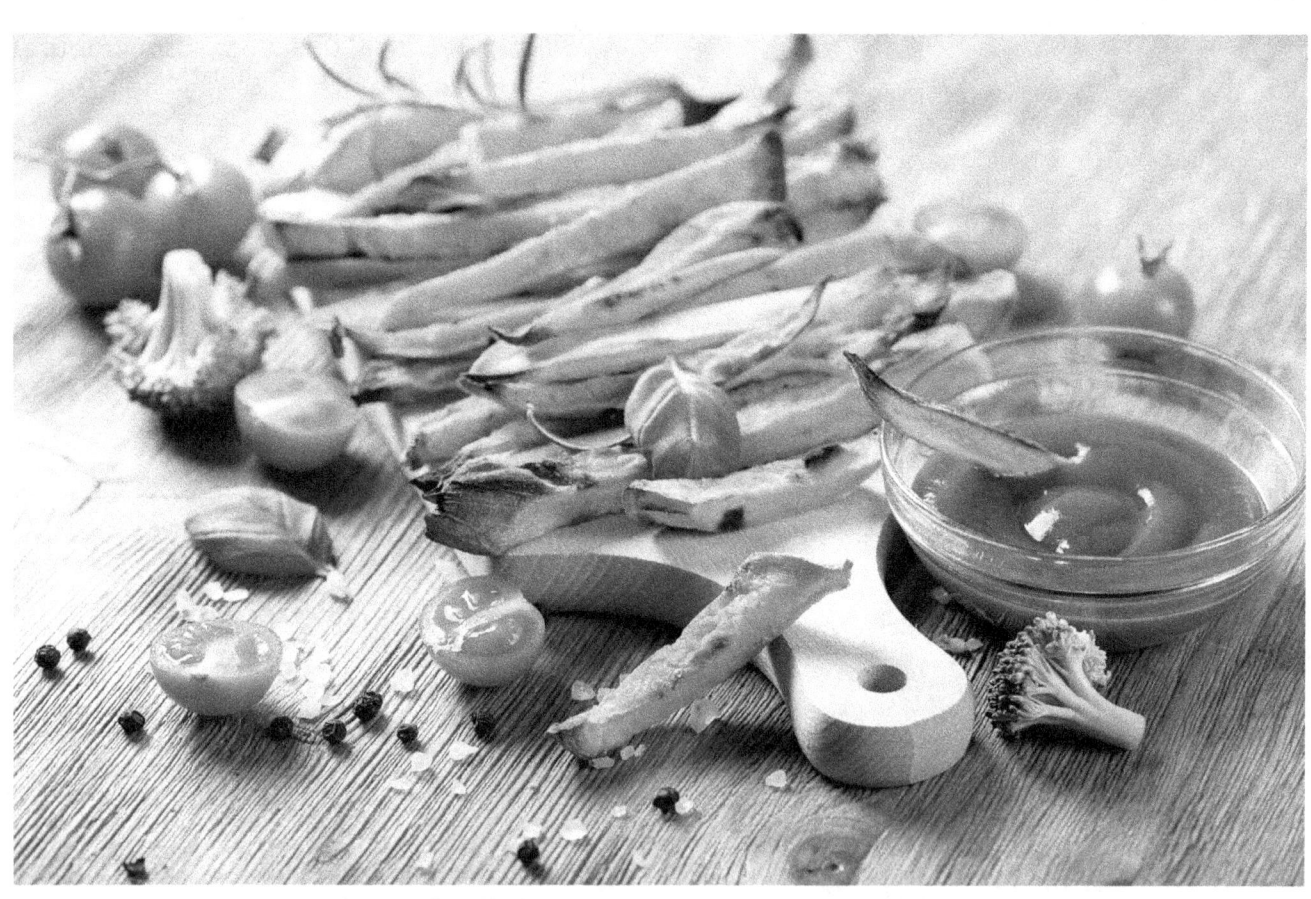

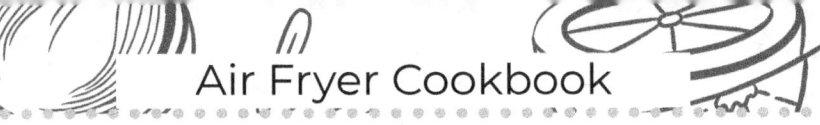

Air Fryer Cookbook

469. PESTO TOMATOES

PREPARATION: 5 MIN   **COOKING:** 10 MIN   **SERVINGS:** 4

INGREDIENTS

- Large heirloom tomatoes – 3, cut into ½ inch thick slices.
- Pesto – 1 cup
- Feta cheese – 8 oz. cut into ½ inch thick slices
- Red onion – ½ cup, sliced thinly
- Olive oil – 1 tbsp.

Nutrition: Calories 480 Fat 41.9g Carbs 13g Protein 15.4g

DIRECTIONS

1. Spread some pesto on each slice of tomato. Top each tomato slice with a feta slice and onion and drizzle with oil. Arrange the tomatoes onto the greased rack and spray with cooking spray.
2. Arrange the drip pan in the bottom of the Air Fryer Oven cooking chamber. Heat at 390°F. Set the time for 14 minutes and press "Start".
3. When Cooking Time is complete, remove the rack from the Air Fryer Oven. Serve warm.

470. SEASONED POTATOES

PREPARATION: 10 MIN   **COOKING:** 15 MIN   **SERVINGS:** 4

INGREDIENTS

- Russet potatoes – 2, scrubbed
- Butter – ½ tbsp. melted
- Garlic & herb blend seasoning – ½ tsp.
- Garlic powder – ½ tsp.
- Salt, as required

Nutrition: Calories 176 Fat 2.1g Carbs 34.2g Protein 3.8g

DIRECTIONS

1. In a bowl, mix all of the spices and salt. With a fork, prick the potatoes. Coat the potatoes with butter and sprinkle with spice mixture. Arrange the potatoes onto the cooking rack. Arrange the drip pan in the bottom of the Air Fryer Oven cooking chamber.
2. Set the temperature to 400°F. Set the time for 40 minutes and press "Start." Insert the cooking rack in the center position. Once cooking is done, remove the tray from the Air Fryer Oven. Serve hot.

471. SPICY ZUCCHINI

PREPARATION: 5 MIN   **COOKING:** 20 MIN   **SERVINGS:** 4

INGREDIENTS

- Zucchini – 1 lb. cut into ½-inch thick slices lengthwise
- Olive oil – 1 tbsp.
- Garlic powder – ½ tsp.
- Cayenne pepper – ½ tsp.
- Salt and ground black pepper, as required

Nutrition: Calories 67 Fat 5g Carbs 5.6g Protein 2g

DIRECTIONS

1. Put all of the ingredients into a bowl and toss to coat well. Arrange the zucchini slices onto a cooking tray. Arrange the drip pan in the bottom of the Air Fryer Oven cooking chamber.
2. Set the temperature to 400°F. Set the time for 12 minutes and press "Start." Insert the cooking tray in the center position. Once cooking is done, remove the tray from the Air Fryer Oven. Serve hot.

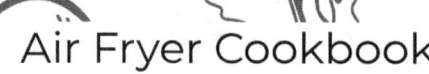

Air Fryer Cookbook

472. SEASONED YELLOW SQUASH

PREPARATION: 5 MIN   **COOKING:** 10 MIN   **SERVINGS:** 4

INGREDIENTS

- Large yellow squash – 4, cut into slices
- Olive oil – ¼ cup
- Onion – ½, sliced
- Italian seasoning – ¾ tsp.
- Garlic salt – ½ tsp.
- Seasoned salt – ¼ tsp

Nutrition: Calories 113 Fat 9g Carbs 8.1g Protein 4.2g

DIRECTIONS

1. In a bowl, mix all the ingredients together. Place the veggie mixture in the greased cooking tray. Arrange the drip pan in the bottom of the Air Fryer Oven cooking chamber.
2. Set the temperature to 400°F. Set the time for 10 minutes and press "Start". Insert the cooking tray in the center position. After 4-5 minutes turn the vegetables. Once cooking is done, remove the tray from the Air Fryer Oven. Serve hot.

473. BUTTERED ASPARAGUS

PREPARATION: 5 MIN   **COOKING:** 10 MIN   **SERVINGS:** 4

INGREDIENTS

- Put all of the ingredients into a bowl and toss to coat well. Arrange the asparagus onto a cooking tray. Arrange the drip pan in the bottom of the Air Fryer Oven cooking chamber.
- Set the temperature to 350°F. Set the time for 10 minutes and press "Start."
- After 4-5 minutes turn the asparagus. Once cooking is done, remove the tray from Air Fryer Oven. Serve hot.

Nutrition: Calories 64 Fat 4g Carbs 5.9g Protein 3.4g

DIRECTIONS

1. Put all of the ingredients into a bowl and toss to coat well. Arrange the asparagus onto a cooking tray. Arrange the drip pan in the bottom of the Air Fryer Oven cooking chamber.
2. Set the temperature to 350°F. Set the time for 10 minutes and press "Start."
3. After 4-5 minutes turn the asparagus. Once cooking is done, remove the tray from Air Fryer Oven. Serve hot.

474. BUTTERED BROCCOLI

PREPARATION: 5 MIN   **COOKING:** 15 MIN   **SERVINGS:** 4

INGREDIENTS

- Broccoli florets – 1 lb.
- Butter – 1 tbsp. melted
- Red pepper flakes – ½ tsp. crushed
- Salt and ground black pepper, as required

Nutrition: Calories 55 Fat 3g Carbs 6.1g Protein 2.3g

DIRECTIONS

1. Gather all of the ingredients in a bowl and toss to coat well. Place the broccoli florets in the rotisserie basket and attach the lid. Arrange the drip pan in the bottom of the Air Fryer Oven cooking chamber.
2. Set the temperature to 400°F. Fix the time for 15 minutes and press "Start."
3. Arrange the rotisserie basket, on the rotisserie spit.
4. When Cooking Time is complete, remove from the Air Fryer Oven. Serve immediately.

475. SEASONED CARROTS WITH GREEN BEANS

PREPARATION: 5 MIN **COOKING:** 10 MIN **SERVINGS:** 4

INGREDIENTS

- Green beans – ½ lb. trimmed
- Carrots – ½ lb. peeled and cut into sticks
- Olive oil – 1 tbsp.
- Salt and ground black pepper, as required

Nutrition: Calories 94 Fat 4.8g Carbs 12.7g Protein 2g

DIRECTIONS

1. Gather all the ingredients into a bowl and toss to coat well. Place the vegetables in the rotisserie basket and attach the lid. Arrange the drip pan in the bottom of the Air Fryer Oven cooking chamber.
2. Set the temperature to 400°F. Set the time for 10 minutes and press "Start".
3. When Cooking Time is completer, emove from the Air Fryer Oven. Serve hot.

476. SWEET POTATO WITH BROCCOLI

PREPARATION: 5 MIN **COOKING:** 20 MIN **SERVINGS:** 4

INGREDIENTS

- Medium sweet potatoes – 2, peeled and cut in 1-inch cubes
- Broccoli head – 1, cut in 1-inch florets
- Vegetable oil – 2 tbsps.
- Salt and ground black pepper, as required

Nutrition: Calories 170 Fat 7.1g Carbs 25.2g Protein 2.9g

DIRECTIONS

1. Grease a baking dish that will fit in the Air Fryer Oven. Gather all of the ingredients into a bowl and toss to coat well. Place the veggie mixture into the prepared baking dish in a single layer.
2. Arrange the drip pan in the bottom of the Air Fryer Oven cooking chamber. Select "Roast" and then adjust the temperature to 415°F. Set the time for 20 minutes and press "Start".
3. Turn the vegetables every few minutes. When Cooking Time is complete, remove the baking dish from the Air Fryer Oven. Serve hot.

477. SEASONED VEGGIES

PREPARATION: 5 MIN **COOKING:** 12 MIN **SERVINGS:** 4

INGREDIENTS

- Baby carrots – 1 cup
- Broccoli florets – 1 cup
- Cauliflower florets – 1 cup
- Olive oil – 1 tbsp.
- Italian seasoning – 1 tbsp.
- Salt and ground black pepper, as required

Nutrition: Calories 66 Fat 4.7 Carbs 5.7g Protein 1.4g

DIRECTIONS

1. Gather all of the ingredients into a bowl and toss to coat well. Place the vegetables in the rotisserie basket and attach the lid. Arrange the drip pan in the bottom of the Air Fryer Oven cooking chamber.
2. Choose "Air Fry" and then set the temperature to 380°F. Set the time for 18 minutes and press "Start". Then, close the door and touch "Rotate".
3. When the display shows "Add Food" arrange the rotisserie basket, on the rotisserie spit. Then, close the door and touch "Rotate". When Cooking Time is complete, press the red lever to release the rod. Remove from the Air Fryer Oven. Serve.

Air Fryer Cookbook

478. POTATO GRATIN

PREPARATION: 5 MIN   **COOKING:** 20 MIN   **SERVINGS:** 4

INGREDIENTS

- Large potatoes – 2, sliced thinly
- Cream – 5½ tbsps.
- Eggs – 2
- Plain flour – 1 tbsp.
- Cheddar cheese – ½ cup, grated

DIRECTIONS

1. Arrange the potato cubes onto the greased rack. Arrange the drip pan in the bottom of the Air Fryer Oven cooking chamber. Choose "Air Fry" and then set the temperature to 355°F. Set the time for 10 minutes and press "Start". When the display shows "Add Food" insert the cooking rack in the center position.
2. Meanwhile, in a bowl, add cream, eggs and flour and mix until a thick sauce form. Once cooking is done, remove the tray from the Air Fryer Oven. Divide the potato slices into 4 lightly greased ramekins evenly and top with the egg mixture, followed by the cheese. Arrange the ramekins on top of a cooking rack.
3. Again, select "Air Fry" and then adjust the temperature to 390°F. Set the time for 10 minutes and press "Start". When the display shows "Add Food" insert the cooking rack in the center position. When Cooking Time is complete, remove the ramekins from the Air Fryer Oven. Serve warm.

Nutrition: Calories 233 Fat 8g Carbs 31.g Protein 9.7g

479. GARLIC EDAMAME

PREPARATION: 5 MIN   **COOKING:** 10 MIN   **SERVINGS:** 4

INGREDIENTS

- Olive oil
- 1 (16 oz.) bag frozen edamame in pods
- salt and freshly ground black pepper
- ½ tsp. garlic salt
- ½ tsp. red pepper flakes (optional)

DIRECTIONS

1. Spray a fryer basket lightly with olive oil.
2. In a medium bowl, add the frozen edamame and lightly spray with olive oil. Toss to coat.
3. In a bowl, combine together the garlic salt, salt, black pepper, and red pepper flakes (if using). Add the mixture to the edamame and toss until evenly coated.
4. Place half the edamame in the fryer basket. Do not overfill the basket.
5. Air fry for 5 minutes at 360°F. Shake the basket and cook until the edamame is starting to brown and get crispy, 3 to 5 more minutes.
6. Repeat with the remaining edamame and serve immediately.
7. Pair It With: These make a nice side dish to almost any meal.
8. Air Fry Like A Pro: If you use fresh edamame, reduce the air fry time by 2 to 3 minutes to avoid overcooking. Air-fried edamame do not retain their crisp texture, so it's best to eat them right after cooking.

Nutrition: Calories 100 Fat 3g Carbs 9g Protein 8g

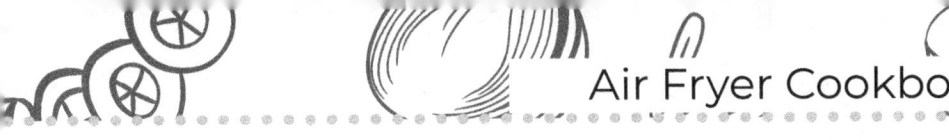

480. EGG ROLL PIZZA STICKS

PREPARATION: 5 MIN   **COOKING:** 40 MIN   **SERVINGS:** 4

INGREDIENTS

- Olive oil
- 8 pieces reduced-fat string cheese
- 8 egg roll wrappers
- 24 slices turkey pepperoni
- Marinara sauce, for dipping (optional)

DIRECTIONS

1. Spray a fryer basket lightly with olive oil. Fill a small bowl with water.
2. Place each egg roll wrapper diagonally on a work surface. It should look like a diamond.
3. Place 3 slices of turkey pepperoni in a vertical line down the center of the wrapper.
4. Place 1 mozzarella cheese stick on top of the turkey pepperoni.
5. Fold the top and bottom corners of the egg roll wrapper over the cheese stick.
6. Fold the left corner over the cheese stick and roll the cheese stick up to resemble a spring roll. Dip a finger in the water and seal the edge of the roll
7. Repeat with the rest of the pizza sticks.
8. Place them in the fryer basket in a single layer, making sure to leave a little space between each one. Lightly spray the pizza sticks with oil.
9. Air fry at 362°F until the pizza sticks are lightly browned and crispy, about 5 minutes.
10. These are best served hot while the cheese is melted. Accompany with a small bowl of marinara sauce, if desired.

Nutrition: Calories 362 Fat 8g Carbs 40g Protein 23g

481. CAJUN ZUCCHINI CHIPS

PREPARATION: 10 MIN   **COOKING:** 15 MIN   **SERVINGS:** 4

INGREDIENTS

- Olive oil
- 2 large zucchinis, cut into ⅛-inch-thick slices
- 2 tsp.s Cajun seasoning

DIRECTIONS

1. Spray a fryer basket lightly with olive oil.
2. Put the zucchini slices in a medium bowl and spray them generously with olive oil.
3. Sprinkle the Cajun seasoning over the zucchini and stir to make sure they are evenly coated with oil and seasoning.
4. Place slices in a single layer in the fryer basket, making sure not to overcrowd.
5. Air fry for 8 minutes at 365°F. Flip the slices over and air fry until they are as crisp and brown as you prefer, an additional 7 to 8 minutes.
6. Air Fry Like A Pro: In order to achieve the best result, it is important not to overcrowd the fryer basket. The zucchini chips turn out best if there is room for the air to circulate around each slice. You can add Cooking Time if you like very brown and crunchy zucchini chips.

Nutrition: Calories 26 Fat <1g Carbs 5g Protein 2g

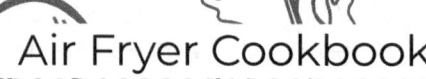
Air Fryer Cookbook

482. CRISPY OLD BAY CHICKEN WINGS

PREPARATION: 10 MIN **COOKING:** 15 MIN **SERVINGS:** 4

INGREDIENTS

- Olive oil
- 2 tbsp. Old Bay seasoning
- 2 tsp.s baking powder
- 2 tsp.s salt
- 2 lb. chicken wings

Nutrition: Calories 501 Fat 36g Carbs 1g Protein 42g

DIRECTIONS

1. Spray a fryer basket lightly with olive oil.
2. In a big resealable bag, combine together the Old Bay seasoning, baking powder, and salt.
3. Pat the wings dry with paper towels. Place the wings in the zip-top bag, seal, and toss with the seasoning mixture until evenly coated.
4. Place the seasoned wings in the fryer basket in a single layer. Lightly spray with olive oil.
5. Air fry for 7 minutes at 375°F. Turn the wings over, lightly spray them with olive oil, and air fry until the wings are crispy and lightly browned, 5 to 8 more minutes. Using a meat thermometer, check to make sure the internal temperature is 165°F or higher.

483. CINNAMON AND SUGAR PEACHES

PREPARATION: 10 MIN **COOKING:** 13 MIN **SERVINGS:** 4

INGREDIENTS

- Olive oil
- 2 tbsp. sugar
- ¼ tsp. ground cinnamon
- 4 peaches, cut into wedges

Nutrition: Calories 67 Fat <1g Carbs 17g Protein 1g

DIRECTIONS

1. Spray a fryer basket lightly with olive oil.
2. In a bowl, combine the cinnamon and sugar. Add the peaches and toss to coat evenly.
3. Place the peaches in a single layer in the fryer basket on their sides.
4. Air fry for 5 minutes at 365°F. Turn the peaches skin side down, lightly spray them with oil, and air fry until the peaches are lightly brown and caramelized, 5 to 8 more minutes.
5. Make it Even Lower Calorie: Use a zero-calorie sugar substitute such as NutraSweet or monk fruit sweetener instead of granulated sugar.
6. Air Fry Like A Pro: These do not get truly crispy, but rather they remain soft, sweet, and caramelized. They are truly delightful and make a wonderful dessert option.

484. CHICKEN WINGS WITH PROVENCAL HERBS IN AIR FRYER

PREPARATION: 15 MIN **COOKING:** 20 MIN **SERVINGS:** 4

INGREDIENTS

- 2 lb. chicken wings
- Provencal herbs
- Extra virgin olive oil
- Salt
- Ground pepper

DIRECTIONS

1. Put the chicken wings in a bowl, clean and chopped.
2. Add a few threads of oil, salt, ground pepper and sprinkle with Provencal herbs.
3. Link well and let macerate a few minutes.
4. Put the wings in the basket of the Air Fryer.
5. Select 360°F for 20 minutes.
6. From time to time remove so that they are done on all their sides
7. Serve hot

Nutrition: Calories 160 Fat 6g Carbs 8g Protein 13g

485. SPICED CHICKEN WINGS IN AIR FRYER

PREPARATION: 15 MIN **COOKING:** 30 MIN **SERVINGS:** 4

INGREDIENTS

- 2 lb. chicken wings
- Salt
- Ground pepper
- Extra virgin olive oil
- Spices

DIRECTIONS

1. Clean the wings and chop, throw the tip and place in a bowl the other two parts of the wings that have more meat.
2. Season and add some extra virgin olive oil threads.
3. Sprinkle with spices, put spices for roast chicken that they sell as is in supermarkets, in regular spice cans.
4. Leave for 30 minutes to rest in the refrigerator.
5. Put the wings in the basket of the Air Fryer and select 360°F, about 30 minutes. From time to time, shake the basket so that the wings move and are made all over their sides
6. Serve hot

Nutrition: Calories 170 Fat 6g Carbs 8g Protein 15g

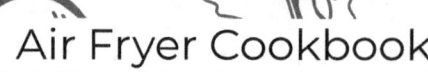
Air Fryer Cookbook

486. ROSTI (SWISS POTATOES)

PREPARATION: 10 MIN **COOKING:** 15 MIN **SERVINGS:** 4

INGREDIENTS

- 250g peeled white potatoes
- 1 tbsp. finely chopped chives
- Freshly ground black pepper
- 1 tbsp. of olive oil
- 2 tbsp. of sour cream

Nutrition: Calories 253g Fat 11.7g Carbs 25.2g Protein 2.5g

DIRECTIONS

1. Preheat the Air Fryer to 180°C. Grate the thick potatoes in a bowl and add three quarters of the chives and salt and pepper to taste. Mix it well.
2. Grease the pizza pan with olive oil and spread the potato mixture evenly through the pan. Press the grated potatoes against the pan and spread the top of the potato cake with some olive oil.
3. Place the pizza pan inside the fryer basket and insert it into the Air Fryer. Set the timer to 15 mins and fry the rosti until it has a nice brownish color on the outside and is soft and well done inside.
4. Cut the rosti into 4 quarters and place each quarter on a plate. Garnish with a spoonful of sour cream. Spread the remaining of the scallions over the sour cream and add a touch of ground pepper.

487. BAKED PARSLEY

PREPARATION: 5 MIN **COOKING:** 5 MIN **SERVINGS:** 4

INGREDIENTS

- 1 stick parsley
- 1 prize salt

Nutrition: Calories 15 Fat 0g Carbs 2g Protein 2g

DIRECTIONS

1. Free the fresh parsley from the coarse stalks and bake it in the Air Fryer for 5 minutes at 350°F.
2. Drain and sprinkle with a little salt.

488. DUCK THIGHS FROM THE AIR FRYER

PREPARATION: 5 MIN **COOKING:** 50 MIN **SERVINGS:** 4

INGREDIENTS

- 2 pcs. Duck legs
- 1 tsp. salt
- 1 tsp. spice mixture (for ducks and geese)
- 1 tsp. olive oil

Nutrition: Calories 25 Fat 28g Carbs 0g Protein 19g

DIRECTIONS

1. Wash the duck legs and pat dry. Mix the oil with the salt and the spice mixture and rub the duck legs around with it.
2. Place the spiced duck legs on the hot Air Fryer's rack and cook at 400°F in 40 minutes. After 20 minutes, turn the legs once.
3. Serve hot

489. CHOPPED BONDIOLA

PREPARATION: 5 MIN **COOKING:** 20 MIN **SERVINGS:** 4

INGREDIENTS

- 2 lb. Bondiola in pieces
- Bread crumbs
- 2 eggs
- Seasoning to taste

Nutrition: Calories 340 Fat 12g Carbs 11g Protein 18g

DIRECTIONS

1. Cut the bondiola into small pieces, add seasonings to taste.
2. Whisk the eggs in a bowl
3. Pass the seasoned bondiola in the eggs and then in the breadcrumbs
4. Place it in the Air Fryer at 360°F for 20 minutes, turn after 10 minutes
5. Serve hot

490. ZUCCHINI CURRY

PREPARATION: 5 MIN **COOKING:** 8-10 MIN **SERVINGS:** -

INGREDIENTS

- 2 Zucchinis, Washed & Sliced
- 1 Tbsp. Olive Oil
- Pinch Sea Salt
- Curry Mix, Pre-Made

Nutrition: Calories 100 Fat 1g Carbs 4g Protein 2g

DIRECTIONS

1. Turn on your Air Fryer to 390°F
2. Combine your zucchini slices, salt, oil, and spices.
3. Put the zucchini into the Air Fryer, cooking for 8 to 10 minutes.
4. You can serve alone or with sour cream.

491. HEALTHY CARROT FRIES

PREPARATION: 5 MIN **COOKING:** 8-10 MIN **SERVINGS:** -

INGREDIENTS

- 5 Large Carrots
- 1 Tbsp. Olive Oil
- ½ Tsp. Sea Salt

DIRECTIONS

1. Heat your Air Fryer to 390°F, and then wash and peel your carrots. Cut them in a way to form fries.
2. Combine your carrot sticks with your olive oil and salt, coating evenly.
3. Place them into the Air Fryer, cooking for twelve minutes. If they're not as crispy as you desire, then cook for 2 to 3 more minutes.
4. Serve with sour cream, ketchup or just with your favorite main dish.

Nutrition: Calories 140 Fat 3g Carbs 6g Protein 7g

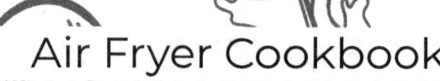
Air Fryer Cookbook

492. SIMPLE STUFFED POTATOES

PREPARATION: 15 MIN **COOKING:** 35 MIN **SERVINGS:** -

INGREDIENTS

- 4 Large Potatoes, Peeled
- 2 Bacon, Rashers
- ½ Brown Onion, Diced
- ¼ Cup Cheese, Grated

Nutrition: Calories 180 Fat 8g Carbs 10g Protein 11g

DIRECTIONS

1. Start by heating your Air Fryer to 350°F.
2. Cut your potatoes in half, and then brush the potatoes with oil.
3. Put it in your Air Fryer, and cook for ten minutes. Brush the potatoes with oil again and bake for another ten minutes.
4. Make a whole in the baked potato to get them ready to stuff.
5. Sauté the bacon and onion in a frying pan. You should do this over medium heat, adding cheese and stir. Remove from heat.
6. Stuff your potatoes, and cook for 4-5 minutes.

493. SIMPLE ROASTED CARROTS

PREPARATION: 5 MIN **COOKING:** 35 MIN **SERVINGS:** -

INGREDIENTS

- 4 Cups Carrots, Chopped
- 1 Tsp. Herbs de Provence
- 2 Tsp.s Olive Oil
- 4 Tbsp. Orange Juice

Nutrition: Calories 125 Fat 2g Carbs 5g Protein 6g

DIRECTIONS

1. Start by preheating your Air Fryer to 320°F.
2. Combine your carrot pieces with your herbs and oil.
3. Cook for 25-28 minutes.
4. Take it out and dip the pieces in orange juice before frying for an additional 7 minutes.

494. BROCCOLI & CHEESE

PREPARATION: 5 MIN **COOKING:** 9 MIN **SERVINGS:** -

INGREDIENTS

- 1 Head Broccoli, Washed & Chopped
- Salt & Pepper to Taste
- 1 Tbsp. Olive oil
- Sharp Cheddar Cheese, Shredded

Nutrition: Calories 170 Fat 5g Carbs 9g Protein 7g

DIRECTIONS

1. Start by putting your Air Fryer to 360°F.
2. Combine your broccoli with your olive oil and sea salt.
3. Place it in the Air Fryer, and cook for 6 minutes.
4. Take it out, and then top with cheese, cooking for another 3 minutes.
5. Serve with your choice of protein.

495. FRIED PLANTAINS

PREPARATION: 5 MIN **COOKING:** 10 MIN **SERVINGS:** 2

INGREDIENTS

- 2 ripe plantains, peeled and cut at a diagonal into ½-inch-thick pieces
- 3 tbsp. ghee, melted
- ¼ tsp. kosher salt

Nutrition: Calories 180 Fat 5g Carbs 10g Protein 7g

DIRECTIONS

1. In a bowl, mix the plantains with the ghee and salt.
2. Arrange the plantain pieces in the Air Fryer basket. Set the Air Fryer to 400°F for 8 minutes. The plantains are done when they are soft and tender on the inside, and have plenty of crisp, sweet, brown spots on the outside.

496. BACON-WRAPPED ASPARAGUS

PREPARATION: 5 MIN **COOKING:** 10 MIN **SERVINGS:** 4

INGREDIENTS

- 1 lb. asparagus, trimmed (about 24 spears)
- 4 slices bacon or beef bacon
- ½ cup Ranch Dressin for serving
- 3 tbsp. chopped fresh chives, for garnish

Nutrition: Calories 241 Fat 22gg Carbs 6g Protein 7g

DIRECTIONS

1. Grease the Air Fryer basket with avocado oil. Preheat the Air Fryer to 400°F.
2. Slice the bacon down the middle, making long, thin strips. Wrap 1 slice of bacon around 3 asparagus spears and secure each end with a toothpick. Repeat with the remaining bacon and asparagus.
3. Place the asparagus bundles in the Air Fryer in a single layer. (If you're using a smaller Air Fryer, cook in batches if necessary.) Cook for 8 minutes for thin stalks, 10 minutes for medium to thick stalks, or until the asparagus is slightly charred on the ends and the bacon is crispy.
4. Serve with ranch dressing and garnish with chives. Best served fresh.

497. AIR FRIED ROASTED CORN ON THE COB

PREPARATION: 5 MIN **COOKING:** 10 MIN **SERVINGS:** 4

INGREDIENTS

- 1 tbsp. vegetable oil
- 4 ears of corn
- Unsalted butter, for topping
- Salt, for topping
- Freshly ground black pepper, for topping

Nutrition: Calories 265 Fat 17g Carbs 29g Protein 5g

DIRECTIONS

1. Rub the vegetable oil onto the corn, coating it thoroughly.
2. Set the temperature of your Air Fryer to 400°F. Set the timer and grill for 5 minutes.
3. Using tongs, flip or rotate the corn.
4. Reset the timer and grill for 5 minutes more.
5. Serve with a pat of butter and a generous sprinkle of salt and pepper.

Air Fryer Cookbook

498. GREEN BEANS & BACON

PREPARATION: 15 MIN **COOKING:** 20 MIN **SERVINGS:** 4

INGREDIENTS

- 3 cups frozen cut green beans
- 1 medium onion, chopped
- 3 slices bacon, chopped
- ¼ cup water
- Kosher salt and black pepper

DIRECTIONS

1. In a 6 × 3-inch round heatproof pan, combine the frozen green beans, onion, bacon, and water. Toss to combine. Place the saucepan in the basket.
2. Set the Air Fryer to 375°F for 15 minutes.
3. Raise the Air Fryer temperature to 400°F for 5 minutes. Season the beans with salt and pepper to taste and toss well.
4. Remove the pan from the Air Fryer basket and cover with foil. Let it rest for 5 minutes then serve.

Nutrition: Calories 230 Fat 10g Carbs 14g Protein 17g

499. AIR FRIED HONEY ROASTED CARROTS

PREPARATION: 5 MIN **COOKING:** 25 MIN **SERVINGS:** 2

INGREDIENTS

- 3 cups baby carrots
- 1 tbsp. extra-virgin olive oil
- 1 tbsp. honey
- Salt
- Freshly ground black pepper
- Fresh dill (optional)

DIRECTIONS

1. In a bowl, combine honey, olive oil, carrots, salt, and pepper. Make sure that the carrots are thoroughly coated with oil. Place the carrots in the Air Fryer basket.
2. Set the temperature of your Air Fryer to 390°F. Set the timer and roast for 12 minutes, or until fork-tender.
3. Remove the Air Fryer drawer and release the Air Fryer basket. Pour the carrots into a bowl, sprinkle with dill, if desired, and serve.

Nutrition: Calories 140 Fat 3g Carbs 7g Protein 9g

500. AIR FRIED ROASTED CABBAGE

PREPARATION: 5 MIN **COOKING:** 10 MIN **SERVINGS:** 4

INGREDIENTS

- 1 head cabbage, sliced in 1-inch-thick ribbons
- 1 tbsp. olive oil
- salt and freshly ground black pepper
- 1 tsp. garlic powder
- 1 tsp. red pepper flakes

DIRECTIONS

1. In a bowl, combine the olive oil, cabbage, salt, pepper, garlic powder, and red pepper flakes. Make sure that the cabbage is thoroughly coated with oil. Place the cabbage in the Air Fryer basket.
2. Set the temperature of your Air Fryer to 350°F. Set the timer and roast for 4 minutes.
3. Using tongs, flip the cabbage. Reset the timer and roast for 3 minutes more.

Nutrition: Calories 100 Fat 1g Carbs 3g Protein 3g

501. BURRATA-STUFFED TOMATOES

PREPARATION: 5 MIN　　**COOKING:** 40 MIN　　**SERVINGS:** 4

INGREDIENTS

- 4 medium tomatoes
- ½ tsp. fine sea salt
- 4 (2 oz.) Burrata balls
- Fresh basil leaves, for garnish
- Extra-virgin olive oil, for drizzling

DIRECTIONS

1. Preheat the Air Fryer to 300°F.
2. Scoop out the tomato seeds and membranes using a melon baller or spoon. Sprinkle the insides of the tomatoes with the salt. Stuff each tomato with a ball of Burrata.
3. Put it in the fryer and cook for 5 minutes, or until the cheese has softened.
4. Garnish with olive oil and basil leaves. Serve warm.

Nutrition: Calories 108 Fat 7g Carbs 5g Protein 6g

502. BROCCOLI WITH PARMESAN CHEESE

PREPARATION: 5 MIN　　**COOKING:** 5 MIN　　**SERVINGS:** 4

INGREDIENTS

- 1 lb. broccoli florets
- 2 tsp.s minced garlic
- 2 tbsp. olive oil
- ¼ cup grated or shaved Parmesan cheese

DIRECTIONS

1. Preheat the Air Fryer to 360°F. In a bowl, mix together the broccoli florets, garlic, olive oil, and Parmesan cheese.
2. Place the broccoli in the Air Fryer basket in a single layer and set the timer and steam for 4 minutes.

Nutrition: Calories 130 Fat 3g Carbs 5g Protein 4g

503. CARAMELIZED BROCCOLI

PREPARATION: 5 MIN　　**COOKING:** 10 MIN　　**SERVINGS:** 4

INGREDIENTS

- 4 cups broccoli florets
- 3 tbsp. melted ghee or butter-flavored coconut oil
- 1½ tsp.s fine sea salt or smoked salt
- Mayonnaise, for serving (optional; omit for egg-free)

DIRECTIONS

1. Grease the basket with avocado oil. Preheat the Air Fryer to 400°F. Place the broccoli in a large bowl. Drizzle it with the ghee, toss to coat, and sprinkle it with the salt.
2. Transfer the broccoli to the Air Fryer basket and cook for 8 minutes, or until tender and crisp on the edges.

Nutrition: Calories 120 Fat 2g Carbs 4g Protein 3g

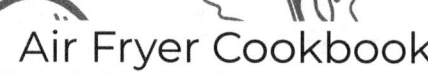
Air Fryer Cookbook

504. BRUSSELS SPROUTS WITH BALSAMIC OIL

PREPARATION: 5 MIN   **COOKING:** 15 MIN   **SERVINGS:** 4

INGREDIENTS

- ¼ tsp. salt
- 1 tbsp. balsamic vinegar
- 2 cups Brussels sprouts, halved
- 3 tbsp. olive oil

DIRECTIONS

1. Preheat the Air Fryer for 5 minutes. Mix all ingredients in a bowl until the zucchini fries are well coated.
2. Place in the Air Fryer basket. Close and cook for 15 minutes for 350°F.

Nutrition: Calories 82 Fat 6.8g Carbs 2g Protein 1.5g

505. SPICED BUTTERNUT SQUASH

PREPARATION: 10 MIN   **COOKING:** 15 MIN   **SERVINGS:** 4

INGREDIENTS

- 4 cups 1-inch-cubed butternut squash
- 2 tbsp. vegetable oil
- 1 to 2 tbsp. brown sugar
- 1 tsp. Chinese five-spice powder

DIRECTIONS

1. In a bowl, combine the oil, sugar, squash, and five-spice powder. Toss to coat.
2. Place the squash in the Air Fryer basket.
3. Set the Air Fryer to 400°F for 15 minutes or until tender.

Nutrition: Calories 160 Fat 5g Carbs 9g Protein 6g

506. GARLIC THYME MUSHROOMS

PREPARATION: 5 MIN   **COOKING:** 10 MIN   **SERVINGS:** 4

INGREDIENTS

- 3 tbsp. unsalted butter, melted
- 1 (8 oz.) package button mushrooms, sliced
- 2 cloves garlic, minced
- 3 sprigs fresh thyme leaves
- ½ tsp. fine sea salt

DIRECTIONS

1. Grease the basket with avocado oil. Preheat the Air Fryer to 400°F.
2. Place all the ingredients in a medium-sized bowl. Use a spoon or your hands to coat the mushroom slices.
3. Put the mushrooms in the basket in one layer; work in batches if necessary. Cook for 10 minutes, or until slightly crispy and brown. Garnish with thyme sprigs before serving.
4. Reheat in a warmed up 350°F Air Fryer for 5 minutes, or until heated through.

Nutrition: Calories 82 Fat 9g Carbs 1g Protein 1g

507. ZUCCHINI PARMESAN CHIPS

PREPARATION: 10 MIN   **COOKING:** 10 MIN   **SERVINGS:** 10

INGREDIENTS

- ½ tsp. paprika
- ½ C. grated parmesan cheese
- ½ C. Italian breadcrumbs
- 1 lightly beaten egg
- 2 thinly sliced zucchinis

DIRECTIONS

1. Use a very sharp knife or mandolin slicer to slice zucchini as thinly as you can. Pat off extra moisture. Beat egg with a pinch of pepper and salt and a bit of water.
2. Combine paprika, cheese, and breadcrumbs in a bowl. Dip slices of zucchini into the egg mixture and then into breadcrumb mixture. Press gently to coat.
3. With olive oil cooking spray, mist coated zucchini slices. Place into your Air Fryer in a single layer. Set temperature to 350°F, and set time to 8 minutes. Sprinkle with salt and serve with salsa.

Nutrition: Calories 130 Fat 2g Carbs 5g Protein 3g

508. JICAMA FRIES

PREPARATION: 10 MIN   **COOKING:** 5 MIN   **SERVINGS:** 4

INGREDIENTS

- 1 tbsp. dried thyme
- ¾ C. arrowroot flour
- ½ large Jicama
- Eggs

DIRECTIONS

1. Sliced jicama into fries.
2. Whisk eggs together and pour over fries. Toss to coat.
3. Mix a pinch of salt, thyme, and arrowroot flour together. Toss egg-coated jicama into dry mixture, tossing to coat well.
4. Spray the Air Fryer basket with olive oil and add fries. Set temperature to 350°F, and set time to 5 minutes. Toss halfway into the cooking process.

Nutrition: Calories 211 Fat 19g Carbs 16g Protein 9g

509. LEMON BELL PEPPERS

PREPARATION: 5 MIN   **COOKING:** 20 MIN   **SERVINGS:** 4

INGREDIENTS

- 1 ½ lb. Mixed bell peppers; halved and deseeded
- 2 tbsp. Lemon juice
- 2 tbsp. Balsamic vinegar
- 2 tsp. Lemon zest, grated
- Parsley; chopped.

DIRECTIONS

1. Put the peppers in your Air Fryer's basket and cook at 350°f for 15 minutes.
2. Peel the bell peppers, mix them with the rest of the ingredients, toss and serve

Nutrition: Calories 151 Fat 2g Carbs 5g Protein 5g

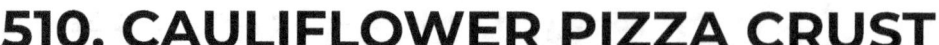

Air Fryer Cookbook

510. CAULIFLOWER PIZZA CRUST

PREPARATION: 5 MIN **COOKING:** 20 MIN **SERVINGS:** 6

INGREDIENTS

- 1(12-oz.) Steamer bag cauliflower
- 1 large egg.
- ½ cup shredded sharp cheddar cheese.
- 2 tbsp. Blanched finely ground almond flour
- 1 tsp. Italian blend seasoning

Nutrition: Calories 230 Fat 14.2g Carbs 10g Protein 14.9g

DIRECTIONS

1. Cook cauliflower according to package. Take out from bag and place into a paper towel to remove excess water. Place cauliflower into a large bowl.
2. Add almond flour, cheese, egg, and italian seasoning to the bowl and mix well
3. Cut a piece of parchment to fit your Air Fryer basket. Press cauliflower into 6-inch round circle. Place into the Air Fryer basket. Adjust the temperature to 360°F and set the timer for 11 minutes. After 7 minutes, flip the pizza crust
4. Add preferred toppings to pizza. Place back into Air Fryer basket and cook an additional 4 minutes or until fully cooked and golden. Serve immediately.

511. SAVOY CABBAGE AND TOMATOES

PREPARATION: 5 MIN **COOKING:** 20 MIN **SERVINGS:** 4

INGREDIENTS

- 2 spring onions; chopped.
- 1 savoy cabbage, shredded
- 1 tbsp. Parsley; chopped.
- 2 tbsp. Tomato sauce
- Salt and black pepper to taste.

Nutrition: Calories 163 Fat 4g Carbs 6g Protein 7g

DIRECTIONS

1. In a pan that fits your Air Fryer, mix the cabbage the rest of the ingredients except the parsley, toss, put the pan in the fryer and cook at 360°f for 15 minutes
2. Divide between plates and serve with parsley sprinkled on top.

512. CAULIFLOWER STEAK

PREPARATION: 5 MIN **COOKING:** 10 MIN **SERVINGS:** 4

INGREDIENTS

- 1 medium head cauliflower
- ¼ cup blue cheese crumbles
- ¼ cup hot sauce
- ¼ cup full-fat ranch dressing
- 2 tbsp. Salted butter; melted.

Nutrition: Calories 122 Fat 8.4g Carbs 7.7g Protein 4.9g

DIRECTIONS

1. Remove cauliflower leaves. Slice the head in ½-inch-thick slices.
2. In a small bowl, mix hot sauce and butter. Brush the mixture over the cauliflower.
3. Place each cauliflower steak into the Air Fryer, working in batches if necessary. Adjust the temperature to 400°F and set the timer for 7 minutes
4. When cooked, edges will begin turning dark and caramelized. To serve, sprinkle steaks with crumbled blue cheese. Drizzle with ranch dressing.

513. TOMATO, AVOCADO AND GREEN BEANS

PREPARATION: 5 MIN   **COOKING:** 20 MIN   **SERVINGS:** 4

INGREDIENTS

- ¼ lb. Green beans, trimmed and halved
- 1 avocado, peeled, pitted and cubed
- 1 pint mixed cherry tomatoes; halved
- 2 tbsp. Olive oil

DIRECTIONS

1. In a pan that fits your Air Fryer, mix the tomatoes with the rest of the ingredients, toss.
2. Put the pan in the fryer and cook at 360°F for 15 minutes. Transfer to bowls and serve

Nutrition: Calories 151 Fat 3g Carbs 4g Protein 4g

514. DILL AND GARLIC GREEN BEANS

PREPARATION: 5 MIN   **COOKING:** 20 MIN   **SERVINGS:** 4

INGREDIENTS

- 1 lb. Green beans, trimmed
- ½ cup bacon, cooked and chopped.
- 2 garlic cloves; minced
- 2 tbsp. Dill; chopped.
- Salt and black pepper to taste.

Nutrition: Calories 180 Fat 3g Carbs 4g Protein 6g

DIRECTIONS

1. In a pan that fits the Air Fryer, combine the green beans with the rest of the ingredients, toss.
2. Put the pan in the fryer and cook at 390°F for 15 minutes
3. Divide everything between plates and serve.

515. EGGPLANT STACKS

PREPARATION: 5 MIN   **COOKING:** 15 MIN   **SERVINGS:** 4

INGREDIENTS

- 2 large tomatoes; cut into ¼-inch slices
- ¼ cup fresh basil, sliced
- 4oz. Fresh mozzarella; cut into ½-oz. Slices
- 1 medium eggplant; cut into ¼-inch slices
- 2 tbsp. Olive oil

Nutrition: Calories 195 Fat 12.7g Carbs 12.7g Protein 8.5g

DIRECTIONS

1. In a 6-inch round baking dish, place four slices of eggplant on the bottom. Put a slice of tomato on each eggplant round, then mozzarella, then eggplant. Repeat as necessary.
2. Drizzle with olive oil. Cover dish with foil and place dish into the Air Fryer basket. Adjust the temperature to 350°F and set the timer for 12 minutes.
3. When done, eggplant will be tender. Garnish with fresh basil to serve.

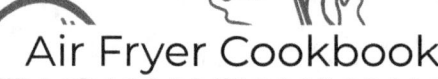

516. AIR FRIED SPAGHETTI SQUASH

PREPARATION: 5 MIN **COOKING:** 50 MIN **SERVINGS:** 4

INGREDIENTS

- ½ large spaghetti squash
- 2 tbsp. Salted butter; melted.
- 1 tbsp. Coconut oil
- 1 tsp. Dried parsley.
- ½ tsp. Garlic powder.

DIRECTIONS

1. Brush shell of spaghetti squash with coconut oil. Place the skin side down and brush the inside with butter. Sprinkle with garlic powder and parsley.
2. Place squash with the skin side down into the Air Fryer basket. Adjust the temperature to 350°F and set the timer for 30 minutes
3. When the timer beeps, flip the squash so skin side is up and cook an additional 15 minutes or until fork tender. Serve warm.

Nutrition: Calories 182 Fat 11.7g Carbs 18.2g Protein 1.9g

517. BEETS AND BLUE CHEESE SALAD

PREPARATION: 5 MIN **COOKING:** 10 MIN **SERVINGS:** 4

INGREDIENTS

- 6 beets, peeled and quartered
- Salt and black pepper to the taste
- ¼ cup blue cheese, crumbled
- 1 tbsp. olive oil

DIRECTIONS

1. Put beets in your Air Fryer, cook them at 350°F for 14 minutes and transfer them to a bowl. Add blue cheese, salt, pepper and oil, toss and serve. Enjoy!

Nutrition: Calories 100 Fat 4g Carbs 10g Protein 5g

518. BROCCOLI SALAD

PREPARATION: 10 MIN **COOKING:** 10 MIN **SERVINGS:** 4

INGREDIENTS

- 1 broccoli head, with separated florets
- 1 tbsp. peanut oil
- 6 cloves of garlic, minced
- 1 tbsp. Chinese rice wine vinegar
- Salt and black pepper to taste

DIRECTIONS

1. In a bowl, mix broccoli half of the oil with salt, pepper and, toss, transfer to your Air Fryer and cook at 350°F for 8 minutes. Halfway through, shake the fryer. Take the broccoli out and put it into a salad bowl, add the rest of the peanut oil, garlic and rice vinegar, mix really well and serve. Enjoy!

Nutrition: Calories 121 Fat 3g Carbs 4g Protein 4g

519. ROASTED BRUSSELS SPROUTS WITH TOMATOES

PREPARATION: 5 MIN **COOKING:** 10 MIN **SERVINGS:** 4

INGREDIENTS

- 1-lb. Brussels sprouts, trimmed
- Salt and black pepper to the taste
- 6 cherry tomatoes, halved
- ¼ cup green onions, chopped
- 1 tbsp. olive oil

DIRECTIONS

1. Season Brussels sprouts with salt and pepper, put them in your Air Fryer and cook at 350°F for 10 minutes. Transfer them to a bowl, add salt, pepper, cherry tomatoes, green onions and olive oil, toss well and serve. Enjoy!

Nutrition: Calories 121 Fat 4g Carbs 11g Protein 4g

520. CHEESY BRUSSELS SPROUTS

PREPARATION: 10 MIN **COOKING:** 10 MIN **SERVINGS:** 4

INGREDIENTS

- 1 lb. Brussels sprouts, washed
- Juice of 1 lemon
- Salt and black pepper to the taste
- 2 tbsp. butter
- 3 tbsp. parmesan, grated

DIRECTIONS

1. Put Brussels sprouts in your Air Fryer, cook them at 350°F for 8 minutes and transfer them to a bowl. Warm up a pan over moderate heat with the butter, then add lemon juice, salt and pepper, whisk well and add to Brussels sprouts. Add parmesan, toss until parmesan melts and serve. Enjoy!

Nutrition: Calories 152 Fat 6g Carbs 8g Protein 12g

521. SWEET BABY CARROTS DISH

PREPARATION: 10 MIN **COOKING:** 10 MIN **SERVINGS:** 4

INGREDIENTS

- 2 cups baby carrots
- A pinch of salt and black pepper
- 1 tbsp. brown sugar
- ½ tbsp. butter, melted

DIRECTIONS

1. In a dish that fits your Air Fryer, mix baby carrots with butter, salt, pepper and sugar, toss, introduce in your Air Fryer and cook at 350°F for 10 minutes. Divide among plates and serve. Enjoy!

Nutrition: Calories 100 Fat 2g Carbs 7g Protein 4g

522. SEASONED LEEKS

PREPARATION: 10 MIN **COOKING:** 10 MIN **SERVINGS:** 4

INGREDIENTS

- 4 leeks, washed, halved
- Salt and black pepper to taste
- 1 tbsp. butter, melted
- 1 tbsp. lemon juice

DIRECTIONS

1. Rub leeks with melted butter, season with salt and pepper, put in your Air Fryer and cook at 350°F for 7 minutes. Arrange on a platter, drizzle lemon juice all over and serve. Enjoy!

Nutrition: Calories 100 Fat 4g Carbs 6g Protein 2g

523. CRISPY POTATOES AND PARSLEY

PREPARATION: 10 MIN **COOKING:** 10 MIN **SERVINGS:** 4

INGREDIENTS

- 1-lb. gold potatoes, cut into wedges
- Salt and black pepper to the taste
- 2 tbsp. olive oil
- Juice from ½ lemon
- ¼ cup parsley leaves, chopped

DIRECTIONS

1. Rub potatoes with salt, pepper, lemon juice and olive oil, put them in your Air Fryer and cook at 350°F for 10 minutes. Divide among plates, sprinkle parsley on top and serve. Enjoy!

Nutrition: Calories 152 Fat 3g Carbs 17g Protein 4g

524. GARLIC TOMATOES

PREPARATION: 10 MIN **COOKING:** 15 MIN **SERVINGS:** 4

INGREDIENTS

- 4 garlic cloves, crushed
- 1-lb. mixed cherry tomatoes
- 3 thyme springs, chopped
- Salt and black pepper to the taste
- ¼ cup olive oil

DIRECTIONS

1. In a bowl, mix tomatoes with salt, black pepper, garlic, olive oil and thyme, toss to coat, introduce in your Air Fryer and cook at 360°F for 15 minutes. Divide tomatoes mix on plates and serve. Enjoy!

Nutrition: Calories 100 Fat 0g Carbs 1g Protein 6g

525. EASY GREEN BEANS AND POTATOES

PREPARATION: 10 MIN **COOKING:** 15 MIN **SERVINGS:** 5

INGREDIENTS

- 2 lb. green beans
- 6 new potatoes, halved
- Salt and black pepper to the taste
- A drizzle of olive oil
- 6 bacon slices, cooked and chopped

DIRECTIONS

1. In a bowl, mix green beans with potatoes, salt, pepper and oil, toss, transfer to your Air Fryer and cook at 390°F for 15 minutes. Divide among plates and serve with bacon sprinkled on top. Enjoy!

Nutrition: Calories 374 Fat 15g Carbs 28g Protein 12g

526. GREEN BEANS AND TOMATOES

PREPARATION: 10 MIN **COOKING:** 15 MIN **SERVINGS:** 4

INGREDIENTS

- 1 pint cherry tomatoes
- 1 lb. green beans
- 2 tbsp. olive oil
- Salt and black pepper to the taste

DIRECTIONS

1. In a bowl, mix cherry tomatoes with green beans, olive oil, salt and pepper, toss, transfer to your Air Fryer and cook at 400°F for 15 minutes. Divide among plates and serve right away. Enjoy!

Nutrition: Calories 162 Fat 6g Carbs 8g Protein 9g

527. FLAVORED ASPARAGUS

PREPARATION: 5 MIN **COOKING:** 30 MIN **SERVINGS:** 2

INGREDIENTS

- Nutritional yeast
- Olive oil non-stick spray
- One bunch of asparagus

DIRECTIONS

1. Wash asparagus and then cut off the bushy, woody ends. Drizzle asparagus with olive oil spray and sprinkle with yeast. In your Air Fryer, lay asparagus in a singular layer. Cook 8 minutes at 360°F.

Nutrition: Calories 17 Fat 4g Carbs 32g Protein 24g

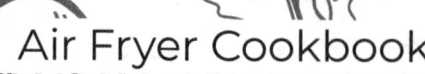

Air Fryer Cookbook

528. SPAGHETTI SQUASH TOTS

PREPARATION: 5 MIN **COOKING:** 5 MIN **SERVINGS:** 10

INGREDIENTS

- ¼ tsp. pepper
- ½ tsp. salt
- 1 thinly sliced scallion
- 1 spaghetti squash

Nutrition: Calories 231 Fat 18g Carbs 3g Protein 5g

DIRECTIONS

1. Wash and cut the squash in lengthwise. Scrape out the seeds. With a fork, remove spaghetti meat by strands and throw out skins. In a clean towel, toss in squash and wring out as much moisture as possible.
2. Place in a bowl and with a knife slice through meat a few times to cut up smaller. Add pepper, salt, and scallions to squash and mix well. Create "tot" shapes with your hands and place in Air Fryer. Spray with olive oil. Cook 15 minutes at 350°F until golden and crispy!

529. CINNAMON BUTTERNUT SQUASH FRIES

PREPARATION: 10 MIN **COOKING:** 10 MIN **SERVINGS:** 2

INGREDIENTS

- 1 pinch of salt
- 1 tbsp. powdered unprocessed sugar
- 2 tsp. cinnamon
- 1 tbsp. coconut oil
- 10 oz. pre-cut butternut squash fries

Nutrition: Calories 175 Fat 8g Carbs 3g Protein 1g

DIRECTIONS

1. In a plastic bag, pour in all ingredients. Coat fries with other components till coated and sugar is dissolved. Spread coated fries into a single layer in the Air Fryer. Cook 10 minutes at 390°F until crispy.

530. CHEESY ROASTED SWEET POTATOES

PREPARATION: 5 MIN **COOKING:** 20 MIN **SERVINGS:** 4

INGREDIENTS

- 2 large sweet potatoes, peeled and sliced
- 1 tsp. olive oil
- 1 tbsp. white balsamic vinegar
- 1 tsp. dried thyme
- ¼ cup grated Parmesan cheese

Nutrition: Calories 100 Fat 3g Carbs 15g Protein 4g

DIRECTIONS

1. In a big bowl, shower the sweet potato slices with the olive oil and toss.
2. Sprinkle with the balsamic vinegar and thyme and toss again.
3. Sprinkle the potatoes with the Parmesan cheese and toss to coat.
4. Roast the slices, in batches, in the Air Fryer basket for 18 to 23 minutes at 375°F, tossing the sweet potato slices in the basket once during cooking, until tender.
5. Repeat with the remaining sweet potato slices. Serve immediately.

Air Fryer Cookbook

531. SALTY LEMON ARTICHOKES

PREPARATION: 15 MIN   **COOKING:** 45 MIN   **SERVINGS:** 2

INGREDIENTS

- 1 lemon
- 2 artichokes
- 1 tsp. kosher salt
- 1 garlic head
- 2 tsp. olive oil

Nutrition: Calories 133 Fat 5g Carbs 21.7g Protein 6g

DIRECTIONS

1. Cut off the edges of the artichokes.
2. Cut the lemon into halves.
3. Peel the garlic head and chop the garlic cloves roughly.
4. Then place the chopped garlic in the artichokes.
5. Sprinkle the artichokes with olive oil and kosher salt.
6. Then squeeze the lemon juice into the artichokes.
7. Wrap the artichokes in the foil.
8. Preheat the Air Fryer to 330°F.
9. Place the wrapped artichokes in the Air Fryer and cook for 45 minutes.
10. When the artichokes are cooked – discard the foil and serve.

532. ASPARAGUS & PARMESAN

PREPARATION: 10 MIN   **COOKING:** 6 MIN   **SERVINGS:** 2

INGREDIENTS

- 1 tsp. sesame oil
- 11 oz asparagus
- 1 tsp. chicken stock
- ½ tsp. ground white pepper
- 3 oz Parmesan

Nutrition: Calories 189 Fat 11.6g Carbs 7.9g Protein 17.2g

DIRECTIONS

1. Wash the asparagus and chop it roughly.
2. Sprinkle the chopped asparagus with the chicken stock and ground white pepper.
3. Then sprinkle the vegetables with the sesame oil and shake them.
4. Place the asparagus in the Air Fryer basket.
5. Cook the vegetables for 4 minutes at 400°F.
6. Meanwhile, shred Parmesan cheese.
7. When the time is over – shake the asparagus gently and sprinkle with the shredded cheese.
8. Cook the asparagus for 2 minutes more at 400°F.
9. After this, transfer the cooked asparagus in the serving plates.
10. Serve and taste it!

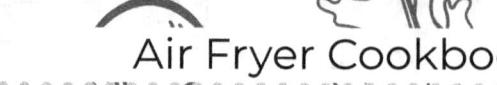
Air Fryer Cookbook

533. CORN ON COBS

PREPARATION: 10 MIN   **COOKING:** 10 MIN   **SERVINGS:** 2

INGREDIENTS

- 2 fresh corn on cobs
- 2 tsp. butter
- 1 tsp. salt
- 1 tsp. paprika
- ¼ tsp. olive oil

Nutrition: Calories 122 Fat 5.5g Carbs 17.6g Protein 3.2g

DIRECTIONS

1. Preheat the Air Fryer to 400°F.
2. Rub the corn on cobs with the salt and paprika.
3. Then sprinkle the corn on cobs with the olive oil.
4. Place the corn on cobs in the Air Fryer basket.
5. Cook the corn on cobs for 10 minutes.
6. When the time is over – transfer the corn on cobs in the serving plates and rub with the butter gently.
7. Serve the meal immediately.

534. ONION GREEN BEANS

PREPARATION: 10 MIN   **COOKING:** 12 MIN   **SERVINGS:** 2

INGREDIENTS

- 11 oz green beans
- 1 tbsp. onion powder
- 1 tbsp. olive oil
- ½ tsp. salt
- ¼ tsp. chili flakes

Nutrition: Calories 145 Fat 7.2g Carbs 13.9g Protein 3.2g

DIRECTIONS

1. Wash the green beans carefully and place them in the bowl.
2. Sprinkle the green beans with the onion powder, salt, chili flakes, and olive oil.
3. Shake the green beans carefully.
4. Preheat the Air Fryer to 400°F.
5. Put the green beans in the Air Fryer and cook for 8 minutes.
6. After this, shake the green beans and cook them for 4 minutes more at 400°F.
7. When the time is over – shake the green beans.
8. Serve the side dish and enjoy!

535. DILL MASHED POTATO

PREPARATION: 10 MIN **COOKING:** 15 MIN **SERVINGS:** 2

INGREDIENTS

- 2 potatoes
- 2 tbsp. fresh dill, chopped
- 1 tsp. butter
- ½ tsp. salt
- ¼ cup half and half

Nutrition: Calories 211 Fat 5.7g Carbs 36.5g Protein 5.1g

DIRECTIONS

1. Preheat the Air Fryer to 390°F.
2. Rinse the potatoes thoroughly and place them in the Air Fryer.
3. Cook the potatoes for 15 minutes.
4. After this, remove the potatoes from the Air Fryer.
5. Peel the potatoes.
6. Mash the potatoes with the help of the fork well.
7. Then add chopped fresh dill and salt.
8. Stir it gently and add butter and half and half.
9. Take the hand blender and blend the mixture well.
10. When the mashed potato is cooked – serve it immediately. Enjoy!

536. CREAM POTATO

PREPARATION: 12 MIN **COOKING:** 20 MIN **SERVINGS:** 2

INGREDIENTS

- 3 medium potatoes, scrubbed
- ½ tsp. kosher salt
- 1 tbsp. Italian seasoning
- 1/3 cup cream
- ½ tsp. ground black pepper

Nutrition: Calories 269 Fat 4.7g Carbs 52.6g Protein 5.8g

DIRECTIONS

1. Slice the potatoes.
2. Preheat the Air Fryer to 365°F.
3. Make the layer from the sliced potato in the Air Fryer basket.
4. Sprinkle the potato layer with the kosher salt and ground black pepper.
5. After this, make the second layer of the potato and sprinkle it with Italian seasoning.
6. Make the last layer of the sliced potato and pour the cream.
7. Cook the scallop potato for 20 minutes.
8. When the scalloped potato is cooked – let it chill to room temperature. Enjoy!

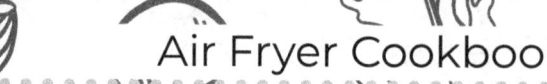
Air Fryer Cookbook

537. CHARD WITH CHEDDAR

PREPARATION: 10 MIN **COOKING:** 11 MIN **SERVINGS:** 2

INGREDIENTS

- 3 oz Cheddar cheese, grated
- 10 oz Swiss chard
- 3 tbsp. cream
- 1 tbsp. sesame oil
- Salt and pepper to taste

DIRECTIONS

1. Wash Swiss chard carefully and chop it roughly.
2. After this, sprinkle chopped Swiss chard with the salt and ground white pepper.
3. Stir it carefully.
4. Sprinkle Swiss chard with the sesame oil and stir it carefully with the help of 2 spatulas.
5. Preheat the Air Fryer to 260°F.
6. Put chopped Swiss chard in the Air Fryer basket and cook for 6 minutes.
7. Shake it after 3 minutes of cooking.
8. Then pour the cream into the Air Fryer basket and mix it up.
9. Cook the meal for 3 minutes more.
10. Then increase the temperature to 400°F.
11. Sprinkle the meal with the grated cheese and cook for 2 minutes more.
12. After this, transfer the meal in the serving plates. Enjoy!

Nutrition: Calories 272 Fat 22.3g Carbs 6.7g Protein 13.3g

538. CHILI SQUASH WEDGES

PREPARATION: 10 MIN **COOKING:** 18 MIN **SERVINGS:** 2

INGREDIENTS

- 11 oz Acorn squash
- ½ tsp. salt
- tbsp. olive oil
- ½ tsp. chili pepper
- ½ tsp. paprika

DIRECTIONS

1. Cut Acorn squash into the serving wedges.
2. Sprinkle the wedges with salt, olive oil, chili pepper, and paprika.
3. Massage the wedges gently.
4. Preheat the Air Fryer to 400°F.
5. Put Acorn squash wedges in the Air Fryer basket and cook for 18 minutes.
6. Flip the wedges into another side after 9 minutes of cooking.
7. Serve the cooked meal hot. Enjoy!

Nutrition: Calories 125 Fat 7.2g Carbs 16.7g Protein 1.4g

539. HONEY CARROTS WITH GREENS

PREPARATION: 7 MIN **COOKING:** 12 MIN **SERVINGS:** 2

INGREDIENTS

- 1 cup baby carrot
- ½ tsp. salt
- ½ tsp. white pepper
- 1 tbsp. honey
- 1 tsp. sesame oil

Nutrition: Calories 83 Fat 2.4g Carbs 16g Protein 0.6g

DIRECTIONS

1. Preheat the Air Fryer to 385°F.
2. Combine the baby carrot with salt, white pepper, and sesame oil.
3. Shake the baby carrot and transfer in the Air Fryer basket.
4. Cook the vegetables for 10 minutes.
5. After this, add honey and shake the vegetables.
6. Cook the meal for 2 minutes.
7. After this, shake the vegetables and serve immediately.

540. SOUTH ASIAN CAULIFLOWER FRITTERS

PREPARATION: 5 MIN **COOKING:** 20 MIN **SERVINGS:** 4

INGREDIENTS

- 1 large chopped into florets cauliflower
- 3 tbsp. of Greek yogurt
- 3 tbsp. of flour
- ½ tsp. of ground turmeric
- ½ tsp. of ground cumin
- ½ tsp. of ground paprika
- 12 tsp. of ground coriander
- ½ tsp. of salt
- ½ tsp. of black pepper

Nutrition: Calories 120 Fat 4g Carbs 14g Protein 7.5g

DIRECTIONS

1. Using a large bowl, add and mix the Greek yogurt, flour, and seasonings properly.
2. Add the cauliflower florets and toss it until it is well covered
3. Heat up your Air Fryer to 390°F.
4. Grease your Air Fryer basket with a nonstick cooking spray and add half of the cauliflower florets to it.
5. Cook it for 10 minutes or until it turns golden brown and crispy, then shake it after 5 minutes. (Repeat this with the other half).
6. Serve and enjoy!

541. SUPREME AIR-FRIED TOFU

PREPARATION: 5 MIN **COOKING:** 50 MIN **SERVINGS:** 4

INGREDIENTS

- 1 block of pressed and sliced into 1-inch cubes of extra-firm tofu
- 2 tbsp. of soy sauce
- 1 tsp. of seasoned rice vinegar
- 2 tsp.s of toasted sesame oil
- 1 tbsp. of cornstarch

Nutrition: Calories 80 Fat 5.8g Carbs 3g Protein 5g

DIRECTIONS

1. Using a bowl, add and toss the tofu, soy sauce, seasoned rice vinegar, sesame oil until it is properly covered.
2. Place it inside your refrigerator and allow to marinate for 30 minutes.
3. Preheat your Air Fryer to 370°F.
4. Add the cornstarch to the tofu mixture and toss it until it is properly covered.
5. Grease your Air Fryer basket with a nonstick cooking spray and add the tofu inside your basket.
6. Cook it for 20 minutes at 370°F, and shake it after 10 minutes. Serve and enjoy!

SWEETS AND DESSERTS

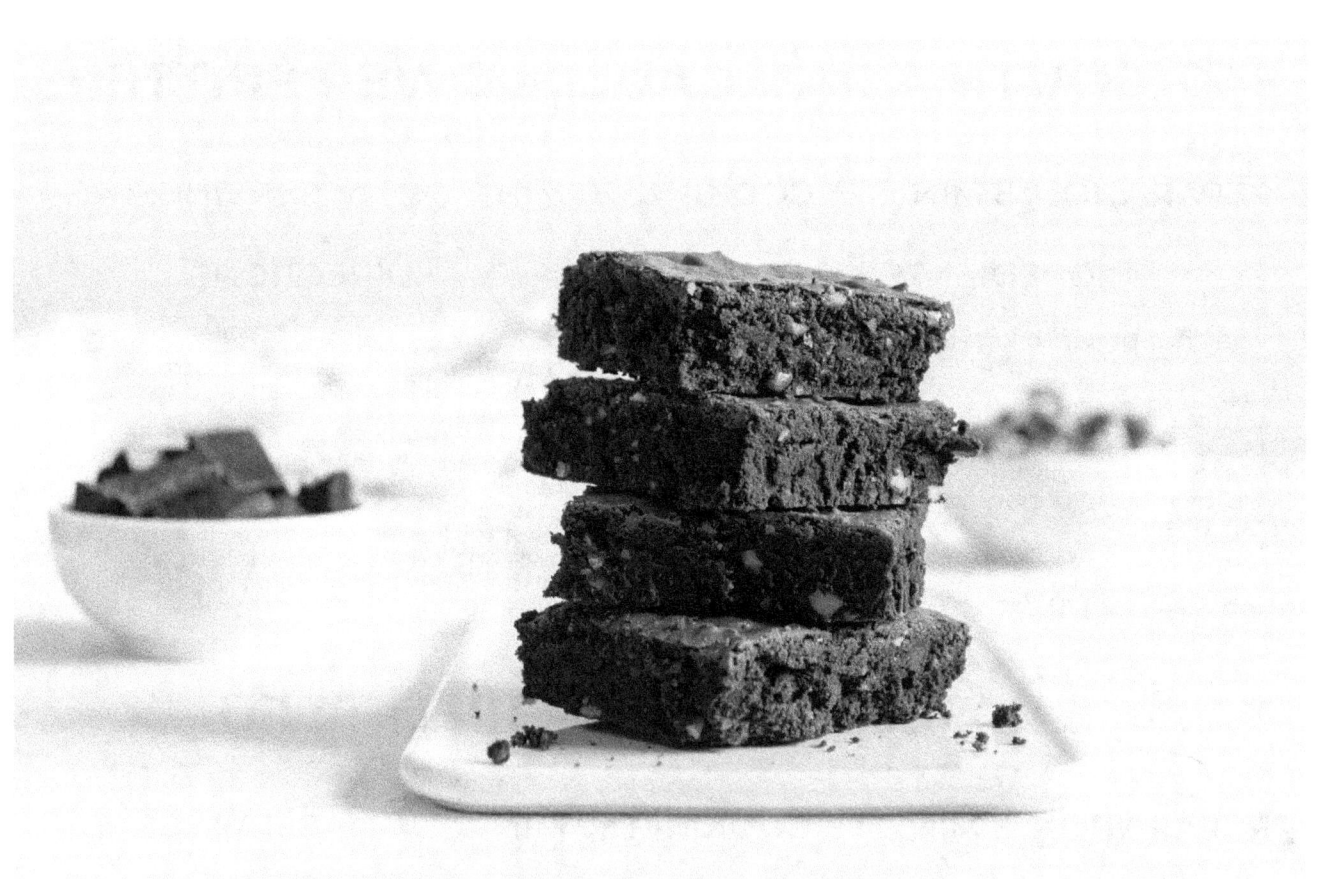

542. LEMON BARS

PREPARATION: 10 MIN **COOKING:** 35 MIN **SERVINGS:** 8

INGREDIENTS

- ½ cup butter, melted
- 1 cup erythritol
- 1 and ¾ cups almond flour
- 3 eggs, whisked
- Juice of 3 lemons

Nutrition: Calories 210 Fat 12g Carbs 4g Protein 8g

DIRECTIONS

1. In a bowl, mix 1 cup flour with half of the erythritol and the butter, stir well and press into a baking dish that fits the Air Fryer lined with parchment paper.
2. Put the dish in your Air Fryer and cook at 350°F for 10 minutes.
3. In the meantime, in a bowl, blend the rest of the flour with the remaining erythritol and the other ingredients and whisk well.
4. Spread this over the crust, put the dish in the Air Fryer once more and cook at 350°F for 25 minutes.
5. Cool down, cut into bars and serve.

543. COCONUT DONUTS

PREPARATION: 5 MIN **COOKING:** 15 MIN **SERVINGS:** 4

INGREDIENTS

- 8 oz. coconut flour
- 1 egg, whisked
- and ½ tbsp. butter, melted
- 4 ounces coconut milk
- 1 tsp. baking powder

Nutrition: Calories 190 Fat 12g Protein 6g Carbs 4g

DIRECTIONS

1. In a bowl, put all of the ingredients and mix well.
2. Shape donuts from this mix, place them in your Air Fryer's basket and cook at 370°F for 15 minutes. Serve warm.

544. BLUEBERRY CREAM

PREPARATION: 4 MIN **COOKING:** 20 MIN **SERVINGS:** 6

INGREDIENTS

- 2 cups blueberries
- Juice of ½ lemon
- 2 tbsp. water
- 1 tsp. vanilla extract
- 2 tbsp. swerve

Nutrition: Calories 123 Fat 2g Carbs 4g Protein 3g

DIRECTIONS

1. In a large bowl, put all ingredients and mix well.
2. Divide this into 6 ramekins, put them in the Air Fryer and cook at 340°F for 20 minutes
3. Cool down and serve.

545. BLACKBERRY CHIA JAM

PREPARATION: 10 MIN **COOKING:** 30 MIN **SERVINGS:** 12

INGREDIENTS

- 3cups blackberries
- ¼ cup swerve
- 4tbsp. lemon juice
- 4tbsp. chia seeds

DIRECTIONS

1. In a pan that suits the Air Fryer, combine all the Ingredients: and toss.
2. Put the pan in the fryer and cook at 300°F for 30 minutes.
3. Divide into cups and serve cold.

Nutrition: Calories 100 Fat 2g Carbs 3g Protein 1g

546. MIXED BERRIES CREAM

PREPARATION: 5 MIN **COOKING:** 30 MIN **SERVINGS:** 6

INGREDIENTS

- 12 oz. blackberries
- 6 oz. raspberries
- 12 oz. blueberries
- ¾ cup swerve
- 2 oz. coconut cream

DIRECTIONS

1. In a bowl, put all the Ingredients: and mix well.
2. Divide this into 6 ramekins, put them in your Air Fryer and cook at 320°F for 30 minutes.
3. Cool down and serve it.

Nutrition: Calories 100 Fat 1g Carbs 2g Protein 2g

547. APPLE CHIPS

PREPARATION: 10 MIN **COOKING:** 20 MIN **SERVINGS:** 2

INGREDIENTS

- 1 apple, sliced thinly
- Salt to taste
- ¼ tsp. ground cinnamon

DIRECTIONS

1. Preheat the Air Fryer to 350°F.
2. Toss the apple slices in salt and cinnamon.
3. Add to the Air Fryer. Cook for 20 minutes
4. Let cool before serving.

Nutrition: Calories 59 Fat 0.2g Carbs 15.6g Protein 0.3g

548. SWEETENED PLANTAINS

PREPARATION: 5 MIN   **COOKING:** 8 MIN   **SERVINGS:** 4

INGREDIENTS

- 2 ripe plantains, sliced
- 2 tsp.s avocado oil
- Salt to taste
- Maple syrup

DIRECTIONS

1. Toss the plantains in oil.
2. Season with salt.
3. Cook in the Air Fryer basket at 400°F for 10 minutes, shaking after 5 minutes.
4. Drizzle with maple syrup before serving.

Nutrition: Calories 125 Fat 0.6g Carbs 32g Protein 1.2g

549. ROASTED BANANAS

PREPARATION: 5 MIN   **COOKING:** 5 MIN   **SERVINGS:** 2

INGREDIENTS

- 2 cups bananas, cubed
- 1 tsp. avocado oil
- 1 tbsp. maple syrup
- 1 tsp. brown sugar
- 1 cup almond milk

DIRECTIONS

1. Coat the banana cubes with oil and maple syrup.
2. Sprinkle with brown sugar.
3. Cook at 375°F in the Air Fryer for 5 minutes.
4. Drizzle milk on top of the bananas before serving.

Nutrition: Calories 107 Fat 0.7g Carbs 27g Protein 1.3g

550. PEAR CRISP

PREPARATION: 10 MIN   **COOKING:** 25 MIN   **SERVINGS:** 2

INGREDIENTS

- 1 cup flour
- 1 stick vegan butter
- 1 tbsp. cinnamon
- ½ cup sugar
- 2 pears, cubed

DIRECTIONS

1. Mix flour and butter to form crumbly texture.
2. Add cinnamon and sugar.
3. Put the pears in the Air Fryer.
4. Pour and spread the mixture on top of the pears.
5. Cook at 350°F for 25 minutes.

Nutrition: Calories 544 Fat 0.9g Carbs 132.3g Protein 7.4g

551. EASY PEARS DESSERT

PREPARATION: 10 MIN **COOKING:** 25 MIN **SERVINGS:** 12

INGREDIENTS

- 6 big pears, cored and chopped
- ½ cup raisins
- 1 tsp. ginger powder
- ¼ cup coconut sugar
- 1 tsp. lemon zest, grated

DIRECTIONS

1. In a container that fits your Air Fryer, mix pears with raisins, ginger, sugar and lemon zest, stir, introduce in the fryer and cook at 350°F for 25 minutes.
2. Divide into bowls and serve cold.

Nutrition: Calories 200 Fat 3g Carbs 6g Protein 6g

552. VANILLA STRAWBERRY MIX

PREPARATION: 10 MIN **COOKING:** 20 MIN **SERVINGS:** 10

INGREDIENTS

- 2 tbsp. lemon juice
- 2 lb. strawberries
- 4 cups coconut sugar
- 1 tsp. cinnamon powder
- 1 tsp. vanilla extract

DIRECTIONS

1. In a pot that fits your Air Fryer, mix strawberries with coconut sugar, lemon juice, cinnamon and vanilla, stir gently, introduce in the fryer and cook at 350°F for 20 minutes
2. Divide into bowls and serve cold.

Nutrition: Calories 140 Fat 0g Carbs 5g Protein 2g

553. SWEET BANANAS AND SAUCE

PREPARATION: 10 MIN **COOKING:** 20 MIN **SERVINGS:** 4

INGREDIENTS

- Juice of ½ lemon
- 3 tbsp. agave nectar
- 1 tbsp. coconut oil
- 4 bananas, peeled and sliced diagonally
- ½ tsp. cardamom seeds

DIRECTIONS

1. Arrange bananas in a pan that fits your Air Fryer, add agave nectar, lemon juice, oil and cardamom, introduce in the fryer and cook at 360°F for 20 minutes
2. Divide bananas and sauce between plates and serve.

Nutrition: Calories 210 Fat 1g Carbs 8g Protein 3g

554. CINNAMON APPLES AND MANDARIN SAUCE

PREPARATION: 10 MIN **COOKING:** 20 MIN **SERVINGS:** 4

INGREDIENTS

- 4 apples, cored, peeled and cored
- 2 cups mandarin juice
- ¼ cup maple syrup
- 2 tsp.s cinnamon powder
- 1 tbsp. ginger, grated

DIRECTIONS

1. In a pot that fits your Air Fryer, mix apples with mandarin juice, maple syrup, cinnamon and ginger, introduce in the fryer and cook at 365°F for 20 minutes
2. Divide apples mix between plates and serve warm.

Nutrition: Calories 170 Fat 1g Carbs 6g Protein 4g

555. CHOCOLATE VANILLA BARS

PREPARATION: 10 MIN **COOKING:** 7 MIN **SERVINGS:** 12

INGREDIENTS

- 1 cup sugar free and vegan chocolate chips
- 2 tbsp. coconut butter
- 2/3 cup coconut cream
- 2 tbsp. stevia
- ¼ tsp. vanilla extract

DIRECTIONS

1. Put the cream in a bowl, add stevia, butter and chocolate chips and stir
2. Leave aside for 5 minutes, stir well and mix the vanilla.
3. Transfer the mix into a lined baking sheet, introduce in your Air Fryer and cook at 356°F for 7 minutes.
4. Leave the mix aside to cool down, slice and serve.

Nutrition: Calories 120 Fat 5g Carbs 6g Protein 1g

556. RASPBERRY BARS

PREPARATION: 10 MIN **COOKING:** 6 MIN **SERVINGS:** 12

INGREDIENTS

- ½ cup coconut butter, melted
- ½ cup coconut oil
- ½ cup raspberries, dried
- ¼ cup swerve
- ½ cup coconut, shredded

DIRECTIONS

1. In your food processor, blend dried berries very well.
2. In a bowl that fits your Air Fryer, mix oil with butter, swerve, coconut and raspberries, toss well, introduce in the fryer and cook at 320°F for 6 minutes.
3. Spread this on a lined baking sheet, keep in the fridge for an hour, slice and serve.

Nutrition: Calories 164 Fat 22g Carbs 4g Protein 2g

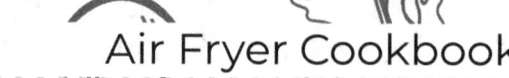

557. COCOA BERRIES CREAM

PREPARATION: 10 MIN **COOKING:** 10 MIN **SERVINGS:** 4

INGREDIENTS

- 3 tbsp. cocoa powder
- 14 oz. coconut cream
- 1 cup blackberries
- 1 cup raspberries
- 2 tbsp. stevia

DIRECTIONS

1. In a bowl, whisk cocoa powder with stevia and cream and stir.
2. Add raspberries and blackberries, toss gently, transfer to a pan that fits your Air Fryer, introduce in the fryer and cook at 350°F for 10 minutes.
3. Divide into bowls and serve cold.

Nutrition: Calories 205 Fat 34g Carbs 6g Protein 2g

558. COCOA PUDDING

PREPARATION: 10 MIN **COOKING:** 20 MIN **SERVINGS:** 2

INGREDIENTS

- 2 tbsp. water
- ½ tbsp. agar
- 4 tbsp. stevia
- 4 tbsp. cocoa powder
- 2 cups coconut milk, hot

DIRECTIONS

1. In a bowl, mix milk with stevia and cocoa powder and stir well.
2. In a bowl, mix agar with water, stir well, add to the cocoa mix, stir and transfer to a pudding pan that fits your Air Fryer.
3. Introduce in the fryer and cook at 356°F for 20 minutes.
4. Serve the pudding cold.

Nutrition: Calories 170 Fat 2g Carbs 4g Protein 3g

559. BLUEBERRY COCONUT CRACKERS

PREPARATION: 10 MIN **COOKING:** 30 MIN **SERVINGS:** 12

INGREDIENTS

- ½ cup coconut butter
- ½ cup coconut oil, melted
- 1 cup blueberries
- 3 tbsp. coconut sugar

DIRECTIONS

1. In a pot that fits your Air Fryer, mix coconut butter with coconut oil, raspberries and sugar, toss, introduce in the fryer and cook at 367°F for 30 minutes
2. Spread on a lined baking sheet, keep in the fridge for a few hours, slice crackers and serve.

Nutrition: Calories 174 Fat 5g Carbs 4g Protein 7g

560. CAULIFLOWER PUDDING

PREPARATION: 10 MIN   **COOKING:** 30 MIN   **SERVINGS:** 4

INGREDIENTS

- 2½ cups water
- 1 cup coconut sugar
- 2 cups cauliflower rice
- 2 cinnamon sticks
- ½ cup coconut, shredded

DIRECTIONS

1. In a pot that fits your Air Fryer, mix water with coconut sugar, cauliflower rice, cinnamon and coconut, stir, introduce in the fryer and cook at 365°F for 30 minutes
2. Divide pudding into cups and serve cold.

Nutrition: Calories 203 Fat 4g Carbs 9g Protein 4g

561. SWEET VANILLA RHUBARB

PREPARATION: 10 MIN   **COOKING:** 10 MIN   **SERVINGS:** 4

INGREDIENTS

- 5 cups rhubarb, chopped
- 2 tbsp. coconut butter, melted
- 1/3 cup water
- 1 tbsp. stevia
- 1 tsp. vanilla extract

DIRECTIONS

1. Put rhubarb, ghee, water, stevia and vanilla extract in a pan that fits your Air Fryer, introduce in the fryer and cook at 365°F for 10 minutes
2. Divide into small bowls and serve cold.

Nutrition: Calories 103 Fat 2g Carbs 6g Protein 2g

562. SHORTBREAD FINGERS

PREPARATION: 10 MIN   **COOKING:** 12 MIN   **SERVINGS:** 12

INGREDIENTS

- 6 oz. Butter
- 2.6 oz. Caster sugar
- 9 oz. Plain flour

DIRECTIONS

1. Mix flour with sugar and butter in a bowl.
2. Knead this shortbread dough well until smooth.
3. Make 4-finger shapes out of this dough and place them in the Air Fryer basket.
4. Air fry for 12 minutes at 350°F
5. Flip the shortbread cookies after 6 minutes then resume cooking
6. Serve.

Nutrition: Calories 204 Fat 12g Carbs 22.2g Protein 2.3g

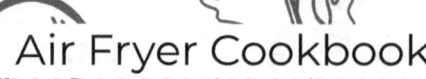
Air Fryer Cookbook

563. FRUIT CRUMBLE PIE

PREPARATION: 10 MIN **COOKING:** 15 MIN **SERVINGS:** 6

INGREDIENTS

- 6 oz. Plain flour
- 1 oz. Butter
- 1 oz. Caster sugar
- 1 medium red apple, peeled and diced
- medium plums, diced
- 1 oz. Frozen berries, diced
- 1 tsp. cinnamon

DIRECTIONS

1. Toss all the fruits into the Air Fryer Basket
2. Whisk flour with sugar and butter to make a crumble
3. Spread this crumble over the fruits evenly
4. Select 15 minutes of cooking time at 350°F, then press "start."
5. Once the Air Fryer beeps, remove the basket
6. Slice and serve.

Nutrition: Calories 149 Fat 4.8g Carbs 26.3g Protein 1.9g

564. CHOCOLATE MUG CAKE

PREPARATION: 7 MIN **COOKING:** 13 MIN **SERVINGS:** 3

INGREDIENTS

- ½ cup of cocoa powder
- ½ cup stevia powder
- 1 cup coconut cream
- 1 package cream cheese, room temperature
- 1 tbsp. Vanilla extract
- 1 tbsp. Butter

DIRECTIONS

1. Preheat the Air Fryer for 5 minutes at 350°F.
2. In a mixing bowl, combine all the listed ingredients using a hand mixer until fluffy.
3. Pour into greased mugs.
4. Place the mugs in the fryer basket and bake for 13 minutes at 350°F.
5. Serve when cool.

Nutrition: Calories 744 Fat 69.7g Carbs 4g Protein 13.9g

Air Fryer Cookbook

565. FRIED PEACHES

PREPARATION: 2 H 10M   **COOKING :** 15 MIN   **SERVINGS:** 4

INGREDIENTS

- 4 Ripe peaches
- 1½ cup flour
- Salt to taste
- 4 egg yolks
- 3/4 cups cold water
- 1 1/2 tbsp. Olive oil
- tbsp. Brandy
- 4 egg whites
- Cinnamon/sugar mix

Nutrition: Calories 306 Carbs 12g Protein 10g

DIRECTIONS

1. Mix flour, egg yolks, and salt in a mixing bowl.
2. Slowly mix in water, then add brandy.
3. Set the mixture aside for 2 hours and meanwhile cut an x at the bottom of each peach.
4. Boil some water and fill a large bowl with water and ice.
5. Boil each peach for about a minute, then plunge them in the ice bath.
6. The peels should fall off the peach.
7. Beat the egg whites and mix into the batter.
8. Dip each peach in the mix to coat. Pour the coated peach into the oven rack/basket.
9. Place the rack on the middle-shelf of the Air Fryer oven.
10. Set temperature to 360°F and set time to 10 minutes.
11. Prepare a plate with cinnamon/sugar mix, roll peaches in the mix and serve.

566. APPLE DUMPLINGS

PREPARATION: 7 MIN   **COOKING:** 25 MIN   **SERVINGS:** 4

INGREDIENTS

- tbsp. Melted coconut oil
- puff pastry sheets
- 1 tbsp. Brown sugar
- tbsp. Raisins
- small apples, peeled and cored

Nutrition: Calories 367 Ffat 7g Carbs 5g Protein 2g

DIRECTIONS

1. Preheat your Air Fryer oven to 356°F
2. Mix apples with raisins and sugar
3. Place a bit of apple mixture into puff pastry sheets and brush sides with melted coconut oil.
4. Place into the Air Fryer. Cook 25 minutes, turning halfway through. Remove from the oven when golden.

Air Fryer Cookbook

567. APPLE PIE

PREPARATION: 5 MIN **COOKING:** 30 MIN **SERVINGS:** 4

INGREDIENTS

- ½ tsp. Vanilla extract
- 1 beaten egg
- 1 large apple, chopped
- 1 pillsbury Pie crust
- 1 tbsp. Butter
- 1 tbsp. Ground cinnamon
- 1 tbsp. Raw sugar
- tbsp. Sugar
- tsp. Lemon juice
- Baking spray

DIRECTIONS

1. Lightly grease baking pan of Air Fryer oven with cooking spray.
2. Spread the pie crust on the bottom of the pan up to the sides.
3. In a bowl, mix vanilla, sugar, cinnamon, lemon juice, and apples and pour on top of the pie crust.
4. Top apples with butter slices, then cover apples with the other pie crust.
5. Prick the pie's top with a knife.
6. Spread beaten egg on top of crust and sprinkle sugar.
7. For 30 minutes, cook on 350°F.
8. Remove when tops are browned.
9. Serve and enjoy.

Nutrition: Calories 372 Fat 19g Carbs 5g Protein 4.2g

568. CINNAMON ROLLS

PREPARATION: 2 H **COOKING:** 15 MIN **SERVINGS:** 8

INGREDIENTS

- 1 lb. vegan bread dough
- ¾ cup coconut sugar
- 1 and ½ tbsp. cinnamon powder
- 2 tbsp. vegetable oil

DIRECTIONS

1. Roll dough on a floured working surface, shape a rectangle and brush with the oil.
2. In a bowl, mix cinnamon with sugar, stir, sprinkle this over dough, roll into a log, seal well and cut into 8 pieces.
3. Leave rolls to rise for 2 hours, place them in your Air Fryer's basket, cook at 350°F for 5 minutes, flip them, cook for 4 minutes more and transfer to a platter.

Nutrition: Calories 170 Fat 1g Carbs 7g Protein 6g

569. CHERRIES AND RHUBARB BOWLS

PREPARATION: 10 MIN   **COOKING:** 35 MIN   **SERVINGS:** 4

INGREDIENTS

- 2 cups cherries, pitted and halved
- 1 cup rhubarb, sliced
- 1 cup apple juice
- 2 tbsp. sugar
- ½ cup raisins.

DIRECTIONS

1. In a pot that fits your Air Fryer, combine the cherries with the rhubarb and the other ingredients, toss, cook at 330°F for 35 minutes, divide into bowls, cool down and serve.

Nutrition: Calories 212 Fat 8g Carbs 13g Protein 7g

570. PUMPKIN BOWLS

PREPARATION: 10 MIN   **COOKING:** 15 MIN   **SERVINGS:** 4

INGREDIENTS

- 2 cups pumpkin flesh, cubed
- 1 cup heavy cream
- 1 tsp. cinnamon powder
- 3 tbsp. sugar
- 1 tsp. nutmeg, ground

DIRECTIONS

1. In a pot that fits your Air Fryer, combine the pumpkin with the cream and the other ingredients, introduce in the fryer and cook at 360°F for 15 minutes.
2. Divide into bowls and serve.

Nutrition: Calories 212 Fat 5g Carbs 15g Protein 7g

571. APPLE JAM

PREPARATION: 10 MIN   **COOKING:** 25 MIN   **SERVINGS:** 4

INGREDIENTS

- 1 cup water
- ½ cup sugar
- 1-lb. apples, cored, peeled and chopped
- ½ tsp. nutmeg, ground

DIRECTIONS

1. In a pot that suits your Air Fryer, mix the apples with the water and the other ingredients, toss, introduce the pan in the fryer and cook at 370°F for 25 minutes.
2. Blend a bit using an immersion blender, divide into jars and serve.

Nutrition: Calories 204 Fat 3g Carbs 12g Protein 4g

572. YOGURT AND PUMPKIN CREAM

PREPARATION: 10 MIN **COOKING:** 30 MIN **SERVINGS:** 4

INGREDIENTS

- 1 cup yogurt
- 1 cup pumpkin puree
- 2 eggs, whisked
- 2 tbsp. sugar
- ½ tsp. vanilla extract

DIRECTIONS

1. In a large bowl, mix the puree and the yogurt with the other ingredients, whisk well, pour into 4 ramekins, put them in the Air Fryer and cook at 370°F for 30 minutes.
2. Cool down and serve.

Nutrition: Calories 192 Fat 7g Carbs 12g Protein 4g

573. RAISINS RICE MIX

PREPARATION: 10 MIN **COOKING:** 25 MIN **SERVINGS:** 6

INGREDIENTS

- 1 cup white rice
- 2 cups coconut milk
- 3 tbsp. sugar
- 1 tsp. vanilla extract
- ½ cup raisins

DIRECTIONS

1. In the Air Fryer's pan, combine the rice with the milk and the other ingredients, introduce the pan in the fryer and cook at 320°F for 25 minutes.
2. Divide into bowls and serve warm.

Nutrition: Calories 132 Fat 6g Carbs 11g Protein 7g

574. ORANGE BOWLS

PREPARATION: 10 MIN **COOKING:** 10 MIN **SERVINGS:** 4

INGREDIENTS

- 1 cup oranges, peeled and cut into segments
- 1 cup cherries, pitted and halved
- 1 cup mango, peeled and cubed
- 1 cup orange juice
- 2 tbsp. sugar

DIRECTIONS

1. In the Air Fryer's pan, mix the oranges with the cherries and the other ingredients, toss and cook at 320°F for 10 minutes.
2. Divide into bowls and serve cold.

Nutrition: Calories 191 Fat 7g Carbs 14g Protein 4g

575. STRAWBERRY JAM

PREPARATION: 10 MIN   **COOKING:** 25 MIN   **SERVINGS:** 8

INGREDIENTS

- 1 lb. strawberries, chopped
- 1 tbsp. lemon zest, grated
- 1 and ½ cups water
- ½ cup sugar
- ½ tbsp. lemon juice

DIRECTIONS

1. In the Air Fryer's pan, mix the berries with the water and the other ingredients, stir, introduce the pan in your Air Fryer and cook at 330°F for 25 minutes.
2. Divide into bowls and serve cold.

Nutrition: Calories 202 Protein 7g Fat 8g Carbs 6g

---

576. CARAMEL CREAM

PREPARATION: 10 MIN   **COOKING:** 15 MIN   **SERVINGS:** 4

INGREDIENTS

- 1 cup heavy cream
- 3 tbsp. caramel syrup
- ½ cup coconut cream
- 1 tbsp. sugar
- ½ tsp. cinnamon powder

DIRECTIONS

1. In a bowl, mix the cream with the caramel syrup and the other ingredients, whisk, divide into small ramekins, introduce in the fryer and cook at 320°F and bake for 15 minutes.
2. Divide into bowls and serve cold.

Nutrition: Calories 234 Fat 13g Carbs 11g Protein 5g

---

577. WRAPPED PEARS

PREPARATION: 10 MIN   **COOKING:** 15 MIN   **SERVINGS:** 4

INGREDIENTS

- 4 puff pastry sheets
- 14 oz. vanilla custard
- 2 pears, halved
- 1 egg, whisked
- 2 tbsp. sugar

DIRECTIONS

1. Put the puff pastry slices on a clean surface, add spoonful of vanilla custard in the center of each, top with pear halves and wrap.
2. Brush pears with egg, sprinkle sugar and place them in your Air Fryer's basket and cook at 320°F for 15 minutes.
3. Divide parcels on plates and serve.

Nutrition: Calories 200 Fat 7g Carbs 6g Protein 6g

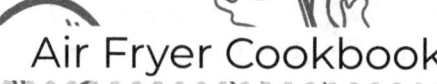
Air Fryer Cookbook

578. PERFECT CINNAMON TOAST

PREPARATION: 10 MIN   **COOKING:** 5 MIN   **SERVINGS:** 6

INGREDIENTS

- 2 tsp. pepper
- 1 ½ tsp. cinnamon
- ½ C. sweetener of choice
- 1 C. coconut oil
- 12 slices whole wheat bread

DIRECTIONS

1. Melt coconut oil and mix with sweetener until dissolved. Mix in remaining ingredients minus bread till incorporated.
2. Spread mixture onto bread, covering all area.
3. Pour the coated pieces of bread into the Oven rack/basket. Place the Rack on the middle-shelf of the Air Fryer oven. Set temperature to 400°F, and set time to 5 minutes.
4. Remove and cut diagonally. Enjoy!

Nutrition: Calories 124 Fat 2g Carbs 5g Protein 0g

579. ANGEL FOOD CAKE

PREPARATION: 5 MIN   **COOKING:** 30 MIN   **SERVINGS:** 12

INGREDIENTS

- ¼ cup butter, melted
- 1 cup powdered erythritol
- 1 tsp. strawberry extract
- 12 egg whites
- 2 tsp.s cream of tartar

DIRECTIONS

1. Preheat the Air Fryer oven for 5 minutes.
2. Blend the cream of tartar and egg whites.
3. Use a hand mixer and whisk until white and fluffy.
4. Add the rest of the ingredients except for the butter and whisk for another minute.
5. Pour into a baking dish.
6. Place in the Air Fryer basket and cook for 30 minutes at 400°F or if a toothpick inserted in the middle comes out clean.
7. Drizzle with melted butter once cooled.

Nutrition: Calories 65 Fat 5g Carbs 6.2g Protein 3.1g

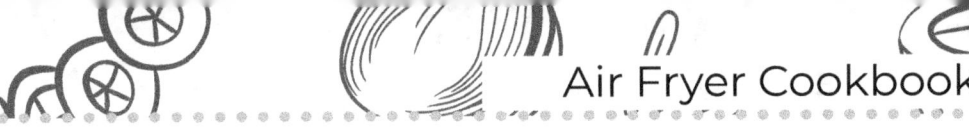

Air Fryer Cookbook

580. APPLE DUMPLINGS

PREPARATION: 10 MIN   **COOKING:** 25 MIN   **SERVINGS:** 4

INGREDIENTS

- 2 tbsp. melted coconut oil
- 2 puff pastry sheets
- 1 tbsp. brown sugar
- 2 tbsp. raisins
- 2 small apples of choice

Nutrition: Calories 367 Fat 7g Carbs 10g Protein 2g

DIRECTIONS

1. Ensure your Air Fryer oven is preheated to 356°F.
2. Core and peel apples and mix with raisins and sugar.
3. Place a bit of apple mixture into puff pastry sheets and brush sides with melted coconut oil.
4. Place into the Air Fryer. Cook 25 minutes, turning halfway through. Will be golden when done.

581. CHOCOLATE DONUTS

PREPARATION: 5 MIN   **COOKING:** 20 MIN   **SERVINGS:** 8-10

INGREDIENTS

- (8 oz.) can jumbo biscuits
- Cooking oil
- Chocolate sauce, such as Hershey's

Nutrition: Calories 181 Fat 98g Carbs 42g Protein 3g

DIRECTIONS

1. Separate the biscuit dough into 8 biscuits and place them on a flat work surface. Use a small circle cookie cutter or a biscuit cutter to cut a hole in the center of each biscuit. You can also cut the holes using a knife.
2. Grease the basket with cooking oil.
3. Place 4 donuts in the Air Fryer oven. Do not stack. Spray with cooking oil. Cook for 4 minutes at 390°F.
4. Open the Air Fryer and flip the donuts. Cook for an additional 4 minutes.
5. Remove the cooked donuts from the Air Fryer oven, then repeat for the remaining 4 donuts.
6. Drizzle chocolate sauce over the donuts and enjoy while warm.

582. APPLE HAND PIES

PREPARATION: 5 MIN   **COOKING:** 8 MIN   **SERVINGS:** 6

INGREDIENTS

- 15 oz. no-sugar-added apple pie filling
- 1 store-bought crust

Nutrition: Calories 278 Fat 10g Carbs 17g Protein 5g

DIRECTIONS

1. Lay out pie crust and slice into equal-sized squares.
2. Place 2 tbsp. filling into each square and seal crust with a fork.
3. Pour into the Oven rack/basket. Place the Rack on the middle-shelf of the Air Fryer oven. Set temperature to 390°F, and set time to 8 minutes until golden in color.

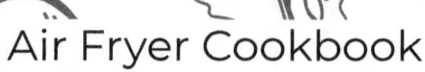

Air Fryer Cookbook

583. SWEET CREAM CHEESE WONTONS

PREPARATION: 5 MIN **COOKING:** 5 MIN **SERVINGS:** 16

INGREDIENTS

- 1 egg with a little water
- Wonton wrappers
- ½ C. powdered erythritol
- 8 oz. softened cream cheese
- Olive oil

DIRECTIONS

1. Mix sweetener and cream cheese together.
2. Lay out 4 wontons at a time and cover with a dish towel to prevent drying out.
3. Place ½ of a tsp. of cream cheese mixture into each wrapper.
4. Dip finger into egg/water mixture and fold diagonally to form a triangle. Seal edges well.
5. Repeat with remaining ingredients.
6. Place filled wontons into the Air Fryer oven and cook 5 minutes at 400°F, shaking halfway through cooking.

Nutrition: Calories 303 Fat 3g Carbs 3g Protein 0.5g

584. FRENCH TOAST BITES

PREPARATION: 15 MIN **COOKING:** 5 MIN **SERVINGS:** 8

INGREDIENTS

- Almond milk
- Cinnamon
- Sweetener
- 3 eggs
- 4 pieces wheat bread

DIRECTIONS

1. Preheat the Air Fryer oven to 360°F.
2. Whisk eggs and thin out with almond milk.
3. Mix 1/3 cup of sweetener with lots of cinnamon.
4. Tear bread in half, ball up pieces and press together to form a ball.
5. Soak bread balls in egg and then roll into cinnamon sugar, making sure to thoroughly coat.
6. Place coated bread balls into the Air Fryer oven and bake 15 minutes.

Nutrition: Calories 289 Fat 11g Carbs 17g Protein 0g

585. CINNAMON SUGAR ROASTED CHICKPEAS

PREPARATION: 5 MIN **COOKING:** 10 MIN **SERVINGS:** 2

INGREDIENTS

- 1 tbsp. sweetener
- 1 tbsp. cinnamon
- 1 cup chickpeas

DIRECTIONS

1. Preheat Air Fryer oven to 390°F.
2. Rinse and drain chickpeas.
3. Mix all ingredients together and add to Air Fryer.
4. Pour into the Oven rack/basket. Place the Rack on the middle-shelf of the Air Fryer oven. Set temperature to 390°F, and set time to 10 minutes.

Nutrition: Calories 111 Fat 19g Carbs 18g Protein 16g

586. BROWNIE MUFFINS

PREPARATION: 10 MIN **COOKING:** 10 MIN **SERVINGS:** 12

INGREDIENTS

- 1 package Betty Crocker fudge brownie mix
- ¼ cup walnuts, chopped
- 1 egg
- 1/3 cup vegetable oil
- 2 tsp.s water

DIRECTIONS

1. Grease 12 muffin molds. Set aside.
2. In a bowl, put all ingredients together.
3. Place the mixture into the prepared muffin molds.
4. Preheat the Air Fryer at 300°F.
5. Arrange the muffin molds in Air Fryer basket and insert in the Air Fryer. Cook for 10 minutes.
6. Place the muffin molds onto a wire rack to cool for about 10 minutes.
7. Carefully, invert the muffins onto the wire rack to completely cool before serving.

Nutrition: Calories 168 Fat 8.9g Carbs 20.8g Protein 2g

587. CHOCOLATE MUG CAKE

PREPARATION: 15 MIN **COOKING:** 13 MIN **SERVINGS:** 1

INGREDIENTS

- ¼ cup self-rising flour
- 5 tbsp. caster sugar
- 1 tbsp. cocoa powder
- 3 tbsp. coconut oil
- 3 tbsp. whole milk

DIRECTIONS

1. In a shallow mug, add all the ingredients and mix until well combined.
2. Preheat the Air Fryer at 392°F.
3. Arrange the mug in Air Fryer basket and insert in the Air Fryer. Cook for 13 minutes.
4. Place the mug onto a wire rack to cool slightly before serving.

Nutrition: Calories 729 Fat 43.3g Carbs 88.8g Protein 5.7g

588. GRILLED PEACHES

PREPARATION: 10 MIN **COOKING:** 10 MIN **SERVINGS:** 2

INGREDIENTS

- 2 peaches, cut into wedges and remove pits
- ¼ cup butter, diced into pieces
- ¼ cup brown sugar
- ¼ cup graham cracker crumbs

DIRECTIONS

1. Arrange peach wedges on Air Fryer oven rack and air fry at 350°F for 5 minutes.
2. In a bowl, put the butter, graham cracker crumbs, and brown sugar together.
3. Turn peaches skin side down.
4. Spoon butter mixture over top of peaches and air fry for 5 minutes more.
5. Top with whipped cream and serve.

Nutrition: Calories 378 Fat 24.4g Carbs 40.5g Protein 2.3g

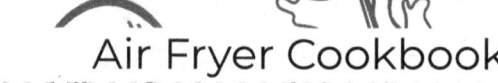
Air Fryer Cookbook

589. SIMPLE & DELICIOUS SPICED APPLES

PREPARATION: 10MIN **COOKING:** 10 MIN **SERVINGS:** 4

INGREDIENTS

- 4 apples, sliced
- 1 tsp. apple pie spice
- 2 tbsp. sugar
- 2 tbsp. ghee, melted

DIRECTIONS

1. Add apple slices into the mixing bowl.
2. Add remaining ingredients on top of apple slices and toss until well coated.
3. Transfer apple slices on Air Fryer oven pan and air fry at 350°F for 10 minutes.
4. Top with ice cream and serve.

Nutrition: Calories 196 Fat 6.8g Carbs 37.1g Protein 0.6g

590. TANGY MANGO SLICES

PREPARATION: 10 MIN **COOKING:** 12 H **SERVINGS:** 6

INGREDIENTS

- 4 mangoes, peel and cut into ¼-inch slices
- 1/4 cup fresh lemon juice
- 1 tbsp. honey

DIRECTIONS

1. In a big bowl, combine together honey and lemon juice and set aside.
2. Add mango slices in lemon-honey mixture and coat well.
3. Arrange mango slices on Air Fryer rack and dehydrate at 135°F for 12 hours.

Nutrition: Calories 147 Fat 0.9g Carbs 36.7g Protein 1.9g

591. PEANUT BUTTER COOKIES

PREPARATION: 10 MIN **COOKING:** 5 MIN **SERVINGS:** 24

INGREDIENTS

- 1 egg, lightly beaten
- 1 cup of sugar
- 1 cup creamy peanut butter

DIRECTIONS

1. In a big bowl, combine sugar, egg, and peanut butter together until well mixed.
2. Spray Air Fryer oven tray with cooking spray.
3. Using ice cream scooper, scoop out cookie onto the tray and flattened them using a fork.
4. Bake cookie at 350°F for 5 minutes.
5. Cook remaining cookie batches using the same temperature.
6. Serve and enjoy.

Nutrition: Calories 97 Fat 5.6g Carbs 10.5g Protein 2.9g

Air Fryer Cookbook

592. DRIED RASPBERRIES

PREPARATION: 10 MIN   **COOKING:** 15 H   **SERVINGS:** 4

INGREDIENTS

- 4 cups raspberries, wash and dry
- 1/4 cup fresh lemon juice

DIRECTIONS

1. Add raspberries and lemon juice in a bowl and toss well.
2. Arrange raspberries on Air Fryer oven tray and dehydrate at 135°F for 12-15 hours.
3. Store in an air-tight container.

Nutrition: Calories 68 Fat 0.9g Carbs 15g Protein 1.6g

593. SWEET PEACH WEDGES

PREPARATION: 10 MIN   **COOKING:** 8 H   **SERVINGS:** 4

INGREDIENTS

- 3 peaches, cut and remove pits and sliced
- 1/2 cup fresh lemon juice

DIRECTIONS

1. Add lemon juice and peach slices into the bowl and toss well.
2. Arrange peach slices on Air Fryer oven rack and dehydrate at 135°F for 6-8 hours.
3. Serve and enjoy.

Nutrition: Calories 52 Fat 0.5g Carbs 11.1g Protein 1.3g

594. AIR FRYER OREO COOKIES

PREPARATION: 5 MIN   **COOKING:** 5 MIN   **SERVINGS:** 9

INGREDIENTS

- Pancake Mix: ½ cup
- Water: ½ cup
- Cooking spray
- Chocolate sandwich cookies: 9 (e.g. Oreo)
- Confectioners' sugar: 1 tbsp., or to taste

DIRECTIONS

1. Blend the pancake mixture with the water until well mixed.
2. Line the parchment paper on the basket of an Air Fryer. Spray nonstick cooking spray on parchment paper. Dip each cookie into the mixture of the pancake and place it in the basket. Make sure they do not touch; if possible, cook in batches.
3. The Air Fryer is preheated to 400°F. Add basket and cook for 4 to 5 minutes; flip until golden brown, 2 to 3 more minutes. Sprinkle the sugar over the cookies and serve.

Nutrition: Calories 77 Fat 2.1g Carbs 13.7g Protein 1.2g

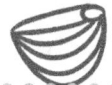
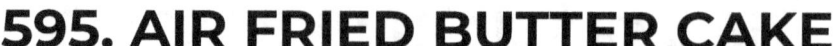

Air Fryer Cookbook

595. AIR FRIED BUTTER CAKE

PREPARATION: 10 MIN   **COOKING:** 15 MIN   **SERVINGS:** 4

INGREDIENTS

- 7 Tbsp. of butter, at ambient temperature
- White sugar: ¼ cup plus 2 tbsp.
- All-purpose flour: 1 ⅔ cups
- Salt: 1 pinch or to taste
- Milk: 6 tbsp.

Nutrition: Calories 470 Fat 22.4g Carbs 59.7g Protein 7.9g

DIRECTIONS

1. Preheat an Air Fryer to 350°F. Spray the cooking spray on a tiny fluted tube pan.
2. Take a large bowl and add ¼ cup butter and 2 tbsp. of sugar in it.
3. Take an electric mixer to beat the sugar and butter until smooth and fluffy. Stir in salt and flour. Stir in the milk and thoroughly combine batter. Move batter to the prepared saucepan; use a spoon back to level the surface.
4. Place the pan inside the basket of the Air Fryer. Set the timer within 15 minutes. Bake the batter until a toothpick comes out clean when inserted into the cake.
5. Turn the cake out of the saucepan and allow it to cool for about five minutes.

596. AIR FRYER S'MORES

PREPARATION: 5 MIN   **COOKING:** 3 MIN   **SERVINGS:** 4

INGREDIENTS

- Four graham crackers (each half split to make 2 squares, for a total of 8 squares)
- 8 Squares of Hershey's chocolate bar, broken into squares
- 4 Marshmallows

Nutrition: Calories 200 Fat 3.1g Carbs 15.7g Protein 2.6g

DIRECTIONS

1. Air Fryers use hot air for cooking food. Marshmallows are light and fluffy, and this should keep the marshmallows from flying around the basket if you follow these steps.
2. Put 4 squares of graham crackers on a basket of the Air Fryer.
3. Place 2 squares of chocolate bars on each cracker.
4. Place back the basket in the Air Fryer and fry on air at 390°F for 1 minute. It is barely long enough for the chocolate to melt. Remove basket from Air Fryer.
5. Top with a marshmallow over each cracker. Throw the marshmallow down a little bit into the melted chocolate. This will help to make the marshmallow stay over the chocolate.
6. Put back the basket in the Air Fryer and fry at 390°F for 2 minutes. (The marshmallows should be puffed up and browned at the tops.)
7. Using tongs to carefully remove each cracker from the basket of the Air Fryer and place it on a platter. Top each marshmallow with another square of graham crackers. Enjoy it right away!

Air Fryer Cookbook

597. AIR FRYER CHOCOLATE CAKE

PREPARATION: 5 MIN **COOKING:** 36 MIN **SERVINGS:** 9

INGREDIENTS

- ½ cups hot water
- 1 tsp. Vanilla
- ¼ cups olive oil
- ½ cups almond milk
- 1 egg
- ½ tsp. Salt
- ¾ tsp. Baking soda
- ¾ tsp. Baking powder
- ½ cups unsweetened cocoa powder
- 2 cups almond flour
- 1 cup brown sugar

DIRECTIONS

1. Preheat your Air Fryer oven to 356°F.
2. Stir all dry ingredients together and then stir in wet ingredients.
3. Add hot water last. The batter should be thin.
4. Pour cake batter into a pan that fits into the fryer.
5. Bake for 35 minutes.

Nutrition: Calories 378 Fat 9g Carbs 5g Protein 4g

598. BANANA BROWNIES

PREPARATION: 4 MIN **COOKING:** 25 MIN **SERVINGS:** 12

INGREDIENTS

- 1/3 cup almond flour
- tsp. Baking powder
- ½ tsp. Baking soda
- ½ tsp. Salt
- 1 over-ripe banana
- 2 large eggs
- ½ tsp. Stevia powder
- ¼ cup coconut oil
- 1 tbsp. Vinegar
- 1/3 cup cocoa powder

DIRECTIONS

1. Preheat the Air Fryer oven for 5 minutes at 350°F.
2. Combine all the listed ingredients in a food processor and pulse until well-combined.
3. Pour into a baking dish that fits in the air fryer.
4. Place in the basket, then cook for 25 minutes, then if a toothpick inserted in the middle comes out clean, take out and let it cool down.

Nutrition: Calories 75 Fat 6.5g Carbs 2g Protein 1.7g

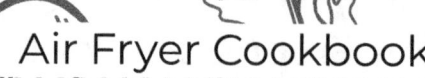
Air Fryer Cookbook

599. AIR FRIED BISCUIT DONUTS

PREPARATION: 7 MIN **COOKING:** 5 MIN **SERVINGS:** 8

INGREDIENTS

- Pinch of allspice
- tbsp. Dark brown sugar
- 1 tsp. Cinnamon
- 1/3 cups granulated sweetener
- tbsp. Melted coconut oil
- 1 can of biscuits

DIRECTIONS

1. Mix allspice, sugar, sweetener, and cinnamon.
2. Take out biscuits from can and with a circle cookie cutter, cut holes from centers, and place into the Air Fryer.
3. Cook 5 minutes at 350°F
4. As batches are cooked, use a brush to coat with melted coconut oil and dip each into sugar mixture. Serve warm!

Nutrition: Calories 209 Fat 4g, Carbs 3g, Protein 0g

600. CHOCOLATE SOUFFLÉ

PREPARATION: 7 MIN **COOKING:** 12 MIN **SERVINGS:** 2

INGREDIENTS

- tbsp. Almond flour
- ½ tsp. Vanilla
- tbsp. Sweetener
- 4 separated eggs
- ¼ cups melted coconut oil
- oz. Of semi-sweet chocolate, chopped

Nutrition: Calories 238 Fat 6g Carbs 4g Protein 1g

DIRECTIONS

1. Preheat the Air Fryer to 330°F.
2. Brush coconut oil and sweetener onto ramekins.
3. Melt coconut oil and chocolate together.
4. Beat egg yolks well, adding vanilla and sweetener.
5. Stir in flour and ensure there are no lumps.
6. Whisk egg whites till they reach peak state and fold them into chocolate mixture.
7. Pour batter into ramekins and place into the Air Fryer oven, then cook for 12 minutes.
8. Serve with powdered sugar dusted on top.

Air Fryer Cookbook

601. SAUCY FRIED BANANAS

PREPARATION: 7 MIN   **COOKING:** 10 MIN   **SERVINGS:** 2

INGREDIENTS

- 1 large egg
- ¼ cup cornstarch
- ¼ cup plain breadcrumbs
- bananas, halved crosswise
- Cooking oil
- Chocolate sauce

Nutrition: Calories 203 Fat 6g Protein 3g

DIRECTIONS

1. Preheat your Air Fryer oven to 350°F.
2. In a small bowl, beat the egg.
3. In another bowl, place the cornstarch.
4. Place the breadcrumbs in a different bowl.
5. Dip the bananas in the cornstarch, then the egg, and then the breadcrumbs.
6. Spray the basket with cooking oil. Place the bananas in the basket and spray them with cooking oil.
7. Cook for 5 minutes.
8. Open the Air Fryer and flip the bananas then cook for an additional 2 minutes.
9. Transfer the bananas to plates.
10. Drizzle the chocolate sauce over the bananas and serve.

602. CRUSTY APPLE HAND PIES

PREPARATION: 7 MIN   **COOKING:** 8 MIN   **SERVINGS:** 6

INGREDIENTS

- 15 oz. no-sugar-added apple pie filling
- 1 store-bought crust

DIRECTIONS

1. Lay out pie crust and slice into equal-sized squares.
2. Place 2 tbsp. Filling into each square and seal crust with a fork
3. Pour into the oven rack/basket.
4. Set temperature to 390°F and set time to 8 minutes until golden in color.

Nutrition: Calories 278 Fat 10g, Carbs 4g Protein 1g

CONCLUSION

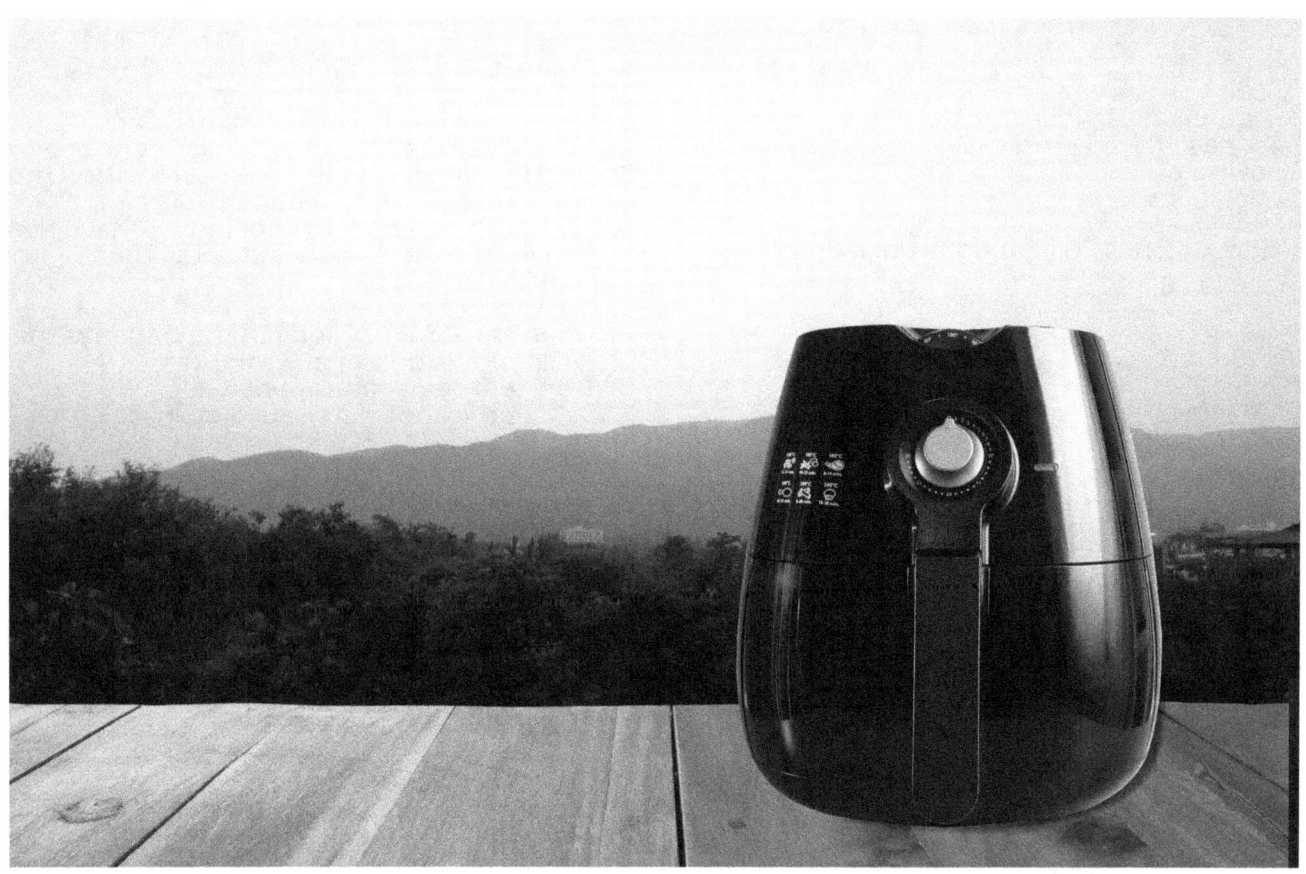

Hopefully, after going through this book and trying out a couple of recipes, you will get to understand the flexibility and utility of the Air Fryers. It is undoubtedly a multipurpose kitchen appliance that I highly recommend to everybody. It allows anyone to enjoy fried foods that are delicious but healthy, cheaper, and more convenient. The use of this kitchen appliance ensures that the making of some of your favorite snacks and meals will be carried out in a stress-free manner without hassling around, which invariably legitimizes its worth and gives you value for your money.

I truly hope that this book will be your all-time guide to understand the basics of the Air Fryer because, with all the recipes mentioned in the book, you can rest assured that it will be something that you and the rest of the people around the world will enjoy for the rest of your lives. You will be able to prepare delicious and flavorsome meals that will not only be easy to carry out but tasty and healthy as well.

However, you should never limit yourself to the recipes solely mentioned in this cookbook. Go on and try new things! Explore new recipes! Experiment with different ingredients, seasonings, and different methods! Create some new recipes and keep your mind open. By so doing, you will be able to get the best out of your Air Fryer.

Happy, healthy eating!

Air Fryer Cookbook

INDEX OF RECIPES

INTRODUCTION	5
HOW TO USE AN AIR FRYER	8
BENEFITS OF AIR FRYING	11
BASIC CARE AND CLEANING	13
HOW TO PREPARE YOUR KITCHEN TO AIR FRY	15
USEFUL TIPS ON HOW TO BEST COOK WITH AN AIR FRYER	17
WHAT ARE THE BEST AND WORST FOOD TO AIR FRY	19
AIR FRYING COOKING CHARTS	21
4-WEEK MEAL PLAN2	4

BREAKFAST 27
1. Zucchini Muffins 28
2. Jalapeno Breakfast Muffins 28
3. Simple Egg Soufflé 28
4. Vegetable Egg Soufflé 29
5. Asparagus Frittata 29
7. Broccoli Stuffed Peppers 30
8. Zucchini Noodles 30
9. Mushroom Frittata 31
10. Blueberry Breakfast Cobbler 31
11. Yummy Breakfast Italian Frittata 32
12. Savory Cheese and Bacon Muffins 32
13. Best Air-Fried English Breakfast 33
14 Sausage and Egg Breakfast Burrito 33
15. French Toast Sticks 34
16. Home-Fried Potatoes 34
17. Homemade Cherry Breakfast Tarts 35
18. Sausage and Cream Cheese Biscuits 35
19. Fried Chicken and Waffles 36
20. Cheesy Tater Tot Breakfast Bake 36
21. BREAKFAST SCRAMBLE CASSEROLE 37
22. Breakfast Grilled Ham and Cheese 37
23. Classic Hash Browns 38
24. Canadian Bacon and Cheese English Muffins 38
25. Radish Hash Browns 39
26. Vegetable Egg Cups 39
27. Spinach Frittata 40
28. Omelet Frittata 40
29. Cheese Soufflés 41
30. Cheese and Red Pepper Egg Cups 41
31. Coconut Porridge with Flax Seed 42
32. Easy Chocolate Doughnut 42
33. Cheesy Spinach Omelet 42
34. Roasted Garlic and Thyme Dipping Sauce 43
35. Cheesy Sausage and Egg Rolls 43
36. Baked Berry Oatmeal 44
37. Broccoli and Cheddar Cheese Quiche 44
38. Egg and Cheese Puff Pastry Tarts 45
39. French Toast 45
40. Grilled Gruyere Cheese Sandwich 46
41. Pancakes 46
42. Breakfast Sandwich 46
43. Egg Muffins 47
44. Bacon & Eggs 47
45. Eggs on the Go 47
46. Protein Banana Bread 48
47. Easy Kale Muffins 48
48. Mozzarella Spinach Quiche 49
49. Fancy Breakfast Quinoa 49
50. Fresh Sautéed Apple 50
51. Perfect Vegetable Roast 50
52. Herb Frittata 51
53. Zucchini Bread 51
54 Blueberry Muffins 52
55. Baked Eggs 52
56. Bagels 53
57. Cauliflower Hash Browns 53
58. Potatoes with Bacon 54
59. Zucchini Squash Mix 54
60. Special Corn Flakes Casserole 55
61. Protein Rich Egg White Omelet 55
62. Shrimp Sandwiches 56
63. Breakfast Soufflé 56
64. Fried Tomato Quiche 56
65. Breakfast Spanish Omelet 57
66. Scrambled Pancake Hash 57
67. Onion Frittata 58
68. Pea Tortilla 58
69. Mushroom Quiches 59
70. Walnuts Pear Oatmeal 59
71. Breakfast Raspberry Rolls 60
72. Bread Pudding 60
73. Cream Cheese Oats 61
74. Bread Rolls 61

SNACKS 62
75. Rolled Salmon Sandwich 63
76. Balsamic Roasted Chicken 63
77. Chicken Capers Sandwich 64
78. Easy Prosciutto Grilled Cheese 64
79. Herb-Roasted Chicken Tenders 64
80. Ground Beef Bowl 65
81. Turmeric Chicken Liver 65
82. Chicken Burgers 65
83. Zucchini Casserole 66
84. Cherry Tuscan Pork Loin 66
85. Moroccan Pork Kebabs 67
86. Banana Chips 67
87. Lemony Apple Bites 67
88. Balsamic Zucchini Slices 68

Air Fryer Cookbook

89. Turmeric Carrot Chips	68
90. Chives Radish Snack	68
91. Lentils Snack	69
92. Air Fried Corn	69
93. Breaded Mushrooms	69
94. Cheesy Sticks with Sweet Thai Sauce	70
95. Bacon Wrapped Avocados	70
96. Hot Chicken Wingettes	71
97. Carrot Crisps	71
98. Quick Cheese Sticks	71
99. Radish Chips	72
100. Herbed Croutons with Brie Cheese	72
101. Stuffed Jalapeno	72
102. Garlicky Bok Choy	73
103. Chia Seed Crackers	73
104. Baked Eggplant Chips	73
105. Flax Seed Chips	74
106. Salted Hazelnuts	74
107. Baguette Bread	75
108. Yogurt Bread	76
109. Sunflower Seed Bread	77
110. Date Bread	77
111. Date & Walnut Bread	78
112. Brown Sugar Banana Bread	78
113. Cinnamon Banana Bread	79
114. Banana & Walnut Bread	79
115. Banana & Raisin Bread	80
116. 3-Ingredients Banana Bread	80
117. Yogurt Banana Bread	81
118. Sour Cream Banana Bread	81
119. Peanut Butter Banana Bread	82
120. Chocolate Banana Bread	82
121. Allspice Chicken Wings	83
122. Friday Night Pineapple Sticky Ribs	83
123. Egg Roll Wrapped with Cabbage and Prawns	84
124. Sesame Garlic Chicken Wings	84
125. Savory Chicken Nuggets with Parmesan Cheese	85
126. Butternut Squash with Thyme	85
127. Chicken Breasts in Golden Crumb	86
128. Yogurt Chicken Tacos	86
129. Flawless Kale Chips	87
130. Vermicelli Noodles & Vegetables Rolls	87
131. Cheese Fish Balls	88
132. Beef Balls with Mixed Herbs	88
133. Roasted Pumpkin Seeds	88
134. Buttery Parmesan Broccoli Florets	89
135. Spicy Chickpeas	89
136. Roasted Peanuts	89
137. Roasted Cashews	90
138. French Fries	90
139. Zucchini Fries	90
140. Spicy Carrot Fries	91
141. Cinnamon Carrot Fries	91
142. Squash Fries	91
143. Avocado Fries	92
144. Dill Pickle Fries	92
145. Mozzarella Sticks	93
146. Tortilla Chips	93

SIDE DISHES	**94**
147. Sky-High Roasted Corn	95
148. Ravishing Air-Fried Carrots with Honey Glaze	95
149. Flaming Buffalo Cauliflower Bites	96
150. Pleasant Air-Fried Eggplant	96
151. Cauliflower Hash	97
152. Asparagus with Almonds	97
153. Zucchini Cubes	98
154. Sweet Potato & Onion Mix	98
155. Spicy Eggplant Cubes	99
156. Roasted Garlic Head	99
157. Wrapped Asparagus	99
158. Baked Yams with Dill	100
159. Honey Onions	100
160. Delightful Roasted Garlic Slices	100
161. Coconut Oil Artichokes	101
162. Roasted Mushrooms	101
163. Mashed Yams	101
164. Cauliflower Rice	102
165. Shredded Cabbage	102
166. Fried Leeks Recipe	102
167. Brussels Sprouts and Tomatoes Mix Recipe	103
168. Radish Hash Recipe	103
169. Broccoli Salad Recipe	103
170. Chili Broccoli	104
171. Parmesan Broccoli and Asparagus	104
172. Butter Broccoli Mix	104
173. Balsamic Kale	105
174. Kale and Olives	105
175. Kale and Mushrooms Mix	105
176. Oregano Kale	106
177. Kale and Brussels Sprouts	106
178. Spicy Olives and Avocado Mix	106
179. Olives, Green beans and Bacon	107
180. Cajun Olives and Peppers	107
181. Crisp Kale	107
182. imple Basil Potatoes	108
183. Sweet Potato Fries	108
184. Crisp & Spicy Cabbage	108
185. Rosemary Potatoes	109
186. Simple Garlic Potatoes	109
187. Crispy Brussels Sprouts	109
188. Flatbread	110
189. Creamy Cabbage	110
190. Vegetable Egg Rolls	111
191. Veggies on Toast	111
192. Jumbo Stuffed Mushrooms	112
193. Mushroom Pita Pizzas	112
194. Spinach Quiche	113
195. Yellow Squash Fritters	113
196. Pesto Gnocchi	114
197. English Muffin Tuna Sandwiches	114
198. Tuna Zucchini Melts	115

Air Fryer Cookbook

199. Shrimp and Grilled Cheese Sandwiches — 115
200. Shrimp Croquettes — 116

POULTRY — 117

201. Turkey Breasts — 118
202. BBQ Chicken Breasts — 118
203. Rotisserie Chicken — 118
204. Honey-Mustard Chicken Breasts — 119
205. Chicken Parmesan Wings — 119
206. Air Fryer Chicken — 119
207. Whole Chicken — 120
208. Honey Duck Breasts — 120
209. Creamy Coconut Chicken — 120
210. Buffalo Chicken Tenders — 121
211. Teriyaki Wings — 121
212. Lemony Drumsticks — 121
213. Parmesan Chicken Tenders — 122
214. Easy Lemon Chicken Thighs — 122
215. Air Fryer Grilled Chicken Breasts — 123
216. Crispy Air Fryer Butter Chicken — 123
217. Light and Airy Breaded Chicken Breasts — 124
218. Chicken Fillets, Brie & Ham — 124
219. Air Fryer Cornish Hen — 124
220. Air Fried Turkey Wings — 125
221. Chicken-Fried Steak Supreme — 125
222. Caesar Marinated Grilled Chicken — 126
223. Cheesy Chicken Tenders — 126
224. Minty Chicken-Fried Pork Chops — 127
225. Bacon Lovers' Stuffed Chicken — 127
226. Air Fryer Turkey Breast — 128
227. Mustard Chicken Tenders — 128
228. Chicken Meatballs — 128
229. Homemade Breaded Nugget in Doritos — 129
230. Chicken Breast — 129
231. Breaded Chicken without Flour — 130
232. Barbecue with Chorizo and Chicken — 130
233. Roasted Thigh — 130
234. Coxinha Fit — 131
235. Rolled Turkey Breast — 131
236. Chicken in Beer — 131
237. Chicken Fillet — 132
238. Chicken with Lemon and Bahian Seasoning — 132
239. Basic BBQ Chicken — 132
240. Basic No Frills Turkey Breast — 133
241. Faire-Worthy Turkey Legs — 133
242. Herb Air Fried Chicken Thighs — 134
243. Quick & Easy Lemon Pepper Chicken — 134
244. Spicy Jalapeno Hassel back Chicken — 134
245. Tasty Hassel back Chicken — 135
246. Western Turkey Breast — 135
247. Lemon Pepper Turkey Breast — 135
248. Tender Turkey Legs — 136
249. Perfect Chicken Breasts — 136
250. Ranch Garlic Chicken Wings — 136
251. Ranch Chicken Thighs — 137
252. Taco Ranch Chicken Wings — 137
253. Simple Cajun Chicken Wings — 137
254. Simple Air Fried Chicken — 138
255. Buffalo Wings — 138
256. Honey Lime Chicken Wings — 138
257. Simple Chicken Drumsticks — 139
258. Healthy Chicken Wings — 139
259. Thai Chicken Thighs — 139
260. Chicken Patties — 140
261. Cajun Seasoned Chicken Drumsticks — 140
262. Honey Garlic Chicken — 140
263. Sriracha Chicken Wings — 141
264. Sweet & Spicy Chicken Wings — 141
265. Ginger Garlic Chicken — 141
266. Salt and Pepper Wings — 142
267. Parmesan Chicken Wings — 142
268. Western Chicken Wings — 142
269. Perfect Chicken Thighs Dinner — 143
270. Perfectly Spiced Chicken Tenders — 143

MEAT — 144

271. Flavorful Steak — 145
272. Easy Rosemary Lamb Chops — 145
273. BBQ Pork Ribs — 145
274. Juicy Steak Bites — 146
275. Greek Lamb Chops — 146
276. Easy Beef Roast — 146
277. Beef Jerky — 147
278. Simple Beef Patties — 147
279. Panko-Breaded Pork Chops — 147
280. Crispy Roast Garlic-Salt Pork — 148
281. Beef Rolls — 148
282. Homemade Corned Beef with Onions — 148
283. Crisp Ribs — 149
284. Roast Beef — 149
285. Basic Pork Chops — 149
286. Breaded Pork Chops — 150
287. Beef and Balsamic Marinade — 150
288. Crispy Brats — 150
289. Basil Pork Chops — 151
290. Beef and Radishes — 151
291. Herbed Pork Chops — 151
292. Beef Tenderloin — 152
293. Honey Mustard Pork Tenderloin — 152
294. Seasoned Pork Chops — 153
295. Crusted Rack of Lamb — 153
296. Lamb Burgers — 154
297. Pork Taquitos — 154
298. Cajun Bacon Pork Loin Fillet — 154
299. Porchetta-Style Pork Chops — 155
300. Apricot Glazed Pork Tenderloins — 155
301. Sweet & Spicy Country-Style Ribs — 156
302. Pork Tenders with Bell Peppers — 156
303. Wonton Meatballs — 157
304. Barbecue Flavored Pork Ribs — 157
305. Easy Air Fryer Marinated Pork Tenderloin — 158
306. Balsamic Glazed Pork Chops — 158

Air Fryer Cookbook

#	Recipe	Page
307.	Perfect Air Fried Pork Chops	159
308.	Rustic Pork Ribs	159
309.	Air Fryer Baby Back Ribs	160
310.	Parmesan Crusted Pork Chops	160
311.	Crispy Dumplings	160
312.	Pork Joint	161
313.	Pork Satay	161
314.	Pork Burgers with Red Cabbage Salad	162
315.	Crispy Mustard Pork Tenderloin	162
316.	Apple Pork Tenderloin	163
317.	Espresso-Grilled Pork Tenderloin	163
318.	Pork and Potatoes	164
319.	Pork and Fruit Kebabs	164
320.	Steak and Vegetable Kebabs	164
321.	Spicy Grilled Steak	165
322.	Greek Vegetable Skillet	165
323.	Light Herbed Meatballs	166
324.	Brown Rice and Beef-Stuffed Bell Peppers	166
325.	Beef and Broccoli	167
326.	Beef and Fruit Stir-Fry	167
327.	Garlic Putter Pork Chops	168
328.	Cajun Pork Steaks	168
329.	Cajun Sweet-Sour Grilled Pork	168
330.	Pork Loin with Potatoes	169
331.	Roasted Char Siew (Pork Butt)	169
332.	Asian Pork Chops	169
333.	Marinated Pork Chops	170
334.	Steak with Cheese Butter	170
335.	Madeira Beef	170
336.	Creamy Pork and Zucchinis	171
337.	Bullet-proof Beef Roast	171
338.	Lamb Burgers	171

FISH AND SEAFOOD 172

#	Recipe	Page
339.	Lemon Butter Scallops	173
340.	Cheesy Lemon Halibut	173
341.	Spicy Mackerel	174
342.	Thyme Scallops	174
343.	Chinese Style Cod	174
344.	Mustard Salmon Recipe	175
345.	Salmon and Orange Marmalade Recipe	175
346.	Tilapia & Chives Sauce	175
347.	Buttery Shrimp Skewers	176
348.	Marinated Salmon Recipe	176
349.	Tasty Grilled Red Mullet	176
350.	Garlicky-Grilled Turbot	177
351.	Char-Grilled Spicy Halibut	177
352.	Swordfish with Charred Leeks	177
353.	Breaded Coconut Shrimp	178
354.	Breaded Cod Sticks	178
355.	Cajun Salmon	178
356.	Cajun Shrimp	179
357.	Codfish Nuggets	179
358.	Creamy Salmon	179
359.	Crumbled Fish	180
360.	Easy Crab Sticks	180
361.	Fried Catfish	180
362.	Grilled Sardines	181
363.	Zucchini with Tuna	181
364.	Caramelized Salmon Fillet	181
365.	Deep Fried Prawns	182
366.	Mussels with Pepper	182
367.	Monkfish with Olives and Capers	182
368.	Shrimp, Zucchini and Cherry Tomato Sauce	183
369.	Salmon with Pistachio Bark	183
370.	Salted Marinated Salmon	183
371.	Sautéed Trout with Almonds	184
372.	Rabas	184
373.	Honey Glazed Salmo	184
374.	Sweet & Sour Glazed Salmon	185
375.	Ranch Tilapia	185
376.	Breaded Flounder	185
377.	Simple Haddock	186
378.	Breaded Hake	186
379.	Sesame Seeds Coated Tuna	186
380.	Cheese and Ham Patties	187
381.	Air-Fried Seafood	187
382.	Fish with Chips	187
383.	Crumbly Fishcakes	188
384.	Bacon Wrapped Shrimp	188
385.	Crab Legs	188
386.	Fish Sticks	189
387.	Crusty Pesto Salmon	189
388.	Salmon Patties	189
389.	Buttery Cod	190
390.	Sesame Tuna Steak	190
391.	Lemon Garlic Shrimp	190
392.	Foil Packet Salmon	191
393.	Foil Packet Lobster Tail	191
394.	Avocado Shrimp	191
395.	Citrusy Branzini on the Gril l	192
396.	Cajun-Seasoned Lemon Salmon	192
397.	Grilled Salmon Fillets	192
398.	Cheesy Breaded Salmon	193
399.	Coconut Crusted Shrimp	193
400.	Rice Flour Coated Shrimp	193
401.	Buttered Scallops	194
402.	Butter Trout	194
403.	Pesto Almond Salmon	194
404.	Garlic Lemon Shrimp	195
405.	Air-Fried Crab Sticks	195
406.	E-Z Catfish	195
407.	Fish Nuggets	196
408.	Grilled Shrimp	196
409.	Honey & Sriracha Tossed Calamari	196
410.	Salmon Croquettes	197
411.	Spicy Cod	197
412.	Air Fried Lobster Tails	198
413.	Air Fryer Salmon	198
414.	Simple Scallops	199
415.	3-Ingredient Air Fryer Catfish	199
416.	Pecan-Crusted Catfish	199
417.	Flying Fish	200

Air Fryer Cookbook

418. Air Fryer Fish Tacos	200
41. Bacon Wrapped Scallops	200
420. Quick Fried Catfish	201
421. Air-Fried Herbed Shrimp	201
422. Wild Caught Salmon	201
BONUS KETO AIR FRYER RECIPES	**202**
423. Crispy Keto Pork Bites	203
424. Keto Air Bread	203
425. Herbed Breakfast Eggs	204
426. Eggs in Zucchini Nests	204
427. Breakfast Liver Pate	205
428. Bread-Free Breakfast Sandwich	205
429. Egg Butter	206
430. Awesome Lemon Bell Peppers	206
431. Creamy Potatoes	206
432. Green Beans and Cherry Tomatoes	207
433. Crispy Brussels Sprouts and Potatoes	207
434. Herbed Tomatoes	207
435. Air Fried Leeks	208
436. Crispy Broccoli	208
437. Garlic-Roasted Bell Peppers	208
438. Asparagus with Garlic	209
439. Instant Lamb Steak with Apples and Pears	209
440. Adobo Chicken	209
441. Tomato & Feta Shrimp	210
442. Roasted Chicken	210
443. Salsa Chicken	211
444. Italian Shredded Chicken	211
445. Zoodle Soup	212
446. Cabbage Soup	212
447. Mojo Chicken	213
448. Spiced Almonds	213
449. Crispy Cauliflower Bites	213
450. Roasted Coconut Carrots	214
451. Baked Potatoes with Bacon	214
452. Walnut & Cheese Filled Mushrooms	214
453. Air-Fried Chicken Thighs	215
454. Simple Buttered Potatoes	215
455. Homemade Peanut Corn Nuts	215
456. Duck Fat Roasted Red Potatoes	216
457. Chicken Wings with Alfredo Sauce	216
458. Crispy Kale Chips	216
459. Crispy Squash	217
460. Ketogenic Mac & Cheese	217
461. Salmon Pie	218
462. Garlic Chicken Stir	218
463. Chicken Stew	219
464. Goulash	219
465. Beef & broccoli	220
466. Ground Beef Mash	220
467. Chicken Casserole	221
468. Chicken Hash	221
VEGETABLES AND VEGETARIAN	**222**
469. Pesto Tomatoes	223
470. Seasoned Potatoes	223
471. Spicy Zucchini	223
472. Seasoned Yellow Squash	224
473. Buttered Asparagus	224
474. Buttered Broccoli	224
475. Seasoned Carrots with Green Beans	225
476. Sweet Potato with Broccoli	225
477. Seasoned Veggies	225
478. Potato Gratin	226
479. Garlic Edamame	226
480. Egg Roll Pizza Sticks	227
481. Cajun Zucchini Chips	227
482. Crispy Old Bay Chicken Wings	228
483. Cinnamon and Sugar Peaches	228
484. Chicken wings with Provencal herbs in Air Fryer	229
485. Spiced Chicken wings in Air Fryer	229
486. Rosti (Swiss potatoes)	230
487. Baked Parsley	230
488. Duck thighs from the Air Fryer	230
489. Chopped Bondiola	231
490. Zucchini Curry	231
491. Healthy Carrot Fries	231
492. Simple Stuffed Potatoes	232
493. Simple Roasted Carrots	232
494. Broccoli & Cheese	232
495. Fried Plantains	233
496. Bacon-Wrapped Asparagus	233
497. Air Fried Roasted Corn on The Cob	233
498. Green Beans & Bacon	234
499. Air Fried Honey Roasted Carrots	234
500. Air Fried Roasted Cabbage	234
501. Burrata-Stuffed Tomatoes	235
502. Broccoli with Parmesan Cheese	235
503. Caramelized Broccoli	235
504. Brussels Sprouts with Balsamic Oil	236
505. Spiced Butternut Squash	236
506. Garlic Thyme Mushrooms	236
507. Zucchini Parmesan Chips	237
508. Jicama Fries	237
509. Lemon bell peppers	237
510. Cauliflower pizza crust	238
511. Savoy cabbage and tomatoes	238
512. Cauliflower steak	238
513. Tomato, avocado and green beans	239
514. Dill and garlic green beans	239
515. Eggplant stacks	239
516. Air Fried Spaghetti Squash	240
517. Beets and Blue Cheese Salad	240
518. Broccoli Salad	240
519. Roasted Brussels Sprouts with Tomatoes	241
520. Cheesy Brussels Sprouts	241
521. Sweet Baby Carrots Dish	241
522. Seasoned Leeks	242
523. Crispy Potatoes and Parsley	242
524. Garlic Tomatoes	242
525. Easy Green Beans and Potatoes	243
526. Green Beans and Tomatoes	243

527. Flavored Asparagus	243
528. Spaghetti Squash Tots	244
529. Cinnamon Butternut Squash Fries	244
530. Cheesy Roasted Sweet Potatoes	244
531. Salty Lemon Artichokes	245
532. Asparagus & Parmesan	245
533. Corn on Cobs	246
534. Onion Green Beans	246
535. Dill Mashed Potato	247
536. Cream Potato	247
537. Chard with Cheddar	248
538. Chili Squash Wedges	248
539. Honey Carrots with Greens	249
540. South Asian Cauliflower Fritters	249
541. Supreme Air-Fried Tofu	249

SWEETS AND DESSERTS — 250

542. Lemon Bars	251
543. Coconut Donuts	251
544. Blueberry Cream	251
545. Blackberry Chia Jam	252
546. Mixed Berries Cream	252
547. Apple Chips	252
548. Sweetened Plantains	253
549. Roasted Bananas	253
550. Pear Crisp	253
551. Easy Pears Dessert	254
552. Vanilla Strawberry Mix	254
553. Sweet Bananas and Sauce	254
554. Cinnamon Apples and Mandarin Sauce	255
555. Chocolate Vanilla Bars	255
556. Raspberry Bars	255
557. Cocoa Berries Cream	256
558. Cocoa Pudding	256
559. Blueberry Coconut Crackers	256
560. Cauliflower Pudding	257
561. Sweet Vanilla Rhubarb	257
562. Shortbread fingers	257
563. Fruit crumble pie	258
564. Chocolate mug cake	258
565. Fried peaches	259
566. Apple dumplings	259
567. Apple pie	260
568. Cinnamon Rolls	260
569. Cherries and Rhubarb Bowls	261
570. Pumpkin Bowls	261
571. Apple Jam	261
572. Yogurt and Pumpkin Cream	262
573. Raisins Rice Mix	262
574. Orange Bowls	262
575. Strawberry Jam	263
576. Caramel Cream	263
577. Wrapped Pears	263
578. Perfect Cinnamon Toast	264
579. Angel Food Cake	264
580. Apple Dumplings	265
581. Chocolate Donuts	265
582. Apple Hand Pies	265
583. Sweet Cream Cheese Wontons	266
584. French Toast Bites	266
585. Cinnamon Sugar Roasted Chickpeas	266
586. Brownie Muffins	267
587. Chocolate Mug Cake	267
588. Grilled Peaches	267
589. Simple & Delicious Spiced Apples	268
590. Tangy Mango Slices	268
591. Peanut Butter Cookies	268
592. Dried Raspberries	269
593. Sweet Peach Wedges	269
594. Air Fryer Oreo Cookies	269
595. Air Fried Butter Cake	270
596. Air Fryer S'mores	270
597. Air Fryer chocolate cake	271
598. Banana Brownies	271
599. Air fried biscuit donuts	272
600. Chocolate soufflé	272
601. Saucy fried bananas	273
602. Crusty apple hand pies	273

CONCLUSION — 274